Reader's Digest

EAT YOURSELF HEALTHY

HOW TO GET THE BEST OUT OF YOUR FOOD

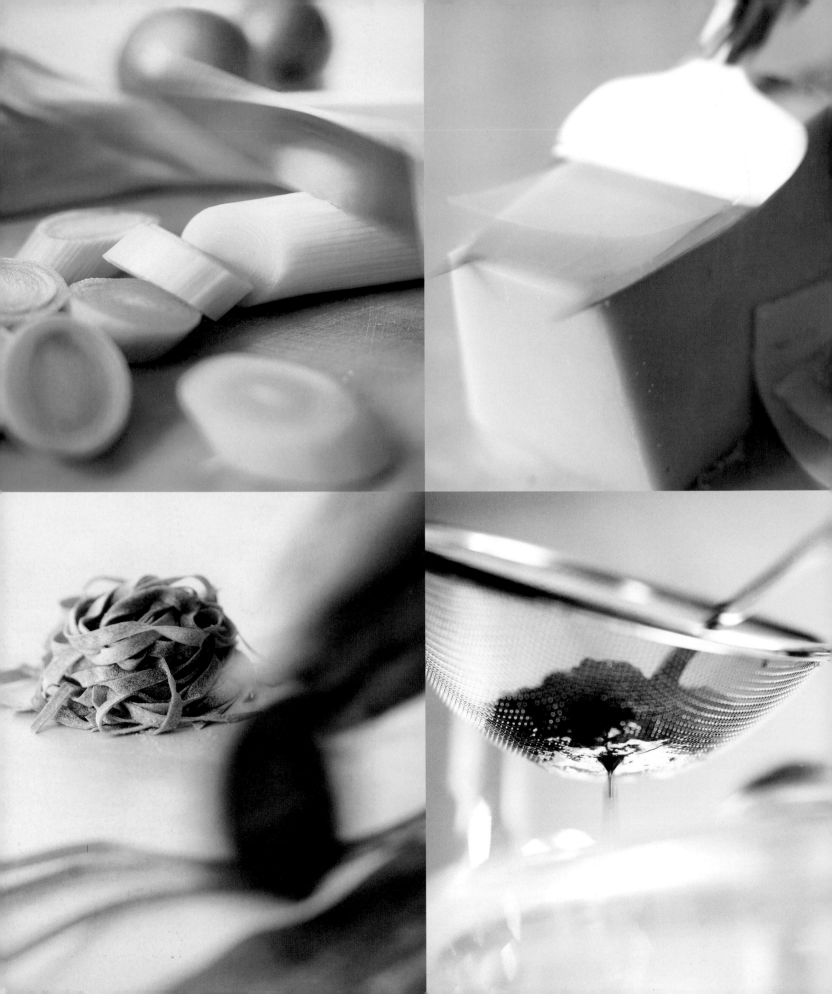

Reader's Digest

EAT YOURSELF HEALTHY

HOW TO GET THE BEST OUT OF YOUR FOOD

Published by the Reader's Digest Association Limited
London • New York • Sydney • Montreal

CONTENTS

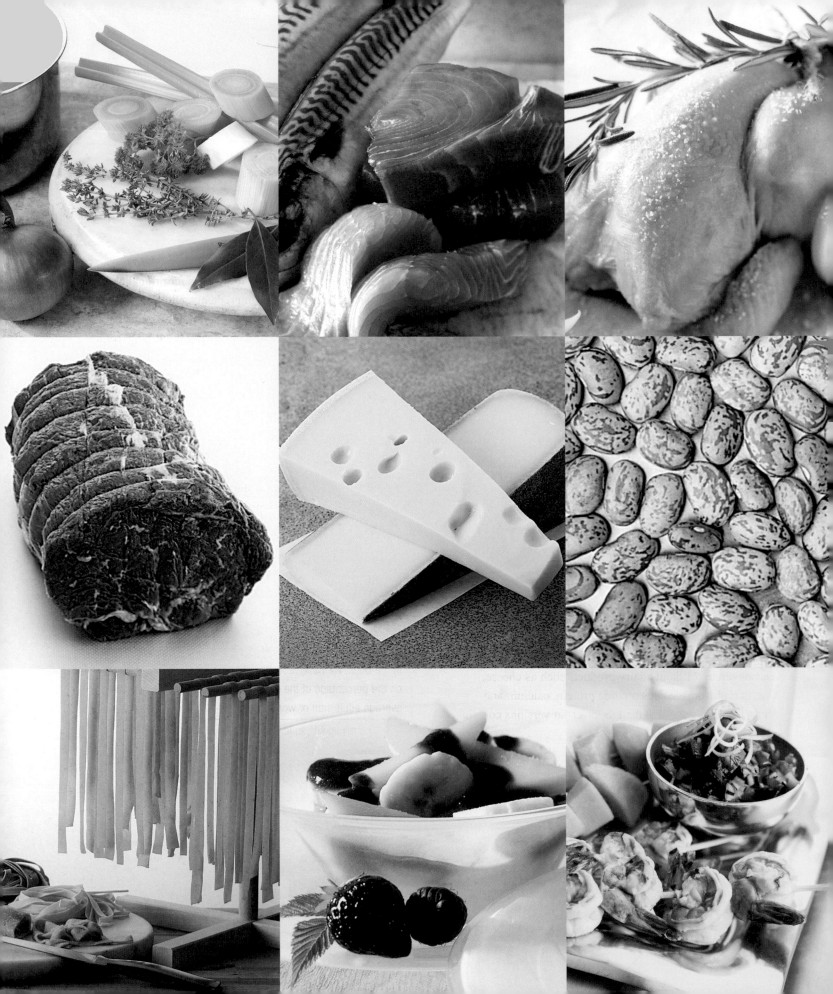

Eating yourself healthy

What we eat has a major impact on our health. If you can get the balance of foods right, you will look and feel your best.

Eating a healthy diet can help you look good, feel great and have lots of energy. Nutrition fads come and go, but the simple keys to eating well remain the same: enjoy a variety of food – no single food contains all the vitamins, minerals, fibre and other essential components you need for health and vitality – and get the balance right by looking at the proportions of the different foods you eat.

Eating all food in moderation may sound boring but it is by far the best and most enjoyable way of ensuring that you do eat yourself healthy. Instead of thinking about foods in terms of treats and sins, look at what you enjoy eating and then use this book to help you to balance your diet so that you can benefit from a variety of all the different types of food. Start to think in terms of food groups, and the main nutrients food provides. Foods like pasta, rice, bread and breakfast cereals provide carbohydrate, fibre, B vitamins and variable amounts of minerals. Fruit and vegetables provide vitamins, particularly those with antioxidant properties, as well as fibre and some carbohydrate. Milk and dairy products such as cheese, yogurt and fromage frais provide protein, calcium and vitamins B_{12}, A and D – though lower-fat versions contain less of the fat soluble vitamins A and D. Meat, poultry, fish and eggs, as well as the vegetarian alternatives such as nuts, beans, peas and lentils, provide protein, minerals such as iron and the B vitamins.

Eat Yourself Healthy is a food bible, a comprehensive but easy-to-access source of nutritional information and delicious recipes to help you to eat a properly balanced diet. Chapter by chapter, it explains what nutrients the key foods provide, introducing less familiar ingredients as well as looking at new, healthier, ways of using more everyday items. At the end of the book, at-a-glance nutritional charts list all the main properties of ingredients, allowing you to compare foods with each other and giving you the confidence to experiment with recipes, exchanging one food in a food group with another. For example, if you choose a recipe for seared tuna and bean salad served with ciabatta bread, you may decide to substitute salmon for the tuna. Or if Mexican pork is your starting point, you may decide to serve a fillet of beef instead of pork.

Overleaf we discuss in more detail what you need from each food group to ensure a healthy balanced diet. Ring the changes, be adventurous and above all enjoy preparing and eating your food, happy in the knowledge that you are eating yourself healthy.

As a guide to the vitamin and mineral content of foods and recipes in the book, we have used the following terms and symbols, based on the percentage of the daily RNI provided by one serving for the average adult man or woman aged 19–49 years

✓✓✓ or excellent	at least 50% (half)
✓✓ or good	25–50% (one-quarter to one-half)
✓ or useful	10–25% (one-tenth to one-quarter)

Note that recipes contribute other nutrients, but the analyses only include those that provide at least 10% RNI per portion. Vitamins and minerals where deficiencies are rare are not included.

ⓥ denotes that a recipe is suitable for vegetarians.

Getting it into proportion

Current guidelines are that most people in the UK should eat more starchy foods, more fruit and vegetables, and less fat, meat products and sugary foods.

It is almost impossible to give exact amounts that you should eat, as every single person's requirements vary, depending on size, age and the amount of energy expended during the day. However, nutrition experts have suggested an ideal balance of the different foods that provide us with energy (calories) and the nutrients needed for health. The number of daily portions of each of the food groups will vary from person to person – for example, an active teenager might need to eat up to 14 portions of starchy carbohydrates every day, whereas a sedentary adult would only require 6 or 7 portions – but the proportions of the food groups in relation to each other should ideally stay the same.

A simple way to get the balance right is to imagine a daily 'plate' divided into the different food groups. On the imaginary 'plate', starchy carbohydrates fill at least one-third of the space, thus constituting the main part of your meals. Fruit and vegetables fill the same amount of space. The remaining third of the 'plate' is divided mainly between protein foods and dairy foods, with just a little space allowed for foods containing fat and sugar. These are the proportions to aim for.

It isn't essential to eat the ideal proportions on the 'plate' at every meal, or even every day – balancing them over a week or two is just as good. The healthiest diet for you and your family is one that is generally balanced and sustainable in the long term.

Our daily plate

Starchy carbohydrate foods: eat 6–14 portions a day

At least 50% of the calories in a healthy diet should come from carbohydrates, and most of that from starchy foods – bread, potatoes and other starchy vegetables, pasta, rice and cereals. For most people in the UK this means doubling current intake. Starchy carbohydrates are the best foods for energy. They also provide protein and essential vitamins and minerals, particularly those from the B group. Eat a variety of starchy foods, choosing wholemeal or wholegrain types whenever possible, because the fibre they contain helps to prevent constipation, bowel disease, heart disease and other health problems.

What is a portion of starchy foods?

Some examples are: 3 tbsp breakfast cereal • 2 tbsp muesli • 1 slice of bread or toast • 1 bread roll, bap or bun • 1 small pitta bread, naan bread or chapatti • 3 crackers or crispbreads • 1 medium-sized potato • 1 medium-sized plantain or small sweet potato • 2 heaped tbsp boiled rice • 2 heaped tbsp boiled pasta.

Fruit and vegetables: eat at least 5 portions a day

Nutrition experts unanimously agree that we would all benefit from eating more fruit and vegetables each day – a total of at least 400 g (14 oz) of fruit and vegetables (edible part) is the target. Fruit and vegetables provide vitamin C for immunity and healing, and other 'antioxidant' vitamins and minerals for protection against cardiovascular disease and cancer. They also offer several 'phytochemicals' that help protect against cancer, and B vitamins, especially folate, which is important for women planning a pregnancy, to prevent birth defects. All of these, plus other nutrients, work together to boost well-being.

Antioxidant nutrients (e.g. vitamins C and beta-carotene, which are mainly derived from fruit and vegetables) and vitamin E help to prevent harmful free radicals in the body initiating or accelerating cancer, heart disease, cataracts, arthritis, general ageing, sun damage to skin, and damage to sperm. Free radicals occur naturally as a by-product of normal cell function, but are also caused by pollutants such as tobacco smoke and over-exposure to sunlight.

What is a portion of fruit or vegetables?

Some examples are: 1 medium-sized portion of vegetables or salad • 1 medium-sized piece of fresh fruit • 6 tbsp (about 140 g/5 oz) stewed or canned fruit • 1 small glass (100 ml/3½ fl oz) fruit juice.

Dairy foods: eat 2–3 portions a day

Dairy foods, such as milk, cheese, yogurt and fromage frais, are the best source of calcium for strong bones and teeth, and important for the nervous system. They also provide some protein for growth and repair, vitamin B_{12}, and vitamin A for healthy eyes. They are particularly valuable foods for young children, who need full-fat versions at least up to age 2. Dairy foods are also especially important for adolescent girls to prevent the development of osteoporosis later in life, and for women throughout life generally.

To limit fat intake, wherever possible adults should choose lower-fat dairy foods, such as semi-skimmed milk and low-fat yogurt.

What is a portion of dairy foods?

Some examples are: 1 medium-sized glass (200 ml/7 fl oz) milk • 1 matchbox-sized piece (40 g/1½ oz) Cheddar cheese • 1 small pot of yogurt • 125 g (4½ oz) cottage cheese or fromage frais.

Protein foods: eat 2–4 portions a day

Lean meat, fish, eggs and vegetarian alternatives provide protein for growth and cell repair, as well as iron to prevent anaemia. Meat also provides B vitamins for healthy nerves and digestion, especially vitamin B_{12}, and zinc for growth and healthy bones and skin.

Only moderate amounts of these protein-rich foods are required. An adult woman needs about 45 g of protein a day and an adult man 55 g, which constitutes about 11% of a day's calories. This is less than the current average intake. For optimum health, we need to eat some protein every day.

What is a portion of protein-rich food?

Some examples are: 3 slices (85–100 g/3–3½ oz) of roast beef, pork, ham, lamb or chicken • about 100 g (3½ oz) grilled offal • 115–140 g (4–5 oz) cooked fillet of white or oily fish (not fried in batter) • 3 fish fingers • 2 eggs (up to 7 a week) • about 140 g/5 oz baked beans • 60 g (2¼ oz) nuts, peanut butter or other nut products.

Foods containing fat: 1–5 portions a day

Unlike fruit, vegetables and starchy carbohydrates, which can be eaten in abundance, fatty foods should not exceed 33% of the day's calories in a balanced diet, and only 10% of this should be from saturated fat. This quantity of fat may seem a lot, but it isn't – fat contains more than twice as many calories per gram as either carbohydrate or protein.

Overconsumption of fat is a major cause of weight and health problems. A healthy diet must contain a certain amount of fat to provide fat-soluble vitamins and essential fatty acids, needed for the development and function of the brain, eyes and nervous system, but we only need a small amount each day – just 25 g is required, which is much less than we consume in our Western diet. The current recommendations from the Department of Health are a maximum of 71 g fat (of this, 21.5 g saturated) for women each day and 93.5 g fat (28.5 g saturated) for men. The best sources of the essential fatty acids are natural fish oils and pure vegetable oils.

What is a portion of fatty foods?

Some examples are: 1 tsp butter or margarine • 2 tsp low-fat spread • 1 tsp cooking oil • 1 tbsp mayonnaise or vinaigrette (salad dressing) • 1 tbsp cream • 1 individual packet of crisps.

Foods containing sugar: 0–2 portions a day

Although many foods naturally contain sugars (e.g. fruit contains fructose, milk lactose), health experts recommend that we limit 'added' sugars. Added sugars, such as table sugar, provide only calories – they contain no vitamins, minerals or fibre to contribute to health, and it is not necessary to eat them at all. But, as the old adage goes, 'a little of what you fancy does you good' and sugar is no exception. Denial of foods, or using them as rewards or punishment, is not a healthy attitude to eating, and can lead to cravings, binges and yo-yo dieting. Sweet foods are a pleasurable part of a well-balanced diet, but added sugars should account for no more than 11% of the total daily carbohydrate intake.

In assessing how much sugar you consume, don't forget that it is a major ingredient of many processed and ready-prepared foods.

What is a portion of sugary foods?

Some examples are: 3 tsp sugar • 1 heaped tsp jam or honey • 2 biscuits • half a slice of cake • 1 doughnut • 1 Danish pastry • 1 small bar of chocolate • 1 small tube or bag of sweets.

Too salty

Salt (sodium chloride) is essential for a variety of body functions, but we tend to eat too much through consumption of salty processed foods, 'fast' foods and ready-prepared foods, and by adding salt in cooking and at the table. The end result can be rising blood pressure as we get older, which puts us at higher risk of heart disease and stroke. Eating more vegetables and fruit increases potassium intake, which can help to counteract the damaging effects of salt.

Alcohol in a healthy diet

In recent research, moderate drinking of alcohol has been linked with a reduced risk of heart disease and stroke among men and women over 45. However, because of other risks associated with alcohol, particularly in excess quantities, no doctor would recommend taking up drinking if you are teetotal. The healthiest pattern of drinking is to enjoy small amounts of alcohol with food, to have alcohol-free days and always to avoid getting drunk. A well-balanced diet is vital because nutrients from food (vitamins and minerals) are needed to detoxify the alcohol.

Water – the best choice

Drinking plenty of non-alcoholic liquid each day is an often overlooked part of a well-balanced diet. A minimum of 8 glasses (which is about 2 litres/3½ pints) is the ideal. If possible, these should not all be tea or coffee, as these are stimulants and diuretics, which cause the body to lose liquids, taking with them water-soluble vitamins. Water is the best choice. Other good choices are fruit or herb teas or tisanes, fruit juices – diluted with water, if preferred – or semi-skimmed milk (full-fat milk for very young children). Fizzy sugary or acidic drinks such as cola are more likely to damage tooth enamel than other drinks.

Notes for the reader

• Use all metric or all imperial measures when preparing a recipe, as the two sets of measurements are not exact equivalents.

• Recipes were tested using metric measures and conventional (not fan-assisted) ovens. Medium eggs were used, unless otherwise specified.

• Can sizes are approximate, as weights can vary slightly according to the manufacturer.

• Preparation and cooking times are only intended as a guide.

The nutritional information in this book is for reference only. The editors urge anyone with continuing medical problems or symptoms to consult a doctor.

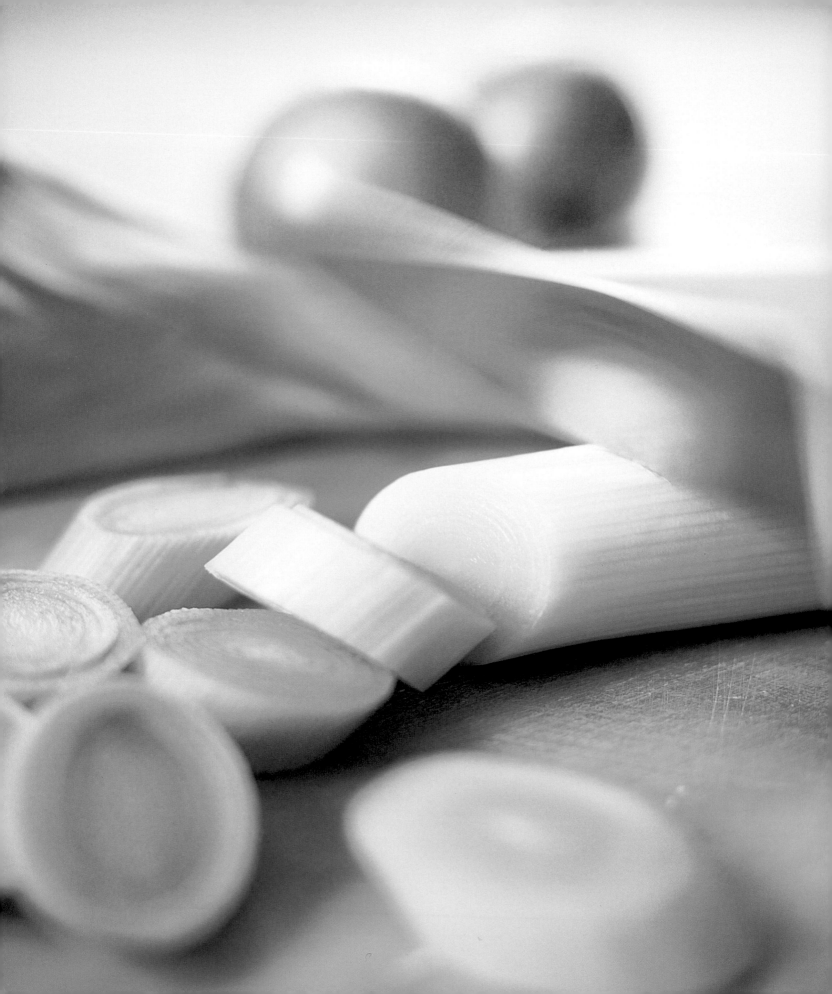

Vital Vegetables

Vegetables bring exciting flavours and textures to every meal. Even better, they are packed with vitamins, minerals, protective compounds and fibre, all vital in a healthy diet. And it's not just a case of long-term benefits, because a vegetable-rich diet makes you feel great every day. Vegetables are the ultimate in versatile ingredients and essential in lots of dishes. They can be stir-fried, steamed, baked or braised as well as boiled. Most also make fabulous salads, which can be as light or as substantial, as simple or as extravagant as you like, served warm or chilled. Fresh produce requires minimum preparation – the less you do to it, the better it is for you.

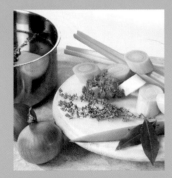

Vegetables in a healthy diet

Making the most of vegetables in main dishes and snacks as well as accompaniments will bring health benefits along with fabulous flavour.

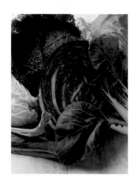

Why are vegetables important?

Vegetables are an essential part of a healthy, well-balanced diet. They are highly nutritious, packed with the vitamins, minerals and other compounds that protect us against illness, and they offer vital dietary fibre. All vegetables are good for us, fresh, frozen or canned.

In cooking, vegetables are indispensable – to create meals in their own right, as ingredients in a wealth of meat-based dishes, and as side dishes to partner fish, poultry and meat courses. They combine perfectly with nuts, grains, seeds and pulses to make delicious vegetarian meals. And adding vegetables improves the nutritional value of convenience foods – always try to serve 2 portions of vegetables with ready-prepared dishes, especially if you eat them often.

Extensive benefits

For any food to make a contribution to health, it needs to be eaten regularly and in quantity. Eating more vegetables – at least 5 portions of fruit and vegetables every day – can have a number of positive benefits.

- A vegetable-rich diet can reduce the risk of heart disease and cancer. In addition to the beneficial antioxidant vitamins and minerals present in vegetables, scientists have now discovered thousands of different plant chemicals, called phytochemicals, that are believed to have dramatic health-giving and health-protecting properties.
- Vegetables are low in sodium and many are naturally high in potassium. Most of us tend to eat too much sodium in the form of salt – much of it in processed and ready-made foods. Potassium works to balance sodium in the body, thus helping to prevent high blood pressure.
- Vegetables contain natural fibre that makes a vital contribution to good digestion and health.
- Vegetables are low in calories and fat, and ideal for making a modest quantity of protein-rich food such as meat, poultry or fish go further.

Valuable antioxidants

Vegetables and fruit are the best food sources of the antioxidants vitamin C and beta-carotene. Along with vitamin E (another antioxidant found in some vegetables), fibre and natural plant chemicals, these work to delay or even prevent oxidative damage caused by free radicals in the body.

- Free radicals cause changes in blood cholesterol and damage to cells, increasing the risk of heart disease and cancer. Similar damage may also increase the risk of other problems, for example eye cataracts.
- In addition to acting as an antioxidant, vitamin C is vital for a healthy immune system and healing. Beta-carotene from plant sources is converted to vitamin A (an antioxidant in its own right) in the body.

Iron-blocking brew

Drinking tea or coffee within 30 minutes of a meal reduces the absorption of iron from food, because the tannin in these drinks binds with the mineral, making it unavailable to the body. Vitamin C has the opposite effect – it enhances iron uptake – so eating or drinking foods with a good vitamin C content promotes iron absorption. Iron from vegetable sources is less easily absorbed than iron from meat, so ensuring a good supply of vitamin C is particularly important in vegetarian or other non-meat meals.

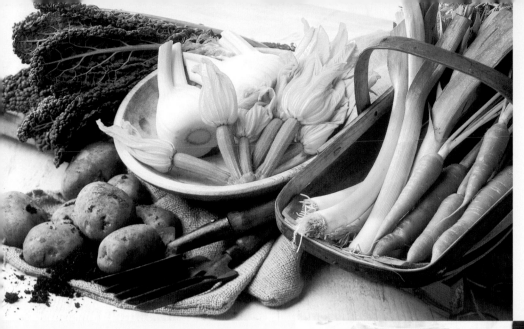

◀ The fresher the better – buy fresh vegetables in prime condition and in quantities that you will use quickly

Frozen vegetables make a valuable nutritional contribution, and they can be combined with fresh produce, for example in delicious stir-fries ▶

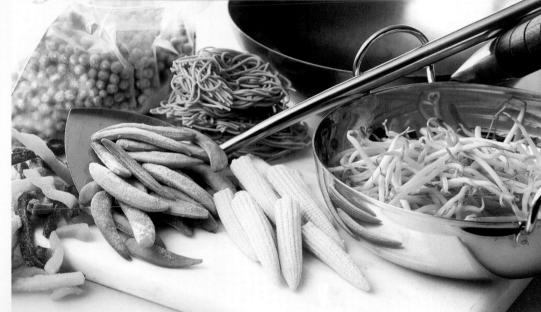

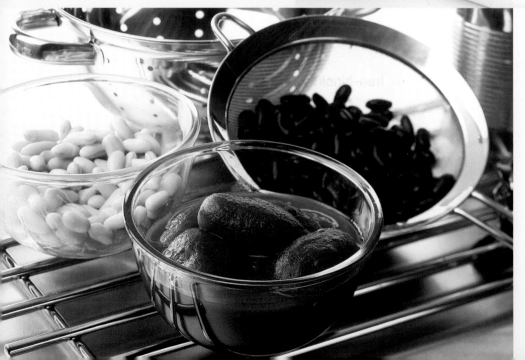

◀ Convenient canned vegetables bring valuable fibre to quick meals, and canned tomatoes provide lycopene, a cancer-fighting carotenoid

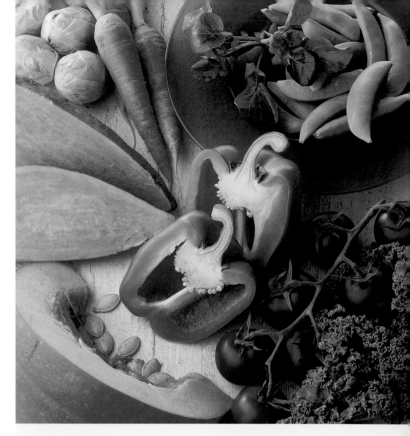

Vegetables for a healthy heart

Recent studies suggest that a raised level of an amino acid known as homocysteine may be closely associated with heart disease and stroke, as high levels of homocysteine can damage the cells that line the arteries. Folic acid is used in the body to convert homocysteine to another amino acid, which is used as a body-building protein, and to other substances that are essential for brain function and DNA production. When insufficient folic acid – and, less importantly, vitamins B_6 and B_{12} – is available to convert the homocysteine, the amino acid builds up in the system.

The best way to obtain the necessary folic acid is to eat foods rich in folates, which are compounds derived from folic acid. Folates are found in many vegetables, particularly dark leafy greens such as spinach and broccoli.

▲ Good for antioxidants – dark leafy greens such as watercress and curly kale, peas, tomatoes, peppers, pumpkin, sweet potatoes, carrots, Brussels sprouts

▼ Good for glucosinolates and sulphur compounds – cruciferous vegetables such as cauliflower, cabbage, broccoli, chard, Brussels sprouts, swede and kohlrabi

Green vegetables for a healthy pregnancy

Women who are trying to conceive are advised to take a folic acid supplement for 3 months before becoming pregnant and through the first 3 months of pregnancy to reduce the risk of spina bifida and related conditions in the baby. In addition to taking supplements, it is advisable to eat plenty of foods that are rich in folates such as leafy green vegetables, broccoli, Brussels sprouts and other brassicas.

Bioactive plants protecting health

Natural plant chemicals, or phytochemicals, are attracting attention for their bioactive properties, which enable them to offer protection against cancer. Much research today is focused on the glucosinolates and sulphur compounds in the brassica family – cabbage and related vegetables, such as broccoli and Brussels sprouts (see page 16). There is also great interest in the phytochemicals found in the onion family and green beans, and in bioflavonoids, the substances responsible for red and blue colours in vegetables. Some bioflavonoids act as antioxidants and also increase enzyme activity, which protects human cells against carcinogens. One of these antioxidants, called quercetin, may be more active in protecting health than vitamins C and E.

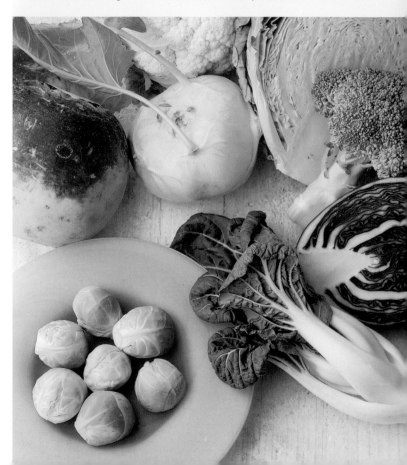

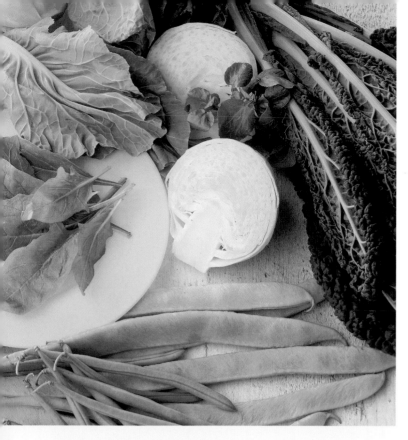

▲ Good for folates – dark leafy greens such as spring greens and watercress, cabbage, beans and spinach

▼ Good for fibre – okra, sweetcorn, fennel, peas and beans

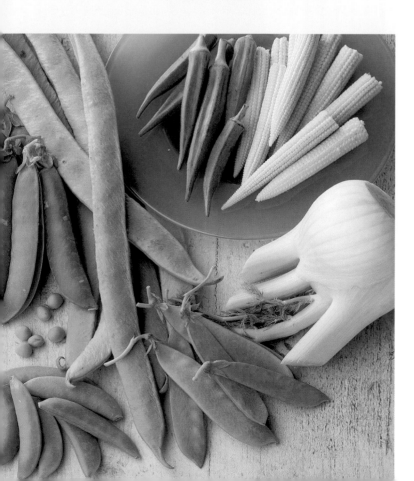

Far more to fibre

Fresh, frozen and canned vegetables all contribute both types of essential dietary fibre. Soluble fibre can help to reduce the risk of heart disease by lowering levels of blood cholesterol. It also helps to control blood sugar levels.

Insoluble fibre softens and adds bulk to food waste passing through the gut. Helping the gut to function efficiently can prevent diverticular disease and control some types of irritable bowel syndrome. Preventing constipation also helps to avoid piles and varicose veins. A fibre-rich diet produces an environment that encourages healthy gut bacteria to grow, suppressing the growth of harmful bacteria. This process also produces a substance that suppresses cancer-cell growth.

Are convenience vegetables good for you?

While vegetables taste best and contain most nutrients when at their freshest, frozen vegetables are also excellent from a nutritional point of view. Many vegetables are frozen within hours of being picked, so they actually retain more nutrients than some 'fresh' produce that is days old before it reaches the consumer. Chilled prepared vegetables are not as rich as whole vegetables in nutrients, particularly vitamins, but they are convenient and still have some value.

Canned vegetables are processed quickly, but the high temperatures involved do reduce the vitamin content. However, they are still a useful source of dietary fibre and some phytochemicals.

Dried vegetables, which are rarely used as a main ingredient in cooking, are not an alternative to fresh produce, as they do not offer the equivalent nutritional benefits.

Vitamin pills or vegetables?

There is still a lot to be learned about exactly how fruit and vegetables actively protect our health, but we do know that the vitamins and minerals in vegetables work with the fibre and phytochemicals to boost vitality and protect against disease. Purified vitamin and mineral tablets cannot offer this advantage. And in any case, why miss out on the pleasures of eating and opt to swallow a pill instead?

Of cabbages and kings

Discover the wide variety of lush leaves and succulent shoots, stalks, stems and sprouts to include in your daily five portions.

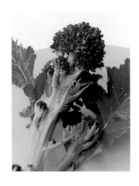

Shoots, stalks and leaves

Here is a mix of favourite vegetables with others that you may not use frequently. They are all shoots from the vegetable plant – some, like asparagus, are in the first stages of growth, while others are fully opened into leafy greens. Average portion sizes are given of the raw vegetable, although the precise quantity may vary according to the type of dish being prepared.

Artichoke, globe (1 head)

In traditional herbal medicine, globe artichokes are used to aid digestion, perhaps due to their slight bitterness, which stimulates digestion. Artichokes contain some calcium.
• Buy heavy, plump and compact heads. They can be stored in the fridge for several days.

Asparagus (5 spears, about 125 g/4½ oz)

Asparagus is an excellent source of folate and green spears are a significant source of vitamin C. The beta-carotene content makes asparagus a useful source of vitamin A, and it offers useful vitamin E. It is known as a potent diuretic.

Eat more brassicas

The brassica group of cruciferous vegetables, which includes cabbage, cauliflower, broccoli, Brussels sprouts, kale, swede and kohlrabi, contains glucosinolates and other sulphur compounds associated with lowering the risk of cancer. They are good sources of vitamin C and among the richest vegetable sources of folates. Eaten regularly, they also contribute appreciable amounts of minerals.

• Buy straight spears with firm tips. Store in the fridge for up to 3 days.

Broccoli (85 g/3 oz)

Broccoli is an excellent source of folate and vitamin C. It provides a useful amount of vitamin E, and the beta-carotene it contains also makes it a useful source of vitamin A.
• Buy firm, upright stalks with compact dark green heads. Store in the fridge for up to 2 days.

Brussels sprouts (85 g/3 oz)

Brussels sprouts provide beta-carotene, and they are an excellent source of folate.
• Buy firm, bright sprouts with tightly packed leaves. Avoid yellowing vegetables. Store in the fridge for up to 3 days.

Cabbages and greens (100 g/3½ oz)

This varied group of vegetables includes red and white cabbages, Chinese leaves, spring greens and Chinese cabbages such as pak choy. The green types are an excellent source of folate and a good source of vitamin C as well as carotenoids.
• Buy crisp, bright vegetables, rejecting any that are wilting, limp or yellowing. Store in the fridge for up to 2 days.

Cauliflower (85 g/3 oz)

Cauliflower contains beneficial sulphur compounds and also provides vitamin C.
• Buy firm heads with a few crisp leaves. Avoid discoloured or slightly soft cauliflower. Store in the fridge for up to 3 days.

Celery (½ small head, about 200 g/7 oz)

Much of celery's flavour is due to its sodium content, which is slightly higher than many vegetables; however, it also contains some potassium which balances this.
• Buy compact heads that are crisp. Avoid damaged or browning vegetables. Store in the fridge for up to a week.

Chicory (1 medium to large head or 2 small heads)

Bitter vegetables such as chicory have traditionally been used to stimulate digestion and aid liver and gall bladder problems.
• Buy firm heads with succulent-looking leaves that are not tinged brown. Store in the fridge for up to 5 days.

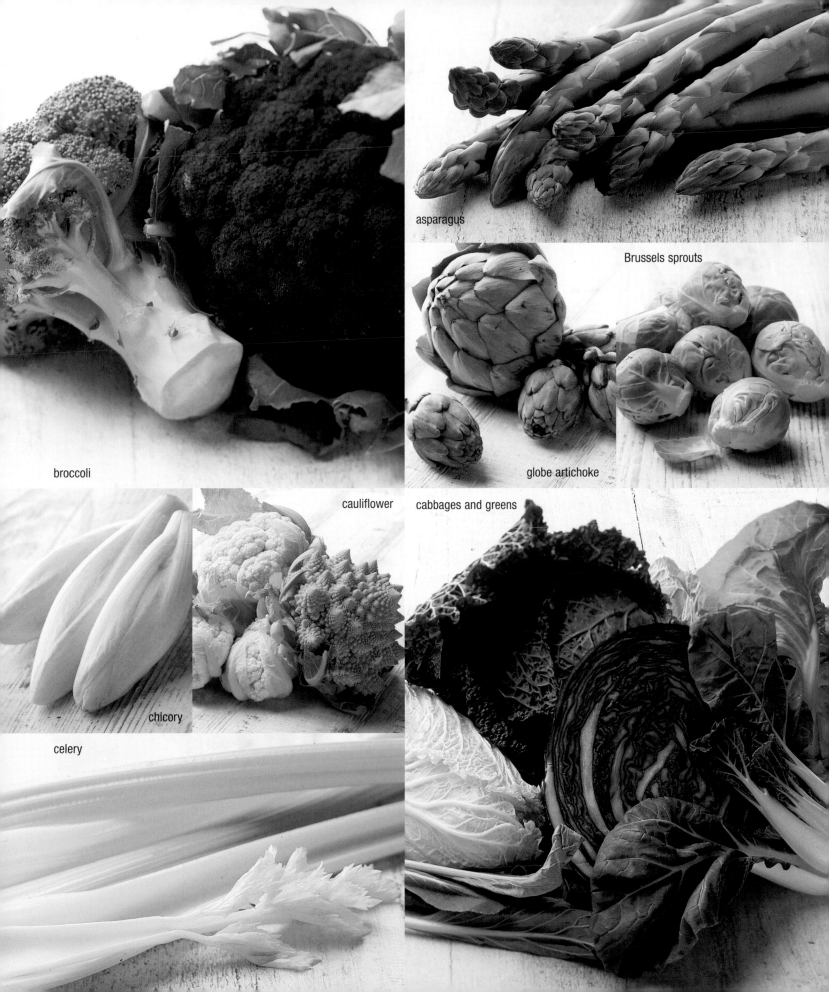

asparagus

Brussels sprouts

broccoli

globe artichoke

cauliflower

cabbages and greens

chicory

celery

Fennel (1 bulb, about 200 g/7 oz)

Fennel contains more phytoestrogen than most vegetables. This phytochemical is believed to help protect against breast and prostate cancers. Fennel is also a good source of potassium, and it is thought to aid digestion and relieve wind and flatulence.

● Buy crisp fennel, and store in the fridge for up to a week.

Kale (100 g/3½ oz)

In common with other dark green, leafy vegetables, kale is as rich in beta-carotene as orange-fleshed vegetables, but the orange colour is masked by the green pigment chlorophyll. In fact, chlorophyll may also help to protect against cancer. Kale is an excellent source of folate, and it contributes vitamin C, iron and calcium.

● Buy dark green leaves that look bright and fresh. Store in the fridge and use as soon as possible, within 2 days.

Kohlrabi (50 g/1¼ oz)

This purple or green-tinged vegetable looks like a root, but it is actually a swollen stem spiked with sprouting stalks and green leaves. Similar to cabbage in flavour, kohlrabi is a good source of vitamin C.

● Buy heavy vegetables that feel firm, and store in the fridge for up to 7 days.

Leek (75 g/2½ oz)

This most useful member of the onion family (see page 24) provides vitamin C, carotenoids and folic acid.

● Buy firm leeks with white bases and bright, lush green tops. Store in the fridge for up to 3 days.

Lettuces and salad leaves (about ¼ head or 1 lettuce heart)

There is a wide variety of salad leaves, including tender round lettuce, and crisp iceberg, cos, Little Gem and romaine. There are frilly varieties, such as Lollo Biondo, and red-tinged leaves, for example Lollo Rosso and Oak Leaf. Lamb's lettuce and frisée (the popular name used for curly endive) are also readily available. Rocket and other strongly flavoured leaves can be mixed in small quantities with more delicate salad leaves. The darker outer leaves contain more vitamins and antioxidants than paler inner leaves.

● Buy whole rather than prepared, torn heads, which will have lost a lot of their vitamin C and folate content. Avoid wilting or brown leaves. Store in the fridge for up to 4 days.

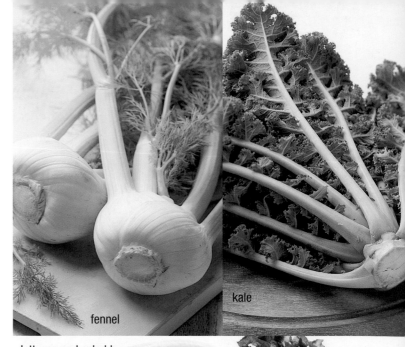

fennel

kale

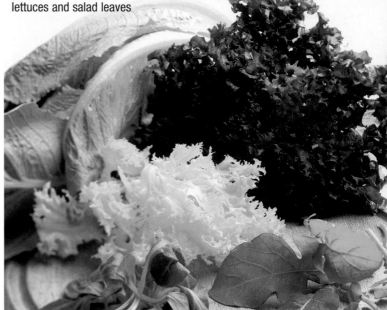

lettuces and salad leaves

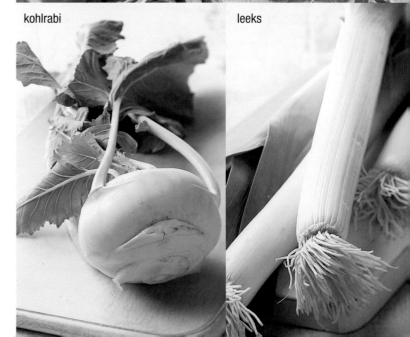

kohlrabi

leeks

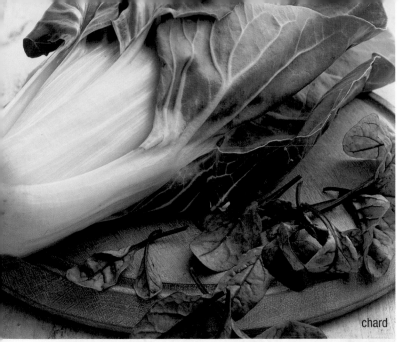
chard

spinach

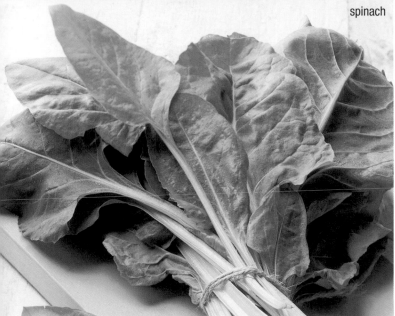

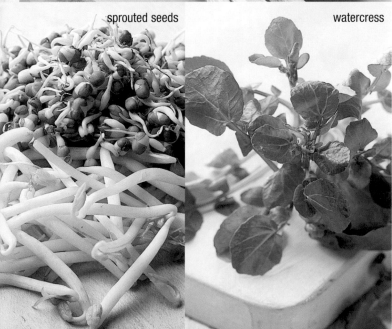
sprouted seeds

watercress

Spinach and chard (200 g/7 oz)

Both of these leafy greens provide vitamin C and folate, and they are the richest sources of a particular type of carotenoid called lutein. Evidence suggests that lutein offers protection against a common cause of blindness in older people. Spinach also makes a useful contribution of iron, and it provides vitamin E. Remember that the chard stalks should be eaten too. Although not offering all the same nutrients as the green leaves, they are a good source of fibre.

● Buy fresh bright leaves. Avoid wilting, yellowing or crushed leaves. Store in the fridge and use within 2 days.

Sprouted seeds (45 g/1½ oz)

The nutritional content varies according to the type of seeds or beans used. Bean sprouts grown from mung beans provide some vitamin C and B vitamins.

● Buy fresh-looking sprouts, avoiding any that are limp and brown or stained. The sprouts should smell pleasantly fresh. Store in the fridge for up to 3 days.

Watercress (1 bunch, about 80 g/scant 3 oz)

Watercress has high levels of carotenoids and offers vitamins C and B_6. It also makes a contribution to mineral intake, providing iron and some zinc, potassium and calcium. Serve watercress raw and in generous portions – for example, as a main ingredient in a salad – to make the most of its nutritional benefits. Use the tender stalks as well as the leaves, as they are tasty and nutritious too.

● Buy glossy, dark green watercress in bunches, if available, rather than ready-trimmed and washed. Avoid yellowed leaves. Store in the fridge and use within 2 days.

Sea vegetables

Seaweed is best known as a popular vegetable in Japanese cooking, but it also features in Western cuisines. British seaweeds include Welsh laverbread and Irish carragheen. Samphire, or glasswort, a salty green vegetable that resembles long, thin, 'jointed' beans, is a shore plant rather than a seaweed. Most types of seaweed are rich in iodine, and they contain other minerals, including calcium, iron, potassium and zinc. Some also have a high sodium content.

For more details on sea vegetables, see page 73.

Picked from the plant

Full of food value and flavour, and with a diversity of exciting textures, these are the ingredients that bring vegetable cuisine to life.

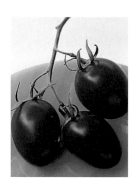

An ABC of vegetable fruits

These bright and varied vegetable fruits are so called because they carry the seeds of the plant on which they grow. In some cases they actually are the seeds – as in peas, for example. Average portion sizes of the raw vegetable are given as a guide.

Aubergine (1 small or ½ large)

Aubergines may be the familiar rich purple or have white, green or striped violet skin, and in shape they may be long and slim, plump ovals or little balls. Aubergines add satisfying bulk to dishes, yet are very low in calories.
● Buy plump, firm vegetables with a smooth, glossy skin. Store in the fridge for up to a week.

Avocado (½ medium)

These are unusual among vegetables in that they have a high fat content, but most of the fat is monounsaturated, so they share the 'good' fat profile of nuts. Avocados also contain vitamin E and the B-group vitamins B_1, B_2 and B_6. They provide a useful source of vitamin C and some folate and potassium, and are extremely low in sodium.
● If bought hard, place in a paper bag and ripen at room temperature. Store ripe avocados in the fridge for up to 2 days.

Broad beans (85 g/3 oz)

Broad beans contain twice as much fibre as green beans and are a good source of quercetin, the phytochemical linked with lowering the risk of heart disease. They also provide beta-carotene, vitamin C and many of the B vitamins.
● Buy plump, fresh-looking pods that feel firm (so you know they will contain good beans). Very large, pale-coloured pods will contain large beans that may be tough, and these will probably need to be skinned after cooking. Store broad beans in the fridge and use within 2 days.

Chillies

Although the many types of hot chillies are used mainly as a spice or flavouring ingredient, there are also milder varieties that are cooked as the main vegetables in a variety of dishes.
● Buy and store as peppers.

Courgette and vegetable marrow (100 g/3½ oz)

Courgettes provide vitamins C and B_6, folate and beta-carotene. It is important to eat the skins as they are the main source of these nutrients. Marrow has a high water content, which means that it provides satisfying bulk with few calories.
● Buy firm vegetables that feel heavy for their size. Store in the fridge for up to 5 days.

Cucumber (¼ medium)

Cucumber is refreshing and distinctive in flavour. It has a high water content and is a mild diuretic.
● Buy green glossy cucumbers that are rigid, and store in the fridge for up to 5 days.

Green beans (85 g/3 oz)

There are many varieties including runner, French and bobby beans. Green beans are a significant source of folate. Runner beans contain the most vitamin C, providing a useful source.
● Buy firm, crisp beans that snap rather than bend – they should be young, tender and a good fresh green colour. Avoid very large, blemished or tired-looking beans. Store in the fridge for up to 5 days.

Mushrooms (50 g/1¾ oz)

Mushrooms contain a good combination of the B vitamins B_2, niacin and pantothenic acid, and they provide copper and potassium. Mushrooms are part of the vast family of fungi. and they are grouped with vegetable fruits of plants because they are the spore-bearing part of the mushroom organism and responsible for dispensing the fungi equivalent of seeds.

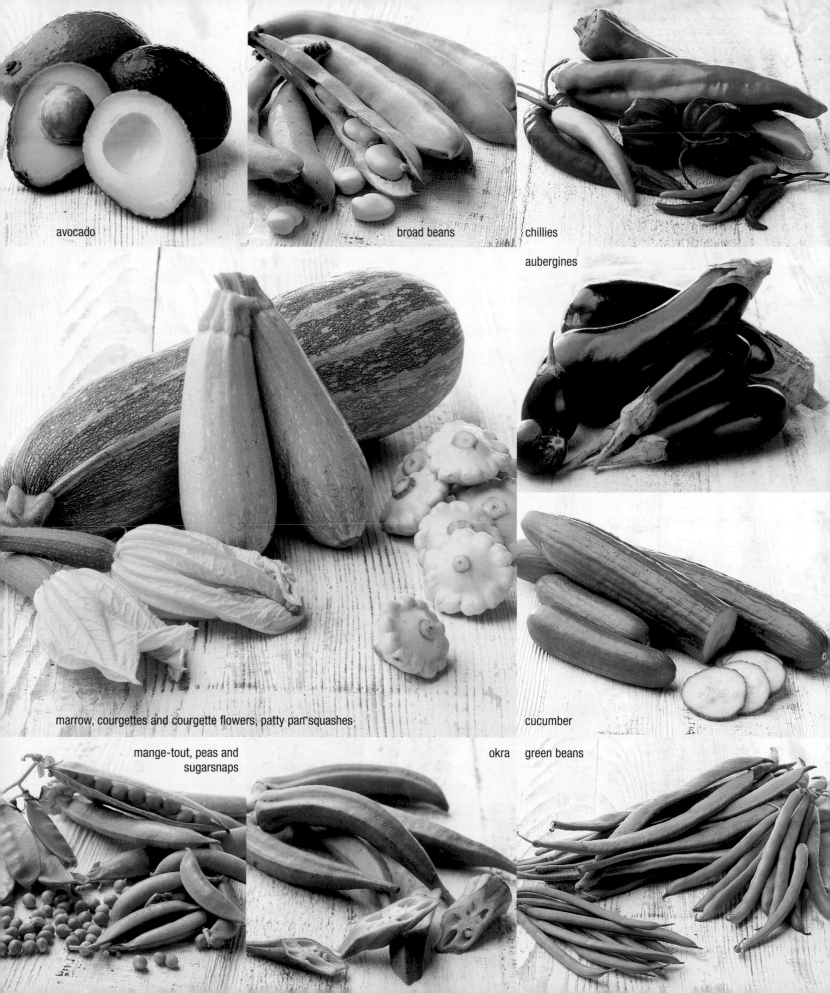

avocado

broad beans

chillies

aubergines

marrow, courgettes and courgette flowers, patty pan squashes

cucumber

mange-tout, peas and
sugarsnaps

okra

green beans

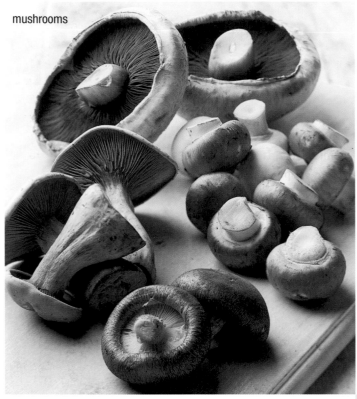

mushrooms

Peas, petit pois, mange-tout and sugarsnap peas (75 g/2½ oz)

Peas are a useful source of vitamin C and fibre, particularly soluble fibre. Mange-tout and sugarsnap peas are richer sources of both vitamin C and fibre because the pods are eaten too. Unusually, peas also contribute B vitamins, in particular B_1, and their protein content is high for a vegetable that also provides a useful amount of folate. Mange-tout are not as good a source of protein as the peas are not developed. In addition, peas are a useful source of iron and zinc. Frozen peas can contain as much vitamin C as fresh peas, and are one of the most nutritious processed foods.

• Fresh pea pods should be bright green and firm. Store in the fridge for up to 5 days. Shell peas just before use.

Pepper (½–1 pepper or 75 g/2½ oz)

These are an excellent source of vitamin C – half a raw pepper provides over twice the RNI of this vitamin. Red peppers are an excellent source of beta-carotene, and all peppers also contain a small amount of vitamin E.

• Buy glossy, crisp and unwrinkled peppers. Store in the fridge for up to 10 days.

• Buy firm, dry mushrooms. Store unwashed in a paper bag in the fridge for up to 5 days.

Okra (85 g/3 oz)

Also known as ladies' fingers, these multi-sided pods provide vitamin C, some carotenoids and folate. They are also a source of calcium and potassium.

• Buy pods that look fresh and feel firm. Avoid limp, wrinkled or blemished pods, and those that look very large and tough. Store in the fridge for up to 3 days.

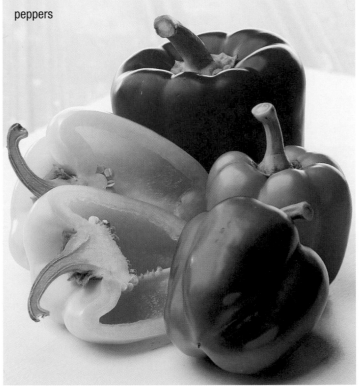

peppers

Cultivated mushrooms

Mushrooms grow rapidly, developing from small buttons, to closed cap, to open and large open mushrooms. As they grow, they darken and become stronger in flavour. Brown cap mushrooms are a different variety, darker and with a slightly stronger flavour. Other common types include delicate oyster and distinctively flavoured shiitake mushrooms.

Pumpkin and other squashes (75 g/2½ oz)

Related to marrows and courgettes, there are many types of squash, from the homely pumpkin to attractively shaped patty pan and spaghetti squash with its pale golden strands of flesh. The nutritional value varies according to type. For example, acorn squash provides some vitamin A, pumpkin supplies a useful amount and butternut squash is an excellent source. Squashes can also be a useful source of vitamin C.

• Buy firm vegetables that are heavy for their size, with hard skins according to variety, preferably whole rather than in cut portions. Store whole hard-skinned squash in a cool, dry, airy place, ideally hanging in a net bag. In the right conditions it will keep for several months. Store cut pieces and squashes with edible skin in the fridge for up to 5 days.

Sweetcorn (1 cob or 85 g/3 oz kernels)

Popular fresh as corn-on-the-cob and frozen or canned as kernels, sweetcorn, a variety of maize, makes a valuable contribution to fibre and folate intake, and also contains vitamins B_1, B_6 and C.

• Buy cobs with firm, plump kernels. Avoid any that look dried and withered. Store in the fridge for up to 5 days.

Tomato (2 medium)

Tomatoes are an excellent source of vitamin C and a good source of vitamin A from beta-carotene. The skin colour is mainly from another carotenoid called lycopene, a powerful antioxidant. Cooking and processing release lycopene from the skin, so there is more in tomato products such as purée, ketchup, passata and canned tomatoes than in raw tomatoes.

• Buy firm, ripe fruit in small quantities and store at room temperature. If tomatoes are refrigerated, let them come to room temperature before eating.

Nuts

Nuts are the fruit seeds of plants contained in hard protective shells. They are high in unsaturated fat, with very small amounts of saturated fat. Coconut is the exception, with a high saturated fat content. Nuts provide vitamin E, folate, phytochemicals, protein and useful amounts of the minerals iron, selenium and zinc (amounts differ according to the type of nut). Nuts are also high in fibre. Eating as little as 30 g (1 oz) of walnuts per day has been shown to reduce harmful levels of blood cholesterol and also to influence the type of cholesterol present, increasing beneficial cholesterol while reducing the harmful type.

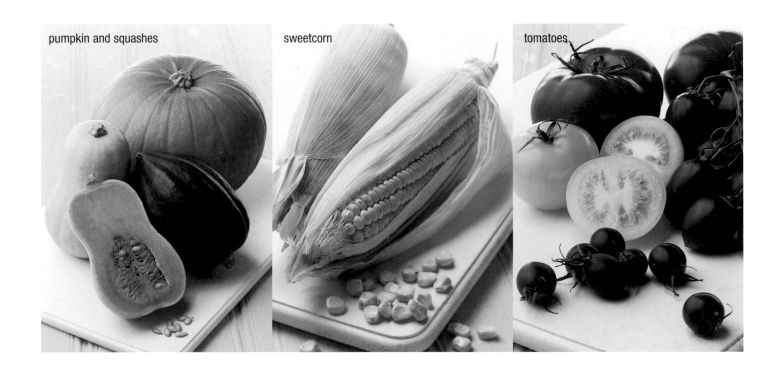

pumpkin and squashes

sweetcorn

tomatoes

Back to your roots

Roots, bulbs and tubers make a satisfying and nutritious contribution to healthy eating.

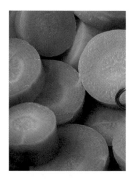

An ABC of roots, bulbs and tubers

The main role of starchy roots and tubers is to provide plenty of good-to-eat complex carbohydrate. Other roots offer complementary nutrients. When eaten regularly and in quantity, these vegetables are beneficial in many ways. Average portion sizes of the raw vegetable are given as a guide.

Beetroot (2 small or 1 large)

Richly coloured beetroot contains potassium and folate as well as iron. It is low in calories and, like other vegetables, provides useful fibre.

● Buy firm, dry beetroot that look plump, but not too big, and feel hard. Remove the leaves, then store in the fridge for up to 5 days. Vacuum-packed cooked beetroot (without vinegar or other acid added) is true to the flavour of freshly boiled, and it has a long shelf life in the sealed pack. Traditionally, freshly harvested beetroot leaves were cooked in the same way as spinach, but it is mainly the root that is used today.

Carrot (55 g/2 oz)

The large amount of beta-carotene and other carotenoids in carrots, particularly in old or main-crop vegetables, make this vegetable an excellent source of vitamin A. The beta-carotene is much better absorbed by the body (and converted into vitamin A) if the carrots are cooked.

● Buy crisp, firm carrots with a good orange colour. If the carrots have tops, these should be bright green and fresh. Store in the fridge for up to a week.

Celeriac (75 g/2½ oz)

With a flavour similar to celery, but lighter, this root is low in sodium and a reasonable source of fibre. It also contains some vitamin C, B_1, folate and potassium.

● Buy firm, heavy celeriac, and store in the fridge or a cool, dark place for up to a week.

Jerusalem artichoke (100 g/3½ oz)

Similar in size and colour to new potatoes, Jerusalem artichokes are high in fibre and contain copper and potassium.

● Buy firm roots and store unwashed as for potatoes.

Onions and their family

Onions, shallots, leeks (see page 18), spring onions, garlic and chives all contain several beneficial phytochemicals. One of these, quercetin, is associated with lower rates of heart disease and stroke. Another, allicin, is believed to assist in lowering blood cholesterol levels, thus preventing blood clots from forming and lowering blood pressure.

● Buy hard, well-shaped onions with dry, papery skins. Avoid any that are soft, discoloured or sprouting. Store in a cool, dark place that is dry and airy. In the right conditions onions will keep for several weeks. Spring onions should be bright and firm – avoid any that look wilted or slightly slimy. Store spring onions in the fridge for up to 5 days.

Parsnip (75 g/2½ oz)

Slightly sweet, full-flavoured parsnips contain some vitamin C. They also provide folate.

● Buy small to medium parsnips. Avoid any that are soft, with wrinkled skin or brown patches. Store in a cool, dark, dry and airy place for up to 10 days.

Potato (1 medium)

There is a wide variety of new, salad and main crop potatoes, and the choice depends on the cooking method. Potatoes are an excellent starchy carbohydrate food. Eaten daily in good quantity, they are a useful source of vitamin C and they also contribute iron and B vitamins. The skin and the area immediately below it contain the most nutrients. New potatoes contain more nutrients than old crop vegetables.

● Buy potatoes loose or in paper bags, if possible. If in polythene bags, avoid any that have been 'sweating' and look moist, and potatoes that are sprouting or green. Remove from polythene bags to a paper bag for storage. Keep potatoes in a cool, dark, dry place for up to 2 weeks. There is no need to wash them before storage.

Radish (50 g/1¾ oz)

Large white radish (mooli or daikon) is now as widely available as the small red radishes familiar in salads. The latter are a useful source of vitamin C.

• Buy firm, bright-skinned radishes; white radish should look moist and fresh. Store in the fridge for up to 5 days.

Swede (75 g/2½ oz)

One of the brassica family, swede offers the same benefits (see page 16) and in addition is a useful source of vitamin C.

• Buy firm swede that looks fresh and feels heavy. Store in the fridge for up to a week or as for potatoes.

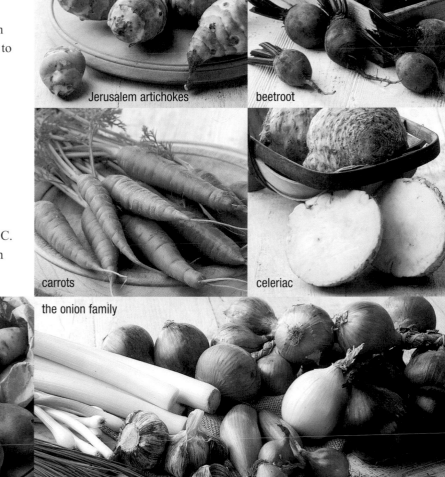

Jerusalem artichokes

beetroot

carrots

celeriac

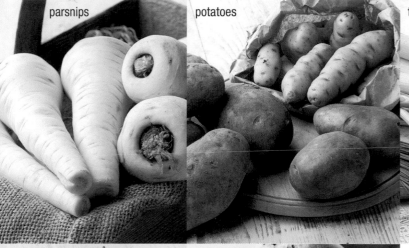

parsnips

potatoes

the onion family

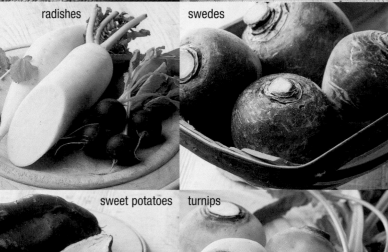

radishes

swedes

sweet potatoes

turnips

Sweet potato (100 g/3½ oz)

Sweet potatoes are a delicious starchy carbohydrate. Orange-fleshed varieties are a good source of beta-carotene, which the body can convert into vitamin A. All sweet potatoes provide vitamins C and E, potassium and fibre.

• Buy firm sweet potatoes with no soft patches. Store in the fridge for up to a week or as for potatoes.

Turnip (75 g/2½ oz)

This slightly peppery root vegetable is similar to swede in vitamin C content.

• Buy hard, crisp turnips that are heavy for their size. If they have green tops, these should be bright and crisp. Store in a cool, dark, airy place, or in the fridge, for up to a week.

Vegetable basics

Enjoy vegetables when they are at their peak of freshness and they will reward you with taste, texture and optimum nutrition.

Speedy turnover – fresh and fast

The vitamins and minerals in vegetables are at peak levels when the produce is first harvested, so buy the freshest possible vegetables, in quantities you will consume quickly. Keep frozen vegetables as back-up for times when you run out of fresh, rather than storing fresh produce for too long.

The fridge is the best storage place for most vegetables. The exceptions are root vegetables, such as potatoes, parsnips and onions, and hard-skinned squashes, which keep best in a cool, dark and dry place.

Golden rules for preparing vegetables

• Prepare as close to cooking or eating as possible. Once cut, oxidation causes loss of vitamin C from vegetables exposed to air – sprinkling with lemon juice helps to reduce this.
• Wash vegetables thoroughly but quickly. Never soak them, because water-soluble vitamins will seep out and then be drained away.

• When possible, eat the peel or skin, as nutrients are often concentrated just under it. The skin also provides fibre.
• Prepare vegetables for boiling or steaming in large pieces rather than cutting them into small cubes or slices. There is then less surface area from which nutrients can be lost.
• When cooking vegetables in water, save the cooking liquid and use it, within a day or two, in soups or sauces.
• Whether boiling, steaming, frying or grilling, be sure not to overcook crisp green and yellow vegetables. Not only does it destroy even more of the vital vitamin content, but it leaves the vegetables limp and flavourless.

Cooking know-how
Boiling

Use the minimum of water and add vegetables to boiling water (rather than covering them with cold water and bringing to the boil), to shorten the time for nutrients to seep out. Pour just enough boiling water over root vegetables to cover them. Never add bicarbonate of soda to the cooking water – it is an old-fashioned method of preserving the vegetable's colour, but it destroys vitamin C. Simmer or boil for the shortest possible time. Drain and serve immediately.

▼ Wash vegetables quickly in a colander under cold running water

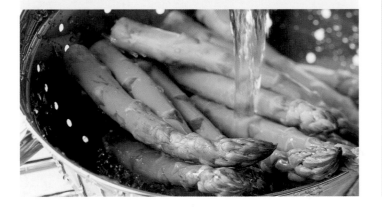

How does cooking affect vitamins and minerals?

Beta-carotene (which is converted into vitamin A by the body) is stable during mild heating, but losses occur at high temperatures.
Vitamin C leaches out during cooking because it is water soluble and it is also heat sensitive, so some is destroyed.
Water-soluble B vitamins are lost if the cooking water is discarded.
Vitamin E is destroyed at high temperature.
Minerals are not destroyed by heating, but they dissolve in water and seep out into the cooking liquid.
Nutrients are lost when food is left standing, kept warm or reheated.

Baked potato wedges

These super-chunky oven chips are a great alternative to deep-fried chips. Preheat the oven to 240ºC (475ºF, gas mark 9) and heat a roasting tin in the oven. Cut scrubbed potatoes (with the skin) into big wedges and place them in a polythene bag. Add 1–2 tbsp sunflower or extra virgin olive oil (or just enough to coat the potatoes lightly) and seasoning to taste (dried herbs and fennel seeds are good too), then shake the bag to coat the potatoes. Tip them into the hot roasting tin and bake for 45–50 minutes, turning once or twice, until the potato wedges are crisp and well browned. Serve hot.

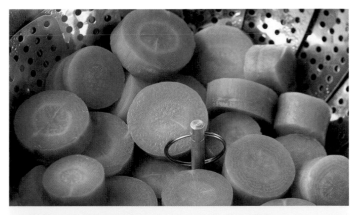

▲ Steam vegetables until they are just tender but still firm

Steaming

This moist method takes slightly longer than boiling, but because the vegetables are not immersed in water there is less loss of water-soluble vitamins and minerals. The maximum vitamins and minerals are retained if the vegetables are sealed in a foil parcel, otherwise some nutrients will be lost by seepage into moisture as the steam condenses and drips back into the pan.

Braising and stewing

Most types of vegetables can be cooked this way, either singly or mixed. Start by cooking those that take longest, and add vegetables that cook quickly towards the end. Use a small amount of liquid and serve it with the vegetables.

Stir-frying

Being quick and using the minimum of liquid and fat, this is a very good method for preserving maximum nutrients. Cut up the vegetables just before cooking. Stir-fry frozen vegetables from frozen. Serve any cooking juices with the vegetables.

Frying

With a non-stick pan and just enough of a monounsaturated or polyunsaturated vegetable oil to prevent the vegetables from sticking to the pan, frying can be a good cooking method for vegetables.

Steaming in foil packets
retains vital nutrients

Grilling

This is good for all sorts of vegetables, particularly peppers, aubergines, mushrooms and courgettes. Brush them with the minimum of oil and cook under a preheated grill. Grilling on a flameproof dish is a useful way of preserving juices.

Baking and roasting

These are perfect methods for preserving water-soluble nutrients and are ideal for a wide variety of vegetables. Roots, vegetable fruits, stalks and shoots all cook well this way. Leafy vegetables can be baked when rolled around a stuffing.

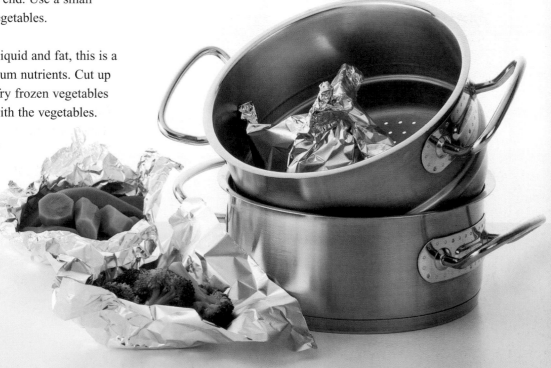

Vegetable stock

Use this light stock as a base for delicate soups and sauces, and in risottos and similar dishes. It will keep in the fridge for up to 5 days or in the freezer for up to 1 month.

Makes about 1.7 litres (3 pints)

15 g (½ oz) butter
225 g (8 oz) leeks, chopped
225 g (8 oz) onions, chopped
1 large bay leaf
several sprigs of fresh thyme
several sprigs of fresh parsley, stalks bruised
225 g (8 oz) carrots, diced
150 g (5½ oz) celery, diced
1 tsp salt
5 black peppercorns

Preparation time: 15 minutes
Cooking time: 1 hour

1 Melt the butter in a large saucepan or stockpot over a moderate heat. Stir in the leeks and onions, then reduce the heat to low. Cover with a tight-fitting lid and leave the vegetables to 'sweat' for 20 minutes without lifting the lid.

2 Tie the herbs together into a bouquet garni. Add it to the pan with the carrots, celery, salt, peppercorns and 2 litres (3½ pints) of cold water. Increase the heat and bring slowly to the boil, skimming the surface if necessary to remove any scum. As soon as the water boils, reduce the heat to low and simmer for 35 minutes.

3 Strain the stock into a large heatproof bowl and set aside to cool. Use immediately, or transfer to tightly sealed jars or freezer containers for storage.

Another idea

• To make a rich roasted vegetable stock, omit the butter and leeks. Increase the quantity of onions to 900 g (2 lb) and carrots to 450 g (1 lb). Instead of sweating the onions as in step 1, roast them with the carrots. Preheat the oven to 220°C (425°F, gas mark 7) and toss the onions and carrots with 1 tbsp extra virgin olive oil in a flameproof casserole. Roast the vegetables for 40 minutes, stirring twice. Add the remaining ingredients and follow steps 2 and 3 to finish the stock. To further enrich the stock, add 10 g (¼ oz) dried porcini mushrooms and 1 tbsp dry sherry with the water.

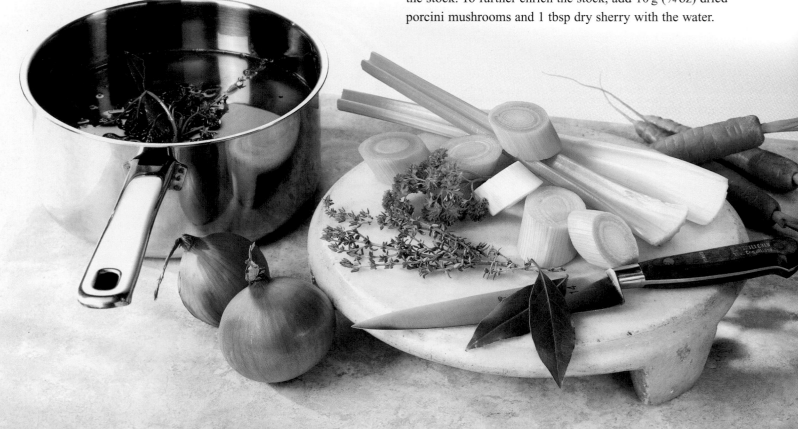

Light mashed potatoes

This plain mash is flavoured with a hint of bay and enriched with a little olive oil instead of butter.

Serves 4

125 ml (4½ fl oz) milk
1 bay leaf
900 g (2 lb) floury potatoes, such as King Edward or Maris Piper, peeled and cut into chunks
2 tbsp extra virgin olive oil
salt and pepper

Preparation time: 15 minutes
Cooking time: 15–20 minutes

1 Place the milk, bay leaf and a pinch of salt in a small saucepan. Heat gently until just boiling, then remove from the heat and set aside to infuse while you cook the potatoes.

2 Place the potatoes in a saucepan and pour over boiling water to cover by 5 cm (2 in). Bring back to the boil, then reduce the heat and cook for 15–20 minutes or until the potatoes are very tender.

3 Drain the potatoes, shaking the colander or sieve to remove any excess water, and return them to the pan. Discard the bay leaf and pour the milk over the potatoes.

4 Mash the potatoes until they are completely smooth. Add the olive oil, then beat in seasoning to taste. Serve immediately.

Some more ideas

• To make a parsley mash, omit the bay leaf used to flavour the milk. Finely chop 55 g (2 oz) parsley – or less if you prefer – and add to the potatoes with the olive oil.

• Dill and lemon mash is excellent with fish or poultry dishes. Replace the bay leaf with the finely grated zest of ½ lemon. Do not strain the zest out of the milk. Beat 4 tbsp finely chopped fresh dill into the mash with the seasoning.

• For a garlic mash, infuse 1 garlic clove, crushed, in the milk instead of the bay leaf. Strain the milk into the potatoes.

• Cardamom sweet potatoes are delicious with grilled or roast poultry or meat, especially pork. Cover 450 g (1 lb) sweet potatoes, cut into 2.5 cm (1 in) dice, with boiling water and add 1 bay leaf and 2 green cardamom pods, crushed. Cook for 10 minutes or until very tender. Drain, reserving 3 tbsp of the cooking liquid; discard the flavourings. Mash until smooth with the reserved liquid, then add a little freshly grated nutmeg and seasoning to taste.

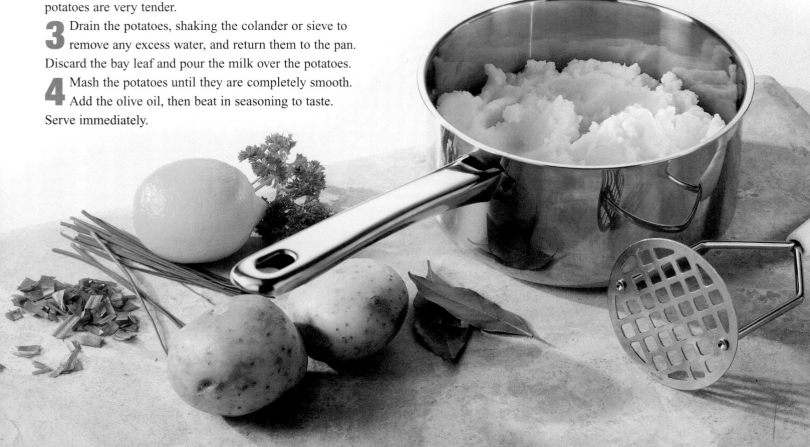

Salads in a healthy diet

With a vast and tempting array of ingredients from all over the world, a salad can be whatever you want it to be.

Why salads are so healthy

Nutritionist experts agree that a varied diet is one of the best routes to good health. Salads are a delicious way to enjoy a wide variety of foods, as they can be prepared from all kinds of fruit and vegetables, along with many other ingredients, so they can offer a broad range of nutrients. And because they are so adaptable, suitable for main meals as well as side dishes, perfect for entertaining and great for everyday family meals, salads can be a regular part of everyone's diet.

Current healthy eating guidelines recommend that we should eat at least 5 portions of fruit and vegetables every day. A salad is an easy and tasty way to help you reach this target. Salad is also very nutritious, because the fruit and vegetables are normally used raw, or only lightly cooked, thus retaining maximum vitamins and minerals – for example, the vitamin C content is higher in raw fruit and vegetables than when they are cooked. An added benefit is that raw foods take more chewing and digesting, so they can help to prevent overeating.

Starchy carbohydrates, such as pasta, rice, starchy grains, bread and potatoes, are another important part of a healthy diet, and they are easy to incorporate into a salad. And with the addition of a moderate amount of protein-rich food, such as meat, chicken, fish, cheese, eggs, nuts or pulses, a salad can become a substantial, well-balanced main dish.

What salad nutrients can do

Because salads can contain such a wide range of ingredients, the nutrients on offer will vary from recipe to recipe. All salads, though, supply lots of vitamins, minerals and dietary fibre from their vegetable and fruit content. Among the key nutrients provided are the antioxidants vitamin C and beta-carotene. Antioxidants help to slow down the production of damaging free radicals. Experts believe that a surplus of these free radicals is one of the major causes of coronary heart disease and cancer.

Eating lots of vitamin C-rich fruit and vegetables has other benefits too, such as increasing the absorption of iron from foods eaten at the same time. And beta-carotene is converted by the body into vitamin A, needed for growth. Vitamin E, another antioxidant vitamin found in some vegetables, helps to keep the skin healthy. Most salad leaves are a good source of folate (a B vitamin), which is important in pregnancy to help prevent birth defects.

Fruit and vegetables contain fibre, which is vital for good health. One type, soluble fibre, helps to regulate the levels of cholesterol and sugar in the blood, and has been shown to improve control of late-onset diabetes. Insoluble fibre (plus water) speeds food through the digestive process, helping to prevent constipation and some diseases. Foods containing soluble fibre are also a good source of oligosaccharides, which are substances that stimulate the growth of beneficial bacteria in the gastro-intestinal tract.

Other ingredients in a fresh salad can provide additional important nutrients, such as omega-3 fatty acids (from oily fish and nuts), iron (from red meat), calcium (from cheese and other dairy products) and zinc (from shellfish).

Salads for all seasons

Salads aren't just for summer – they can be warm and hearty, spicy and cheering, just as appetising in January as in July. By using seasonal ingredients, such as asparagus in May and June, or chicory and pumpkin in the autumn, you will ensure maximum taste and nutrients all year round. And you can ring the changes, whatever the season, with the addition of fresh herbs and flavouring ingredients like garlic, chilli and ginger.

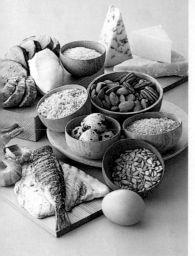

◀ Best for B vitamins – meat, poultry, whole grains, cheese, nuts, seeds, eggs and fish; pulses are another good source

▼ Best for beta-carotene – orange-fleshed melons, pumpkin, carrots, dark green leafy vegetables, tomatoes, red peppers, papaya and mango

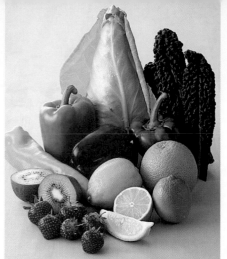

◀ Best for vitamin C – peppers, green leafy vegetables, citrus fruits, strawberries and kiwi fruit; guava, mango and papaya are other good sources

▼ Best for calcium – dark green leafy vegetables, cheese, yogurt dressings, nuts, seeds, and canned fish with bones

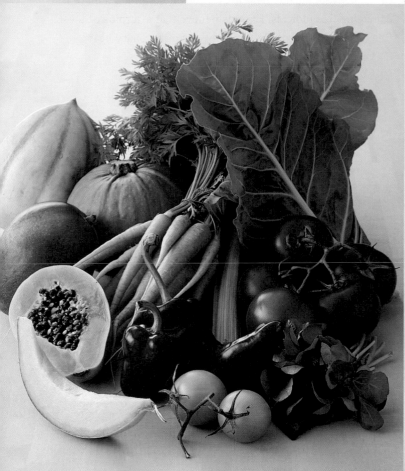

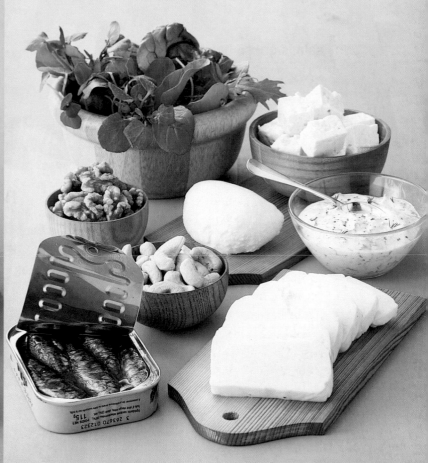

Best for iron – pulses, liver, lean red meat, wholegrains and dried apricots; other good sources include seeds and dark green, leafy vegetables ▶

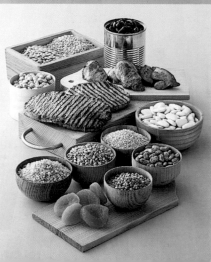

Best for fibre – green leafy vegetables, pears, apples, onions, olives, green beans, dried fruit and fresh berries; other good sources include pulses, whole grains, nuts, asparagus, citrus fruits and mango ▶

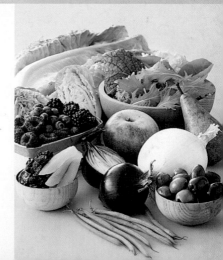

A riot of salad leaves

Savour the full range of salad leaves. From tender pale green to vivid red and purple, they are crisp, tasty, and never boring.

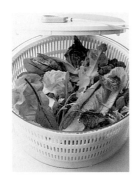

Choosing salad leaves

To be interesting, a leafy salad needs a good mix of colours, flavours and textures. This will also ensure that it is nutritious because, in general, the darker and more bitter leaves tend to have a higher nutrient content than sweet leaves. For example, the darker green (or red) and more strongly flavoured a salad leaf is, the more beta-carotene and other carotenoids it will contain. Also, the dark outer leaves of lettuces may provide up to 50 times more carotenoids than inner, paler leaves. Another way to be sure that leafy salads are nutritious is to make them large. Salad leaves contain such a high proportion of water that you need a lot of them to provide a reasonable amount of nutrients.

Sweet and mild-flavoured leaves

The light, subtle flavour of soft, sweet salad leaves makes them an excellent base for a simple side salad with a tasty vinaigrette, or for salads made with other delicately flavoured ingredients, such as avocado or egg.

Beet greens

Dark green or reddish-green with a red stalk, beet greens taste like a cross between beetroot and spinach – slightly sweet, yet full of flavour. Use young leaves as older ones may be tough. They are rich in carotenoids.

Cos and romaine lettuces

The classic base for a Caesar salad, cos and romaine lettuces have a long, oval head of tightly packed crisp leaves. They are rich in potassium and also contain carotenoids.

Iceberg lettuce

This pale, round, tightly packed lettuce has crisp leaves with a refreshing but bland flavour. It is useful for its texture.

Lamb's lettuce (corn salad, mâche)

These small rosettes of mid-green leaves have a delicious velvety texture and delicate flavour.

Little Gem lettuce

This is a smaller, compact variety of cos lettuce. The rich green outer leaves and delicate yellow inner leaves are crisp, with a sweet flavour. Simply halve or quarter the spear-shaped heads lengthways or separate into individual leaves.

Lollo Rosso lettuce

A non-hearting, loose-leaf lettuce, Lollo Rosso has fringed and crinkled leaves that are tinged deep red at their ends, with a fairly tender yet crisp texture and a bland flavour. It is a useful source of the antioxidant quercetin, which is believed to help to reduce the risk of heart disease.

Oak Leaf lettuce (feuille de chêne)

This loose-leaf lettuce has very attractive serrated, deep bronze leaves and a pleasant mild but distinctive flavour. It is a useful source of the antioxidant quercetin.

Red chard

A member of the beet family, red chard has red stalks and mid to deep-green leaves sometimes tinged with red. It provides fibre, vitamin C, folate and beta-carotene. Use the young leaves in mixed salads to add rich colour.

Round lettuce

With its soft mid-green outer leaves and a slightly crisper, paler heart, this is the traditional 'British lettuce'.

Spinach

Glossy green spinach leaves have a slightly metallic flavour due to their high iron content. The iron is not all absorbed by the body, however, due to the leaf's oxalic acid content. In addition, spinach offers vitamins C and E, folate and a carotenoid called lutein, which aids eye health and may help to protect against lung cancer. Use young leaves raw in salads.

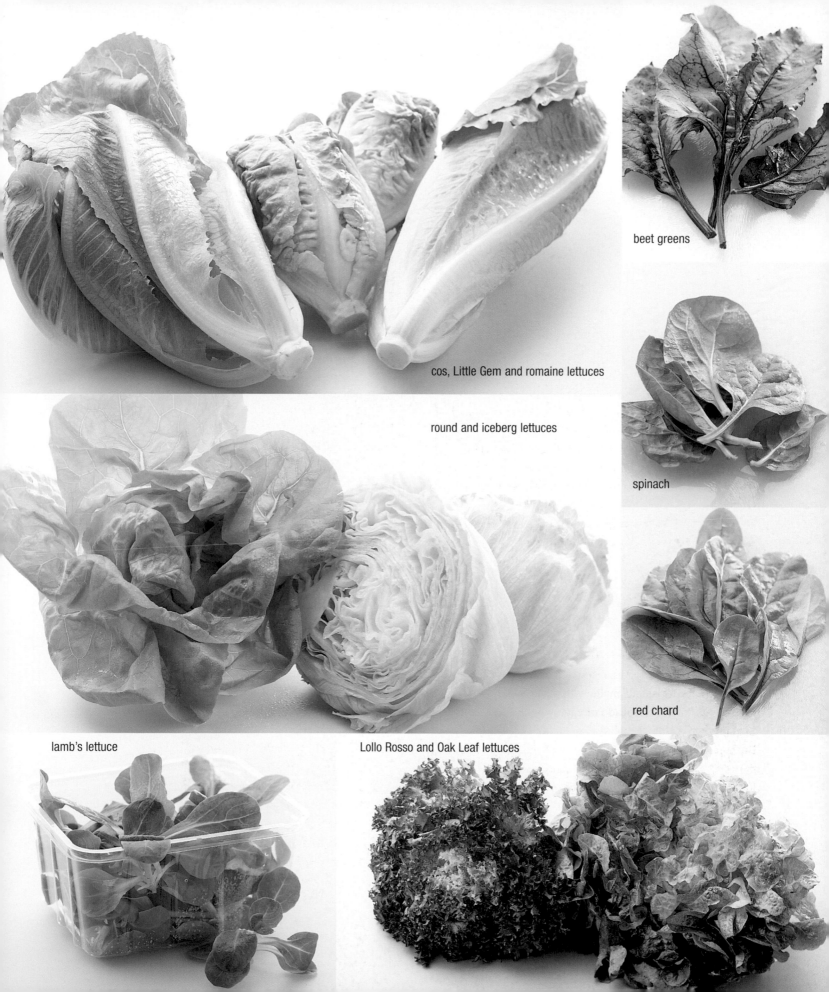

beet greens

cos, Little Gem and romaine lettuces

round and iceberg lettuces

spinach

red chard

lamb's lettuce

Lollo Rosso and Oak Leaf lettuces

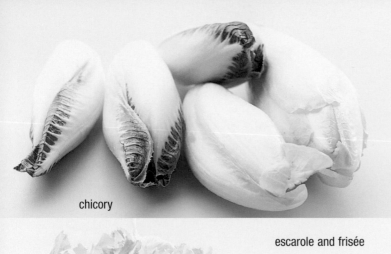

chicory

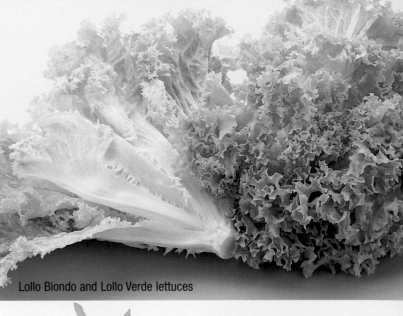

escarole and frisée

Lollo Biondo and Lollo Verde lettuces

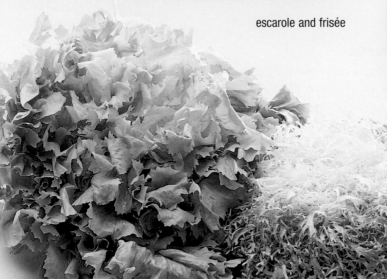

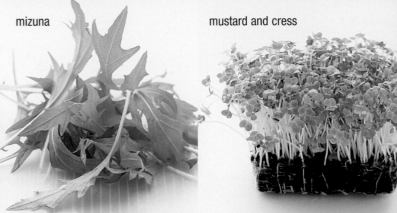

mizuna

mustard and cress

Bitter and strongly flavoured leaves

In general, darker salad leaves have a stronger flavour than pale ones, and just a few sprigs of a peppery green such as watercress or rocket will provide delightful contrast in a salad of sweet leaves.

Chicory

Chicory has small, tightly packed, spear-shaped heads of pale – almost white – leaves tinged with yellow or red at the tips. It has a fairly crisp texture and a pleasantly bitter flavour that can be strong. Cut the head into quarters lengthways or separate into individual leaves. Chicory is in season in autumn and winter, so it is an ideal winter salad ingredient. It can be kept in the fridge for up to 5 days.

Escarole

A broad-leaved kind of frisée, this has crunchy, mid-green outer leaves and a pale heart. The flavour is slightly bitter, less bitter than frisée. It is good mixed with milder salad leaves.

Frisée

The large, round, slightly flattened heads of frisée have finely divided, mid-green leaves with a strong bitter flavour. The paler centre leaves are milder.

Lollo Biondo and Lollo Verde lettuces

These loose-leaf lettuces have a fairly mild flavour (but stronger than the closely related Lollo Rosso). If you grow your own loose-leaf lettuces you can pick individual leaves rather than the whole head.

Mizuna

A recent arrival from the Far East, this deeply divided, pretty green leaf has a strong and peppery flavour. It is rich in the B vitamin folate. Mizuna is in season in winter and can add interest to any winter salad. It goes well with sweet flavours such as dried apricots.

Mustard and cress

Sold in small tubs, this mixture of seedlings of garden cress

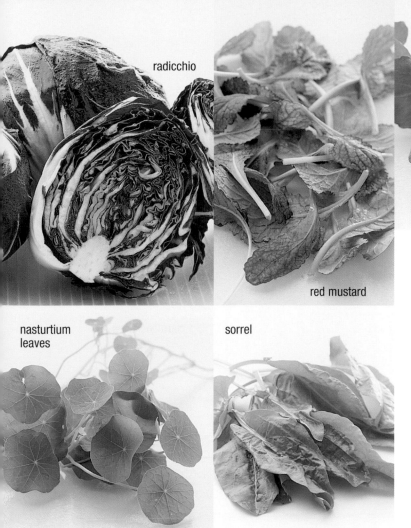

radicchio

red mustard

nasturtium leaves

sorrel

watercress

rocket

Rocket

This popular salad leaf has deep green, elongated frilled leaves with a pungent flavour. It is rich in carotenoids and iron.

Sorrel

Looking something like spinach, sorrel leaves are mid-green and oval or spear shaped. Their flavour is lemony and refreshing, and just a few young leaves will lift a bland salad.

Watercress

The small, glossy, dark green leaves of watercress are rich in vitamin C, folate, iron and other minerals, and carotenoids, and they also offer cancer-fighting glucosinolates. Be sure to use the tender stalks as well as the leaves.

Buying, storing and preparing salad leaves

• Buy the freshest lettuces and salad leaves you can find – the vitamins and minerals are at peak levels when the greens are first harvested. If the leaves have a brown tinge to their edges or are wilted and slimy, don't buy them. Most can be stored in the fridge for up to 4 days, although it is best to use them as soon as possible.

• You may only be able to find some of the less common salad leaves ready-prepared and packed in a cellophane bag, often as part of a mixed salad. Ready-prepared salad leaves should be used within 24 hours, because once cut they begin to lose their vitamin C and B-complex vitamins.

• Give salad leaves a quick wash in cold water, then spin dry in a salad spinner or pat dry in a clean tea-towel. Don't leave them to soak as this will result in the loss of some of the water-soluble vitamins such as C and folate.

• Salad leaves can be trimmed, washed and dried, then kept in the fridge for a few hours before serving, but do not dress them until ready to serve, otherwise the acid in the dressing will make the leaves wilt.

and white mustard (or, sometimes, rape) is mostly used as a garnish or in a sandwich. If eaten in larger quantities, though, it can be a good source of vitamin C and carotenoids.

Nasturtium leaves

With their peppery flavour and nice succulent texture, these make a pretty addition to a mixed leaf salad. They contain phytochemicals, which have antibiotic properties.

Radicchio

A member of the chicory family, radicchio has crisp, deep red and white leaves with a slightly bitter, nutty flavour. It is high in beta-carotene and other cancer-fighting phytochemicals. In season during the autumn, it makes a beautiful addition to a green leaf salad, and is delicious mixed with citrus fruits.

Red mustard

These colourful, mottled red and green leaves have a hot mustardy flavour. If picked as baby leaves, the flavour is milder. Red mustard is a good source of phytochemicals.

Herbs for salads

Fresh herbs can give a wonderful burst of flavour to a salad, and may bring extra nutritional benefits too.

Basil Traditional in a pesto dressing, basil's small leaves have a pungent and delicious flavour. Scatter over any tomato salad, but particularly one with mozzarella cheese.

Chervil A good winter herb, delicate and pretty chervil tastes slightly of aniseed and parsley. It goes well with carrots and other root vegetables.

Chives In common with other members of the onion family, the grass-like leaves of chives are rich in beneficial sulphur compounds and allicin, a phytochemical that helps to prevent heart disease. Snip chives over meat, poultry, fish or leaf salads.

Coriander Powerful, spicy-tasting coriander leaves are an essential ingredient in Oriental and Mexican-style salads. They are decorative too, with their round, frilled-edge petals.

Dill The mild caraway taste of feathery dill leaves works well in seafood, potato and cucumber salads.

Mint With its strong fresh flavour and good green colour, mint is one of the most popular herbs, and is delicious in potato and bean salads as well as with fruits such as melon and mango.

Oregano and marjoram These closely related herbs with very small leaves have a strong flavour, so use them sparingly in tomato salads or warm salads of courgette, aubergine or lamb. They are a traditional flavouring in a Greek salad.

Parsley The classic garnish for savoury dishes, parsley is also a tasty addition to a herb or leaf salad, particularly Italian or flat-leaf parsley. It is a good source of folate, iron and vitamin C.

Purslane A herb from Greece and Turkey, purslane has fleshy, round, mid-green leaves with a mild, fresh flavour. Add a few leaves to a mixed leaf salad or scatter over a potato salad.

Rosemary One of the most aromatic of herbs, needle-like rosemary leaves are best used in warm vegetable, pork, lamb and fish salads. Tarragon The lance-shaped leaves of this herb have a strong aniseed flavour that is perfect in chicken salads.

Thyme Tiny yet very aromatic, thyme leaves are good in potato and bean salads as well as in warm salads with beef and duck.

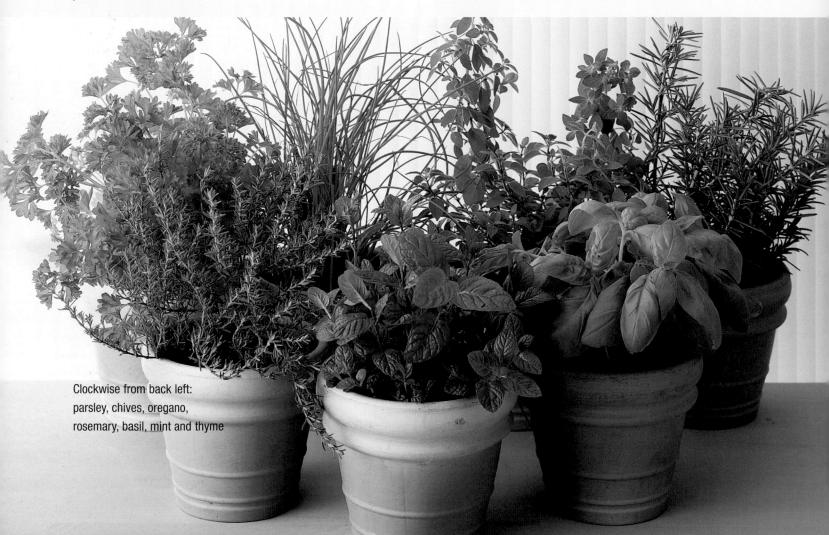

Clockwise from back left:
parsley, chives, oregano,
rosemary, basil, mint and thyme

Dressed in style

A good dressing makes all the difference, complementing the salad, not overwhelming it. It can also add vitamins, calcium and healthy fats to your meal.

The right ingredients

Salads can be dressed simply with fresh fruit juice, or with a vinaigrette or creamy dressing. Vinaigrettes usually consist of an oil base sharpened with vinegar or an acidic fruit juice, plus seasoning and flavourings such as fresh herbs. Creamy dressings are based on mayonnaise, yogurt, fromage frais and so on. Most dressings can be whisked together with a fork, or, in the case of vinaigrette, shaken in a screw-top jar.

Oils

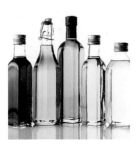

Good-quality oils contain beneficial phytochemicals, so it makes sense to use the best that you can afford. Extra virgin cold-pressed oils are the 'top of the range'. These are produced with minimal heat and refining processes, and thus retain more of their phytochemicals and essential fatty acids. Cheap blended vegetable oils that have been highly refined (the paler the colour, the more refined they are) have little goodness left in them. They may also contain oils high in saturated fat, such as coconut oil.

Choosing the right oil is vital to the success of a dressing. Olive oil is the classic for most vinaigrettes. Olive oil is like wine – different varieties of olive and a different growing region will give the oil its own special properties, and it can be peppery, salty, fruity, creamy and mild, and so on. Some olive oils are so delicious that they can be used alone to dress a salad. Have at least one basic mild extra virgin olive oil and then experiment with others.

Sunflower and groundnut oils are good for lighter salad dressings. Walnut and hazelnut oils work well with salads that include cheese, chicken, celery, spinach, apples and green beans, and can be mixed with olive or another oil to make them go further. Toasted sesame oil, often used in Oriental dressings, has a smoky, nutty flavour. You can also find oils flavoured with herbs and fresh chillies, and these can add extra zest to plain salads.

Keep oils in a cool, dark place to prevent them from oxidising and going rancid. Nut oils are particularly susceptible to oxidisation, so it is best to buy them in small quantities.

Vinegars

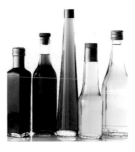

There are many vinegars you can use in salad dressings. The classic is wine vinegar (red or white, with red being slightly more robust in flavour). Sherry vinegar has an even fuller flavour. Richest of all the wine-based vinegars is balsamic, which should be used sparingly. It is so delicious it is often sprinkled over a salad on its own as a dressing. Fruit vinegars are made by steeping fresh fruit, such as raspberries, in white wine vinegar. Sharp and refreshing apple cider vinegar is good in dressings for cheese and ham salads. Rice vinegar, with its delicate flavour, is traditional in Oriental salad dressings.

Creamy dressings

Mayonnaise is the classic base for creamy dressings, but it is high in fat and calories. A healthier alternative can be made with yogurt or by mixing yogurt with mayonnaise. Yogurt (along with other dairy products) is a valuable source of calcium and contains beneficial bacteria that help to maintain a healthy digestive tract. Greek-style yogurt is deliciously rich; bio yogurt is mild and creamy; low-fat plain yogurt has a pleasant tangy flavour.

Other calcium-rich dairy products that make a good base for salad dressings are soured cream, crème fraîche and fromage frais. Even if they are higher in fat than low-fat yogurt, they are still a healthy alternative to mayonnaise. Reduced-fat versions of mayonnaise, Greek-style yogurt, soured cream, crème fraîche and fromage frais are also available, for an even lower fat creamy salad dressing.

Myriad flavourings

Ring the changes with vinaigrettes and creamy dressings by adding different seasonings and flavourings.

● Choose fresh herbs to complement the ingredients in the salad. Try thyme and rosemary for a roast Mediterranean vegetable salad, parsley and mint for a broad bean salad.

● Coarsely ground black pepper, with salt, is the classic seasoning for any dressing, but other spices can enliven a salad dressing too. Try paprika or cayenne pepper in a dressing for seafood and pasta salads; mustard or poppy seeds for leaf

salads; caraway seeds in a creamy dressing for cabbage and root vegetable salads; ground cardamom and coriander for carrot, rice and grain salads. A little curry paste can be mixed into a dressing for a chicken salad.

● Use fresh flavourings such as lemongrass, garlic, chilli and ginger in Oriental salad dressings.

● Add a gentle bit of heat with Dijon mustard, a traditional component of a vinaigrette. Crunchy wholegrain mustard is also delicious.

● Roast a whole head of garlic until soft, then squeeze out the cloves, mash and mix into a creamy yogurt to make a healthy aioli dressing. Fresh garlic, finely chopped or crushed, is another dressing classic.

● Squeeze citrus juices for a tangy fresh flavour – try orange juice for a carrot salad, lime juice for a Thai salad or lemon juice for a Greek salad.

● Give a piquant touch to a dressing for seafood and poultry salads by adding capers.

● Sweeten soy-based Oriental salad dressings with honey or caster sugar.

● Finely chop black olives and mix into a vinaigrette for Mediterranean salads, or use tapenade (black olive paste).

● For seafood salads, flavour and colour a vinaigrette or creamy dressing with sun-dried tomato paste or ketchup.

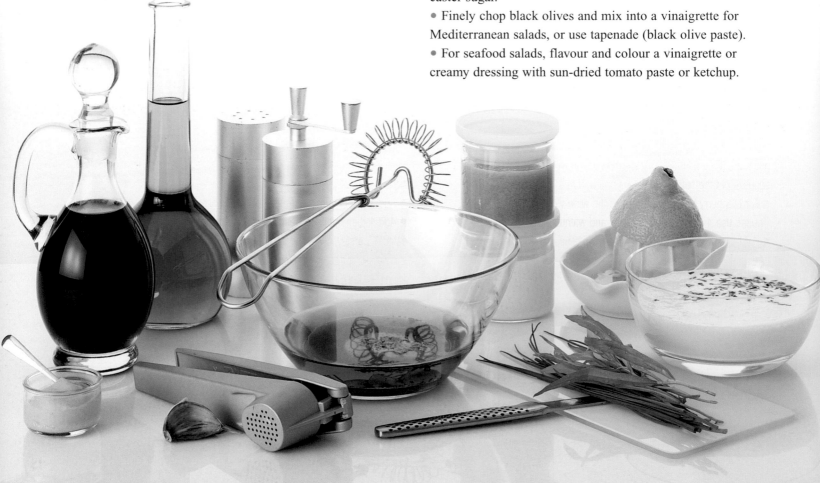

Basic vinaigrette

A vinaigrette can be mixed specially for a salad or it can be made in a larger quantity, to use as required – it will keep in the fridge for several weeks. If made ahead, store it in a screw-top jar and shake well just before using.

Makes about 150 ml (5 fl oz)

120 ml (4 fl oz) extra virgin olive oil
2 tbsp red wine vinegar
1 tsp Dijon mustard or wholegrain mustard
pinch of caster sugar (optional)
salt and pepper

Preparation time: 2 minutes

1 Whisk all the ingredients together in a bowl, adding salt and pepper to taste. Alternatively, put all the ingredients in a screw-top jar, put on the lid and shake well.

Some more ideas

● For herb vinaigrette, add 1 tbsp chopped fresh herbs of your choice, such as tarragon, chives or thyme. If storing the vinaigrette, add the herbs just before using.

● For chilli vinaigrette, add 1–2 seeded and finely chopped fresh red chillies. Replace 1 tbsp of the olive oil with toasted sesame oil, if you like.

● For garlic vinaigrette, add 1–2 finely crushed garlic cloves. For a milder taste, roast 1 bulb of garlic, wrapped in foil, in a preheated 180°C (350°F, gas mark 4) oven for 40 minutes or until tender. Leave until cool, then squeeze out the soft garlic cloves and add to the oil, whisking well.

● For raspberry vinaigrette, replace the wine vinegar with raspberry vinegar. Use 4 tbsp each of olive oil and walnut oil.

● For poppy seed vinaigrette, replace the olive oil with sunflower or groundnut oil and add 1–2 tsp poppy seeds. Use lemon juice instead of vinegar or, for a richer, more robust flavour, use 1 tbsp each of balsamic vinegar and red wine vinegar.

● For an Oriental vinaigrette, replace the wine vinegar with rice vinegar and add 1 tbsp soy sauce. Sweeten with a few drops of clear honey instead of sugar.

Basic creamy dressing

Made with fromage frais or yogurt, this rich, smooth and refreshing dressing is lower in fat than traditional creamy dressings based on mayonnaise. It can be stored in the fridge for 1–2 days.

Makes about 150 ml (5 fl oz)

120 ml (4 fl oz) fromage frais or Greek-style yogurt
1 tbsp lemon juice
2 tsp white wine vinegar
pinch of caster sugar
salt

Preparation time: 2 minutes

1 Put all the ingredients into a bowl, adding salt to taste, and stir together until evenly blended. Taste and add more sugar, salt or lemon juice, if necessary.

2 Cover the bowl with cling film and keep the dressing in the fridge until ready to use.

Some more ideas

● For an even lower fat dressing, use 8%-fat fromage frais and half-fat Greek-style yogurt. The result will still be very creamy.

● Add 1–2 tsp creamed horseradish for beef and smoked mackerel salads.

● Add 1–2 tsp sun-dried tomato paste for seafood salads.

● Add 1 finely chopped shallot for pasta salads. Alternatively, add 1 crushed garlic clove or 1 tsp garlic purée.

● Add 1–2 tsp curry paste for chicken salads.

● Add 1 tbsp chopped fresh herbs, such as coriander, basil (for pasta salads), parsley, chives or tarragon (for chicken salads).

● To make a dip for crudités, add 1–2 tbsp grated Cheddar cheese or crumbled soft blue cheese, such as Roquefort or Dolcelatte.

Chilled leek and avocado soup

Coriander and lime juice accentuate the delicate avocado flavour in this refreshing soup. It is simple yet interesting, and ideal for a summer's dinner-party first course or a light lunch. Do not add the avocado too soon – not only will it discolour slightly, but its flavour will mellow and lose the vital freshness.

Serves 4

1 tbsp extra virgin olive oil

450 g (1 lb) leeks, halved lengthways and thinly sliced

1 garlic clove, finely chopped

750 ml (1¼ pints) vegetable or chicken stock, bought chilled or made with a stock cube or bouillon powder

1 large ripe avocado

125 g (4½ oz) plain low-fat yogurt

1 tbsp lime juice

2 tbsp chopped fresh coriander

salt and pepper

To garnish

8–12 ice cubes (optional)

slices of lime

sprigs of fresh coriander

Preparation and cooking time: 30 minutes, plus cooling and chilling

Each serving provides

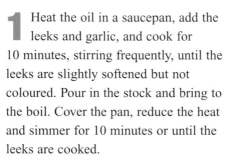

kcal 170, protein 5 g, fat 14 g (of which saturated fat 3 g), carbohydrate 7 g (of which sugars 5 g), fibre 4 g

✓✓	B_6, C, E, potassium
✓	A, B_1, folate

1 Heat the oil in a saucepan, add the leeks and garlic, and cook for 10 minutes, stirring frequently, until the leeks are slightly softened but not coloured. Pour in the stock and bring to the boil. Cover the pan, reduce the heat and simmer for 10 minutes or until the leeks are cooked.

2 Remove the soup from the heat and let it cool slightly, then purée it in a blender or food processor. Alternatively the soup can be puréed in the saucepan with a hand-held blender. Pour the soup into a bowl and leave it to cool, then chill well.

3 Just before serving the soup, prepare the avocado. Halve the avocado and discard the stone. Scoop the flesh from the peel and press through a fine stainless steel or nylon sieve. The avocado can also be puréed in a blender or food processor until smooth, adding a little of the chilled soup to thin the purée and ensure it is completely smooth.

4 Stir the avocado purée into the soup together with the yogurt, lime juice and coriander. Add seasoning to taste, then ladle the soup into 4 bowls. Float 2–3 ice cubes in each bowl, if you wish, then add slices of lime and sprigs of coriander. Serve at once.

Some more ideas

● This soup is also good hot. Purée the hot soup with the avocado and stir in crème fraîche instead of yogurt.

● For a soup with Mexican flavours, cook 1–2 seeded and finely chopped fresh green chillies with the leeks.

● For a simple no-cook avocado soup, blend 2 avocados with 450 ml (15 fl oz) vegetable stock, then add the yogurt and lime juice, and season to taste.

● To make vichyssoise, the classic chilled leek and potato soup, increase the stock to 1 litre (1¾ pints) and cook 2 peeled and sliced potatoes with the leeks. Omit the avocado, lime juice and coriander, and serve sprinkled with snipped fresh chives.

Plus points

● Half an avocado provides a quarter of the recommended daily intake of vitamin B_6 and useful amounts of vitamin E and potassium. Other substances in avocados are good for the skin.

● Leeks provide useful amounts of folate, which is important for proper blood cell formation and development of the nervous system in an unborn baby.

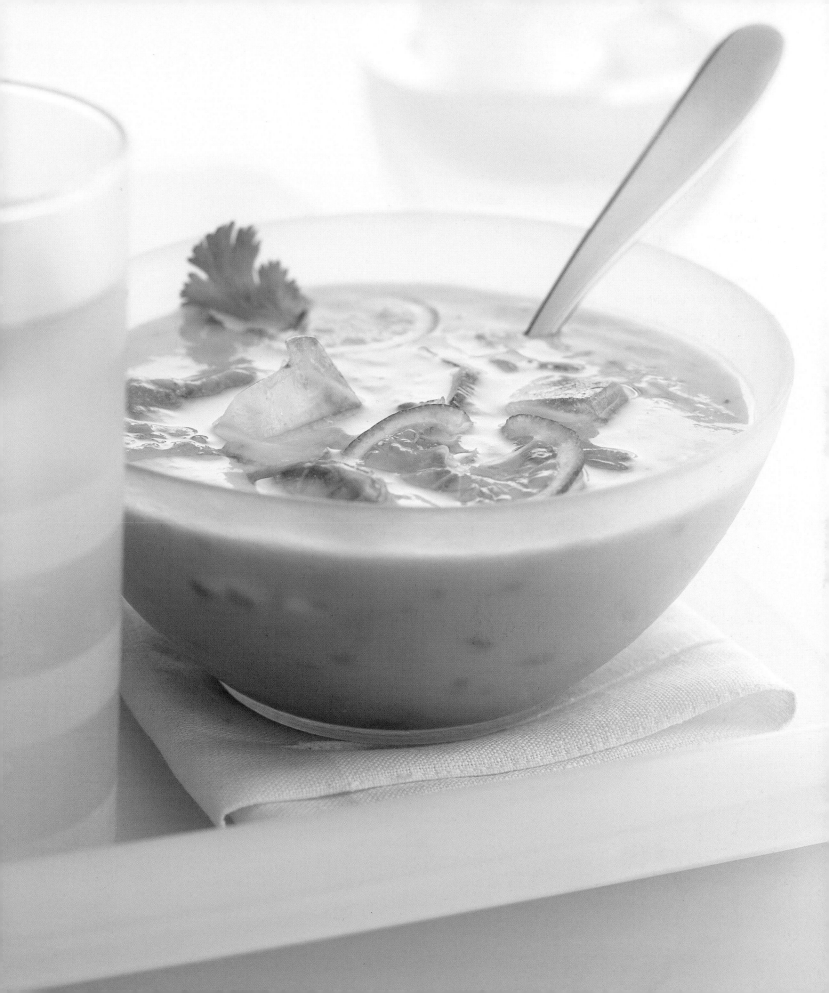

Borscht with crunchy mash

Guaranteed to beat off the winter blues, this hearty beetroot soup is served with creamy mashed potatoes enlivened with crunchy raw vegetables. There are as many types of borscht as there are cooks in Eastern Europe. The soup is often strained and served as a clear broth, but this puréed version retains every gram of goodness.

Serves 4

1 tbsp extra virgin olive oil

1 onion, chopped

1 large carrot

½ tsp lemon juice

1 bulb of fennel

500 g (1 lb 2 oz) raw beetroot

1 litre (1¾ pints) vegetable stock, preferably home-made light or rich (see page 28)

800 g (1¾ lb) floury potatoes, peeled and cut into small cubes

120 ml (4 fl oz) semi-skimmed milk

4 tbsp Greek-style yogurt

2 spring onions, finely chopped

salt and pepper

chopped leaves from the fennel bulb, herb fennel or parsley to garnish

Preparation time: about 35 minutes

Cooking time: about 50 minutes

Each serving provides   Ⓥ

kcal 300, protein 11 g, fat 4 g (of which saturated fat 1 g), carbohydrate 56 g (of which sugars 21 g), fibre 7 g

✓✓✓	A, folate
✓✓	B₁, B₆, C
✓	iron

1 Place the oil in a large saucepan and add the onion. Set aside 55 g (2 oz) of the carrot for the mash, then chop the rest and add it to the pan. Mix well, cover and cook over a moderate heat for 5 minutes to soften the onion.

2 Place the lemon juice in a small bowl. Cut the bulb of fennel into quarters. Finely grate one quarter into the lemon juice and toss well. Finely grate the reserved carrot and add it to the grated fennel. Cover and set aside.

3 Chop the remaining fennel and add to the saucepan. Peel and dice the beetroot, and add it to the pan. Pour in the stock and bring to the boil. Reduce the heat, cover the pan and simmer for about 30 minutes or until all the vegetables are tender.

4 Meanwhile, bring another pan of water to the boil. Add the potatoes and boil for 10 minutes or until very tender. Drain the potatoes well and return them to the pan. Place over a low heat for about 1 minute to dry, shaking the pan occasionally to prevent the potatoes from sticking. Remove from the heat and set aside, covered to keep hot.

5 Purée the soup in a blender or food processor until smooth, or purée in the pan using a hand blender. Return the soup to the pan, if necessary, and reheat. Taste and adjust the seasoning.

6 While the soup is reheating, set the pan of potatoes over a moderate heat and mash until completely smooth, gradually working in the milk. Stir in the yogurt, grated fennel and carrot, spring onions and seasoning to taste.

7 Divide the mashed potato among 4 bowls, piling it up in the centre. Ladle the soup around the mash and sprinkle with chopped fennel or parsley. Serve at once.

Plus points

• Beetroot is a particularly rich source of the B vitamin folate, which may help to protect against heart disease and spina bifida. It also provides useful amounts of iron. The characteristic deep red colour comes from a compound called betacyanin, which has been shown to prevent the growth of tumours in animal studies.

• Adding grated raw vegetables to mashed potatoes is a good way of including them in a hot meal, especially for children.

• Fennel contains phytoestrogen, a naturally occurring plant hormone that encourages the body to excrete excess oestrogen. A high level of oestrogen is associated with increased risk of breast cancer. Fennel also contains useful amounts of folate.

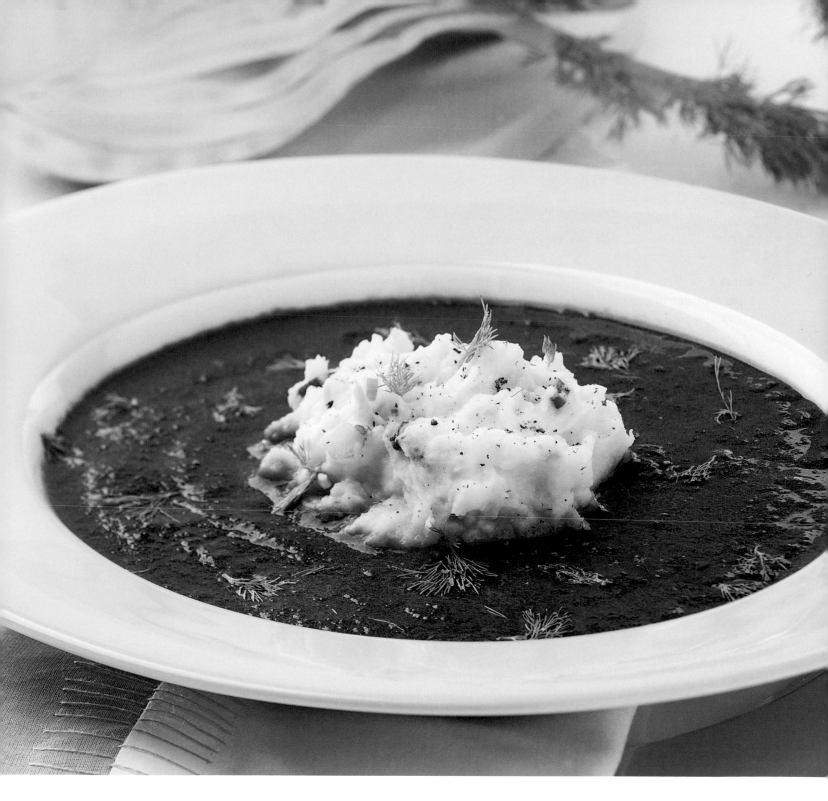

Some more ideas

• Other delicious raw vegetable additions to mashed potatoes are finely chopped celery, grated celeriac, finely shredded red or Savoy cabbage, shredded Brussels sprouts and coarsely chopped spring onions. They all contribute extra vitamins and minerals.

• Serve the borscht chunky instead of puréed, and add 2 tbsp hazelnut oil to the mashed potatoes instead of the yogurt.

• Instead of spooning the borscht around a pile of mash, garnish each bowl of soup simply with 1 tbsp Greek-style yogurt, soured cream or creamed horseradish, then sprinkle with chopped fresh fennel or parsley.

Avocado salad with raspberries

It's a misconception that avocados cannot be enjoyed in a healthy diet because of their high fat content. Yes, they do contain a great deal of fat, but it is the good monounsaturated type. In this salad, the creaminess of avocado is complemented by fresh raspberries and a fruity vinaigrette.

Serves 4

2 avocados

170 g (6 oz) mixed salad leaves, such as frisée, baby chard and lamb's lettuce

100 g (3½ oz) raspberries

sprigs of fresh mint to garnish

Raspberry vinaigrette

2 tbsp extra virgin olive oil

1½ tbsp raspberry vinegar

1 tbsp single cream

finely grated zest of ½ orange

½ tsp orange juice

pinch of caster sugar

salt and pepper

Preparation time: about 10 minutes

Each serving provides

kcal 255, protein 3 g, fat 25 g (of which saturated fat 5 g), carbohydrate 4 g (of which sugars 3 g), fibre 4 g

✓✓✓	B_1, B_6, C, E, niacin
✓	B_2, folate, copper, potassium

1 Put all the ingredients for the raspberry vinaigrette in a large salad bowl, adding salt and pepper to taste, and whisk to mix.

2 Halve the avocados and remove the stone, then peel and dice the flesh. Drop immediately into the dressing and turn to coat, to prevent the avocado from turning brown.

3 Add the salad leaves to the bowl and toss gently with the avocado. Scatter over the raspberries and garnish with mint sprigs. Serve at once.

Some more ideas for avocado salads

• For an Italian-style avocado and mozzarella starter salad, thickly slice each avocado half horizontally and arrange on 4 plates with 140 g (5 oz) sliced mozzarella cheese. Sprinkle with 100 g (3½ oz) sliced sun-dried tomatoes, then drizzle 1 tbsp extra virgin olive oil, or oil from the jar of tomatoes, over each serving. Season with pepper and garnish with fresh basil leaves.

• For an avocado and grapefruit salad, make the vinaigrette as in the main recipe, but replace the raspberry vinegar with pink grapefruit juice and omit the orange juice. Use watercress or rocket, or a mixture of watercress and baby spinach leaves, instead of mixed salad leaves, and 1 large pink grapefruit, peeled, divided into segments and each segment cut in half, instead of raspberries.

Toss the grapefruit with the avocado and leaves.

• Make a tropical avocado and mango salad. Line 4 plates with cos or romaine lettuce leaves. Cut each avocado half horizontally into thin slices and arrange on the plates with 1 thinly sliced, large ripe mango. Scatter 3 chopped spring onions over the top. Drizzle each salad with 1 tbsp extra virgin olive oil and 1–2 tbsp orange juice, and dust lightly with cayenne pepper.

Plus points

• Avocados are high in oleic acid, which helps to lower levels of the 'bad' LDL cholesterol while raising levels of the 'good' HDL cholesterol. Just one avocado provides half the recommended daily intake of vitamin B_6. They also provide useful amounts of vitamin E and potassium.

• Raspberries are an excellent source of vitamin C and also provide useful amounts of vitamin E.

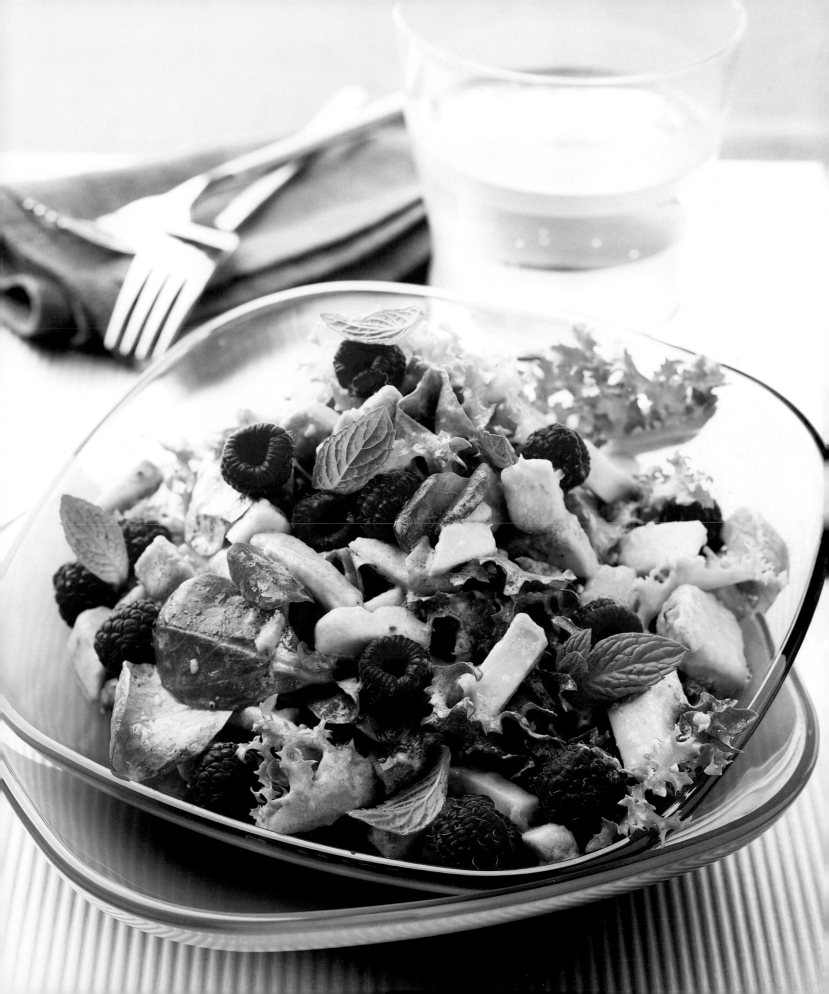

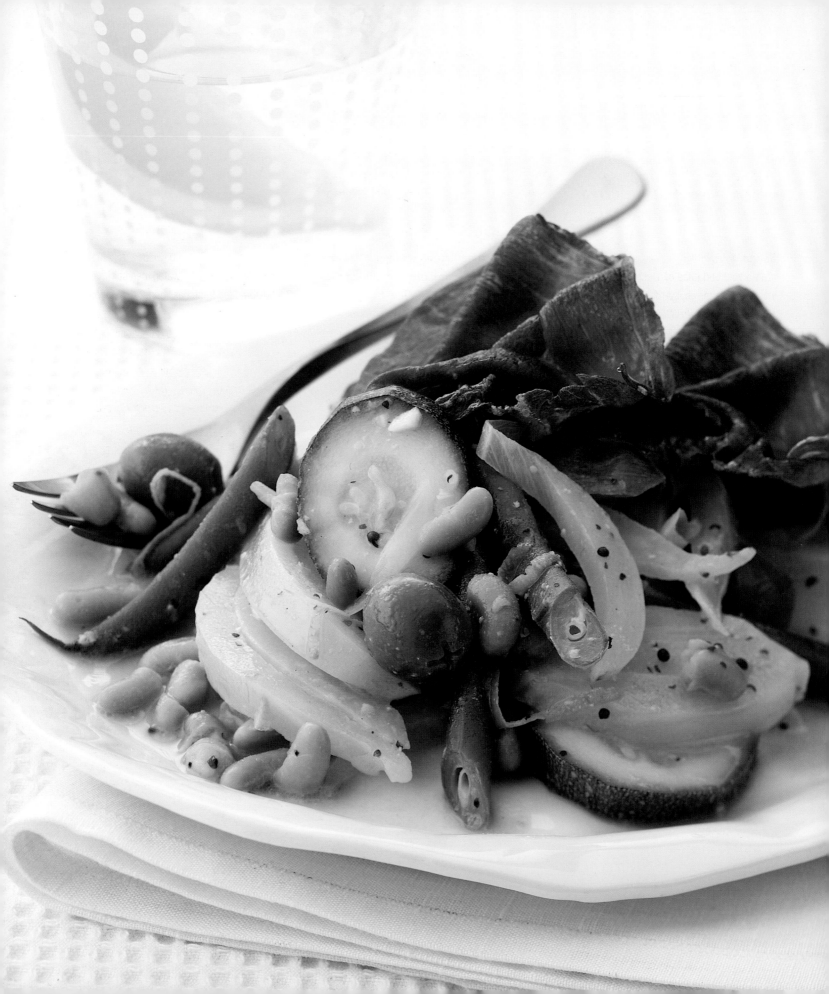

Fennel and bean salad

The pleasant aniseed flavour of fresh fennel combines with flageolet beans, green olives, Parma ham and a fresh orange dressing in this appetising warm salad. Serve it with crusty French bread for a satisfying lunch.

Serves 4

grated zest and juice of 1 small orange

1 tsp wholegrain mustard

1½ tbsp extra virgin olive oil

1 garlic clove, crushed

1 can flageolet beans, about 400 g, drained and rinsed

75 g (2½ oz) stoned green olives

1 large bulb of fennel, about 340 g (12 oz), sliced

150 g (5½ oz) green beans, halved

2 courgettes, about 250 g (8½ oz) in total, sliced

6 slices Parma ham, about 85 g (3 oz) in total, fat removed and slices halved

salt and pepper

Preparation and cooking time: 20–25 minutes

Each serving provides

kcal 221, protein 14 g, fat 10 g (of which saturated fat 2 g), carbohydrate 19 g (of which sugars 7 g), fibre 9 g

✓✓	C, E, folate, potassium
✓	A, B₁, B₆, calcium, zinc

1 Mix together the orange zest and juice, mustard, olive oil and garlic in a gratin or other shallow baking dish. Add the flageolet beans and olives and toss well. Season with salt and pepper to taste, then set aside while preparing the rest of the salad.

2 Bring a pan of salted water to the boil, add the fennel and green beans, and simmer for 1 minute. Add the courgettes and cook for a further 3–4 minutes or until the vegetables are just tender. Meanwhile, preheat the grill to high.

3 Drain the vegetables and toss them with the flageolet beans and olives in the gratin dish. Scrunch up the pieces of Parma ham and arrange on top. Place the dish under the grill and cook for 1–2 minutes, just to warm the ham, then serve immediately.

Another idea

● To make a pepper and cannellini bean salad with omelette strips, combine 1 crushed garlic clove, 1 finely chopped shallot, 2 tbsp extra virgin olive oil, 1 tsp balsamic vinegar, 2 tbsp shredded fresh basil, and salt and pepper to taste in a salad bowl. Whisk to mix. Add 2 red peppers, seeded and roughly chopped, 1 can cannellini beans, about 410 g, drained and rinsed, and 75 g (2½ oz) stoned black olives. Cook 115 g (4 oz) green beans in boiling water for 4 minutes, then drain and refresh under cold running water. Add to the bowl. Beat together 3 large eggs and 3 tbsp water, then stir in 2 tbsp shredded fresh basil and 2 tbsp snipped fresh chives. Heat 1 tbsp extra virgin olive oil in a 20 cm (8 in) non-stick frying pan, pour in the egg mixture and cook for 2–3 minutes or until the omelette is set, lifting the edges so the liquid egg can run onto the pan. Cut the omelette into strips, place on top of the salad and serve.

Plus points

● Bulb fennel was first cultivated by the Egyptians. It provides useful amounts of potassium and folate, as well as phytoestrogen, a naturally occurring plant hormone that may be helpful in protecting against breast cancer.

● Parma ham is the best known of the Italian salted, air-dried prosciuttos (the Italian word for ham). It is very lean, as long as you trim off visible fat, and has a wonderful flavour.

Griddled asparagus and peppers

Here, spears of asparagus, spring onions and peppers are cooked on a ridged cast-iron grill pan, then mixed with oven-baked Parmesan croutons. If you haven't got a ridged grill pan, the vegetables can be sizzled under the grill instead. Serve as a starter, or as a side salad with grilled chicken or griddled tuna.

Serves 4

500 g (1 lb 2 oz) asparagus spears, woody
ends trimmed

2 large red peppers, halved and seeded

225 g (8 oz) spring onions

2 tbsp extra virgin olive oil

shavings of Parmesan cheese, about 15 g
(½ oz) in total, to garnish

Parmesan croutons

2 thick slices of bread, crusts removed
and diced

1 tbsp extra virgin olive oil

30 g (1 oz) Parmesan cheese, freshly grated

salt and pepper

Lemon and basil dressing

2 tbsp lemon juice

2 tbsp extra virgin olive oil

16 fresh basil leaves, torn into pieces

1 garlic clove, very finely chopped

Preparation and cooking time: 40 minutes

Each serving provides ⓥ

kcal 296, protein 12 g, fat 19 g (of which
saturated fat 5 g), carbohydrate 20 g
(of which sugars 11 g), fibre 5 g

✓✓✓	A, B$_1$, B$_6$, C, E, folate
✓✓	niacin, calcium, zinc
✓	B$_2$, iron, potassium

1 Preheat the oven to 180°C (350°F, gas mark 4). Heat a ridged cast-iron grill pan. Put the asparagus, peppers and spring onions in a bowl, add the oil and toss to coat.

2 Arrange the asparagus and peppers in the hot grill pan, in one layer, and cook for 10 minutes or until tender, adding the spring onions after the asparagus and peppers have been cooking for a few minutes. Turn the vegetables frequently so they cook and colour evenly. (You may have to griddle the vegetables in 2 batches, depending on the size of the pan.)

3 Meanwhile, make the croutons. Put the bread in a bowl with the oil and seasoning to taste and toss well. Spread out on a baking tray and bake for about 5 minutes. Sprinkle over the Parmesan cheese and bake for a further 5 minutes or until golden and crisp.

4 Whisk together the dressing ingredients in a salad bowl, adding salt and pepper to taste. Roughly slice the griddled vegetables, add to the bowl and stir to coat with the dressing. Scatter the croutons over the top and garnish with a few shavings of Parmesan. Serve while still warm.

Some more ideas

• For an impressive dinner party starter, leave the griddled asparagus and spring onions whole (omit the peppers) and toss with the dressing. Serve on toasted ciabatta slices with Parmesan shavings scattered over the top.

• To make a griddled mango salad with chilli dressing, peel, stone and slice 1 large mango. Cook on a hot ridged grill pan with 1 red onion and 1 large green pepper, both cut into wedges, for 8–10 minutes or until tender. Chop roughly and put into a bowl with ½ tsp seeded and very finely chopped fresh red chilli, 1 tbsp extra virgin olive oil, 1 tbsp lemon juice and 1 tbsp chopped fresh coriander. Add 45 g (1½ oz) rocket and 25 g (scant 1 oz) cashew nuts, toss well and serve warm.

Plus points

• Parmesan cheese is a good source of protein and a rich source of calcium, needed for strong bones and teeth. Although it has a high fat content, Parmesan also has a very strong and distinctive flavour, so a little goes a long way in a recipe.

• Bread is an important part of a healthy diet as it is a very good source of starchy (complex) carbohydrate. It also contributes vitamins and minerals, particularly calcium, and dietary fibre.

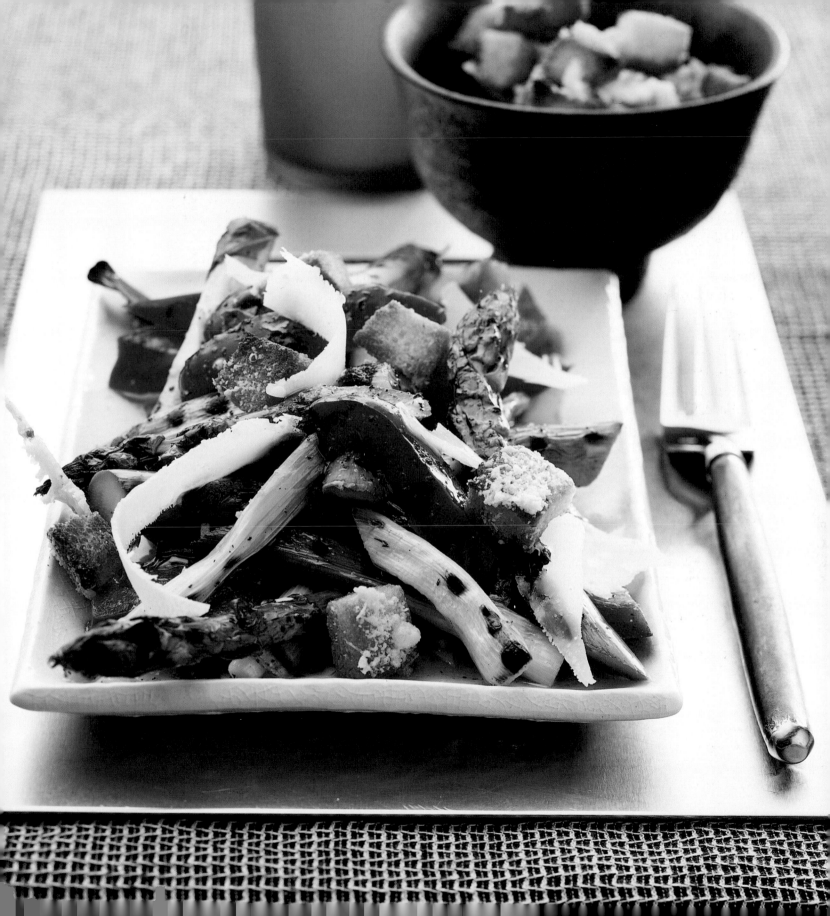

Braised roots with Hunza apricots

Orange juice and caramel-tasting Hunza apricots enhance a comforting mix of traditional root vegetables. This can be served as a light main course, or a side dish for 4, providing warming nourishment on cold winter days.

Serves 2

100 g (3½ oz) dried Hunza apricots
100 g (3½ oz) shallots
100 g (3½ oz) carrots
100 g (3½ oz) swede
100 g (3½ oz) turnips
100 g (3½ oz) celeriac
100 g (3½ oz) parsnips
100 g (3½ oz) sweet potato
100 g (3½ oz) mushrooms
2 tbsp olive oil
200 ml (7 fl oz) vegetable stock
200 ml (7 fl oz) orange juice
black pepper
fresh flat-leaf parsley to garnish

Preparation time: 20 minutes,
  plus overnight soaking
Cooking time: about 1 hour

Each serving provides

kcal 380, protein 8 g, fat 14 g (of which saturated fat 2 g), carbohydrate 59 g (of which sugars 47 g), fibre 14 g

✓✓✓	A, B₁, C, potassium
✓✓	B₆, folate, niacin, calcium, copper, iron
✓	B₂

1 Rinse the Hunza apricots to remove any grit, then place them in a bowl and cover generously with cold water. Leave them to soak for about 8 hours or overnight until rehydrated.

2 Preheat the oven to 180°C (350°F, gas mark 4). Pull apart the shallots, allowing them to fall into their natural segments. If the shallots are large and not segmented, halve them lengthways. Cut the carrots, swede and turnips into 5 cm (2 in) chunks. Cut the celeriac, parsnips and sweet potato into 6 cm (2½ in) chunks. Quarter or halve the mushrooms, depending on size.

3 Heat the oil in a large flameproof casserole and add all of the vegetables, stirring to coat them lightly with the oil. Cook over a high heat, stirring frequently, for 5–10 minutes or until the vegetables are browned.

4 Meanwhile, drain the apricots thoroughly. Using your fingers, tear each apricot open to remove the stone and divide the flesh into quarters.

5 Pour the vegetable stock and orange juice into the casserole and bring to the boil. Add the apricots and season with pepper. Transfer the casserole to the oven and bake for 45–60 minutes or until the vegetables are tender and the liquid has reduced to a reasonably thick sauce. Garnish with parsley and serve, with crusty bread.

Some more ideas

● To make a spicier vegetarian main course dish, add 2 tsp ground cumin and 1 tsp garam masala to the oil before adding the vegetables. Add a drained can of chickpeas, about 425 g, to the casserole before adding the stock. The chickpeas will add protein.

● Onions, cut into wedges, can be used in place of the shallots and canned chopped tomatoes can be used instead of the orange juice. If desired, beef or chicken stock can be used instead of vegetable stock.

● Dried apricots can be used instead of Hunza apricots, but will give a sweeter flavour.

Plus points

● Root vegetables are generally good sources of fibre. Carrots also provide vitamin A as beta-carotene, which is essential for night vision and an important antioxidant.

● People in Hunza, a region in northern Kashmir, are famous for their long lives – and some have put this down to eating apricots. Whether true or not, dried apricots are a good source of fibre and iron and a useful source of vitamin A.

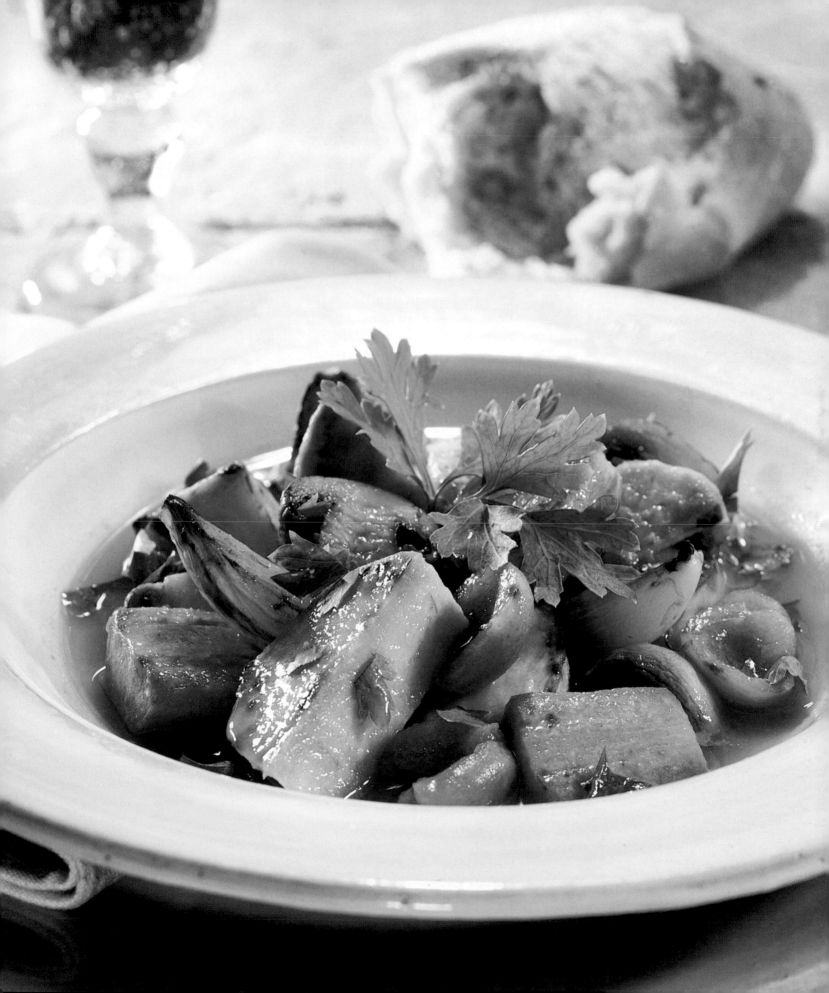

Tofu and vegetable stir-fry

If your family is not tempted by tofu, win them round with this Chinese-style dish. The tofu is glazed with ginger and soy, and served on a bed of garlicky noodles and crisp vegetables tossed with plum sauce. Although the method may look long, the dish is incredibly quick to make and there's very little washing up!

Serves 4

250 g (8½ oz) chilled plain tofu, drained

2 tbsp soy sauce

2 tbsp tomato purée

2 tbsp sunflower oil

3 garlic cloves, crushed

2 cm (¾ in) piece fresh root ginger, peeled and finely chopped

2 sheets medium Chinese egg noodles, about 170 g (6 oz) in total

200 g (7 oz) broccoli florets, thinly sliced

200 g (7 oz) carrots, cut into matchstick strips

1 red pepper, seeded and cut into thin strips

150 ml (5 fl oz) vegetable stock or water

3 tbsp plum sauce

200 g (7 oz) pak choy, stems and leaves separated and thickly sliced

4 spring onions, cut into thin strips about 5 cm (2 in) long

1 tsp sesame seeds (optional)

Preparation time: 15 minutes

Cooking time: 11 minutes

Each serving provides Ⓥ

kcal 360, protein 16 g, fat 13 g (of which saturated fat 2 g), carbohydrate 45 g (of which sugars 11 g), fibre 6 g

✓✓✓	A, C, calcium
✓✓	B_1, B_6, E, folate, copper, iron
✓	B_{12}, potassium, zinc

1 Preheat the grill. Line the grill pan with foil. Using a small knife, mark both sides of the tofu with a criss-cross pattern. Cut the tofu into quarters and place on the foil, spaced apart. Fold up the edges of the foil to make a case.

2 Mix together 1 tbsp soy sauce, 1 tbsp tomato purée, 1 tbsp oil, 1 garlic clove and the ginger, and brush the mixture on the top and base of the tofu squares. Set aside while you prepare the remaining ingredients.

3 Put the noodles in a bowl, cover with boiling water and leave to soak for 5 minutes, or according to the packet instructions.

4 Meanwhile, heat the remaining 1 tbsp oil in a wok or large frying pan. Add the broccoli and stir-fry over a high heat for 2 minutes. Add the carrots, red pepper and remaining 2 cloves of garlic, and stir-fry for 2 minutes. Stir in the stock or water and the remaining 1 tbsp soy sauce and 1 tbsp tomato purée, then mix in the plum sauce. Stir-fry for 1 minute.

5 Drain the noodles and add to the wok together with the pak choy and three-quarters of the spring onions. Stir-fry for 2 minutes or until the pak choy leaves have just wilted. Remove the wok from the heat and keep hot while you cook the tofu.

6 Put the tofu under the grill and cook for 2 minutes. Turn it over and grill the other side for 1 minute. Sprinkle the sesame seeds over and cook for a further 1 minute.

7 Spoon the vegetables and noodles into bowls, place a piece of tofu in the centre of each and garnish with the remaining spring onions. Serve hot.

Plus points

● Tofu is high in protein – pressed tofu contains 15.8% and plain 11.5% – but low in saturated fat. It is also rich in iron and B vitamins and is a useful source of calcium – just 50 g (1¾ oz) provides about 40% of the recommended daily amount of calcium for an adult woman. As the fibre from the soya bean is removed during processing, tofu is very easy to digest.

● Evidence from around the world is accumulating to suggest that eating soya beans and products made from soya beans, such as tofu, may help to reduce the risk of certain cancers, heart disease and osteoporosis as well as reducing symptoms associated with the menopause.

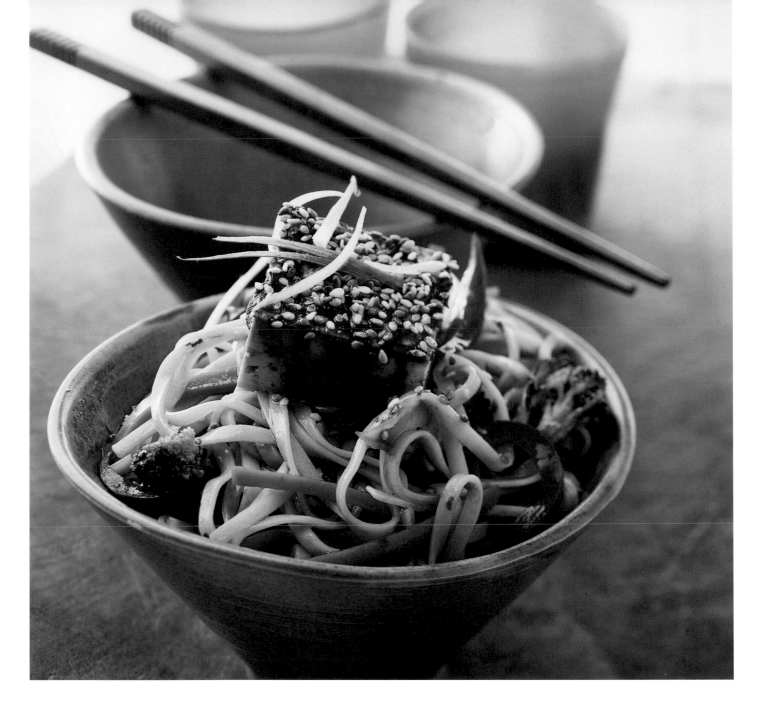

Some more ideas

- For a chicken and green vegetable stir-fry, use 4 skinless boneless chicken breasts (fillets), about 140 g (5 oz) each. Spread the skinned side with the soy and ginger glaze, then grill for 6 minutes on each side. Meanwhile, make the stir-fry, substituting courgettes for the carrots, and a green pepper in place of the red; omit the noodles. Turn the chicken glazed side uppermost and sprinkle with 2 tsp sesame seeds. Grill for 2 more minutes or until lightly browned. Serve the chicken on the vegetables, with plain boiled rice to accompany.

- Instead of plum sauce, use 3 tbsp yellow bean paste or 2 tbsp hoisin sauce. Other flavouring ideas are to replace 2–3 tbsp of the stock with dry sherry, or up to 100 ml (3½ fl oz) stock with white wine.

- Fresh plain tofu, which is the most widely available, is found in the chiller cabinet of most supermarkets. It is suspended in water, so needs to be well drained before use. Firm pressed tofu, which is usually sold in long-life cartons, is equally good for this dish as it holds its shape well. It doesn't absorb flavours as readily, so it is a good idea to marinate it in the soy sauce mixture for 10–15 minutes (or as long as possible) before grilling.

- If pak choy is unavailable, you can use Swiss chard or spinach instead.

Squash and aubergine casserole

This colourful vegetable casserole is finished with a fresh and punchy mixture of parsley, garlic, lemon zest and toasted almonds, and served with fluffy Parmesan polenta. Touches like these can transform a simple vegetable dish into a feast for the eye and palate.

Serves 4

1 tbsp extra virgin olive oil

1 large onion, cut into 8 wedges

12 baby corn

1 small or ½ large butternut squash, about 600 g (1 lb 5 oz), peeled, quartered lengthways, seeded and cut across into 2.5 cm (1 in) slices

1 aubergine, halved lengthways and cut across into 2.5 cm (1 in) slices

1 Romano sweet red pepper, seeded and cut into 1 cm (½ in) pieces

100 ml (3½ fl oz) dry white wine

500 ml (17 fl oz) hot vegetable stock, preferably home-made light or rich (see page 28)

salt and pepper

Topping

2 tbsp slivered almonds

1 garlic clove, finely chopped

finely shredded or coarsely grated zest of 1 lemon

5 tbsp chopped parsley

Parmesan polenta

200 g (7 oz) instant polenta

55 g (2 oz) freshly grated Parmesan cheese

2 tbsp chopped fresh oregano

Preparation time: about 20 minutes

Cooking time: about 45 minutes

1 Heat the oil in a flameproof casserole. Add the onion wedges and baby corn and fry over a moderate heat for 5 minutes, stirring occasionally. Preheat the oven to 180°C (350°F, gas mark 4).

2 Add the slices of butternut squash to the casserole, toss them in the oil and then stir in the aubergine and sweet red pepper. Cover and leave the vegetables to sweat over a low to moderate heat for 10 minutes, turning them twice, until they are lightly tinged golden brown. Pour in the wine, let it sizzle and then stir in the stock. Bring to the boil and add seasoning to taste. Cover the casserole and cook in the oven for 30 minutes.

3 Meanwhile, make the topping. Preheat the grill to high. Spread the slivered almonds on a baking tray and toast under the grill until they are lightly browned. Watch them closely and shake the tray occasionally to ensure the nuts are evenly toasted. Place in a small bowl and mix in the remaining topping ingredients.

4 To prepare the polenta, bring 1 litre (1¾ pints) water to the boil in a large saucepan over a high heat. Gradually whisk in the polenta and continue whisking until the polenta absorbs all the liquid. Reduce the heat to moderate and cook for 5–10 minutes, stirring, until the polenta is thick. Beat in the Parmesan cheese and oregano with seasoning to taste.

5 To serve, spoon the polenta onto plates or into large individual bowls. Ladle the vegetable casserole on top and sprinkle with the topping.

Plus points

- Butternut squash is a good source of beta-carotene, which the body converts into vitamin A. Beta-carotene also works as an antioxidant, helping to prevent free-radical damage that may lead to certain types of cancer and heart disease.
- Sweetcorn provides fibre for keeping the digestive system in good shape.
- Parmesan cheese is a good source of protein and a rich source of calcium for strong bones and teeth. It also contains a high percentage of vitamin B_{12}.

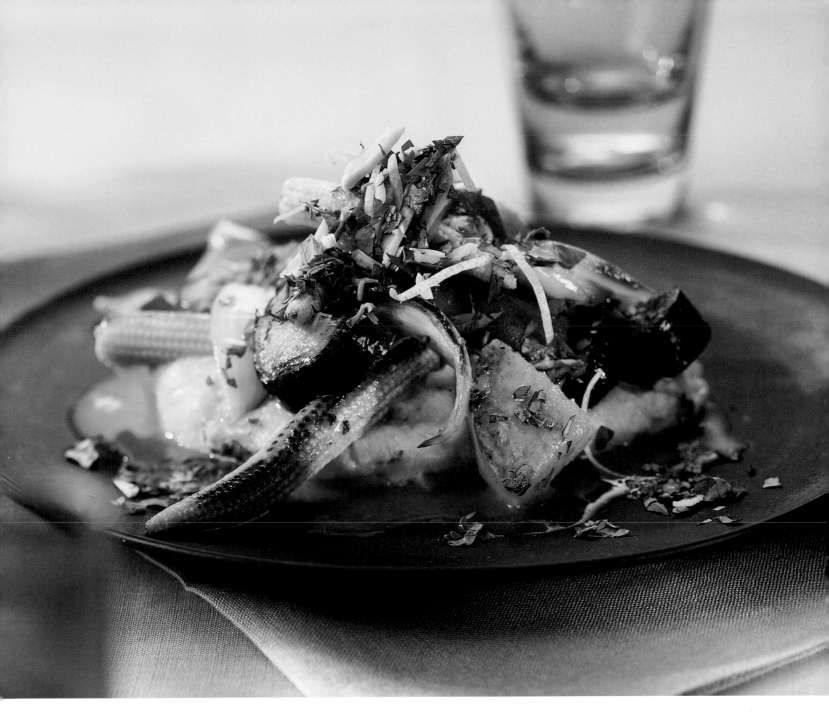

Some more ideas

● Serve the casserole with potato and carrot mash instead of polenta. Cook 450 g (1 lb) potatoes with 250 g (8½ oz) sliced carrots in boiling water until tender, then drain well and mash with 5 tbsp semi-skimmed milk and 30 g (1 oz) butter. Stir in 55 g (2 oz) grated extra mature Cheddar cheese and 2–4 tbsp chopped parsley.

● Pearl barley is another delicious alternative to polenta. It can be cooked in the oven with the vegetable casserole. Put 170 g (6 oz) rinsed pearl barley in a casserole with 1 chopped onion and 1 tsp dried sage. Pour in 600 ml (1 pint) hot vegetable stock, cover and cook in the oven at 180°C (350°F, gas mark 4) for 45–50 minutes or until the stock is absorbed and the barley is tender.

Each serving provides

kcal 440, protein 17 g, fat 14 g (of which saturated fat 4 g), carbohydrate 58 g (of which sugars 14 g), fibre 8 g

✓✓✓	A, C
✓✓	B$_6$, folate, calcium, copper, iron, phosphorus, zinc
✓	B$_1$, B$_{12}$, E

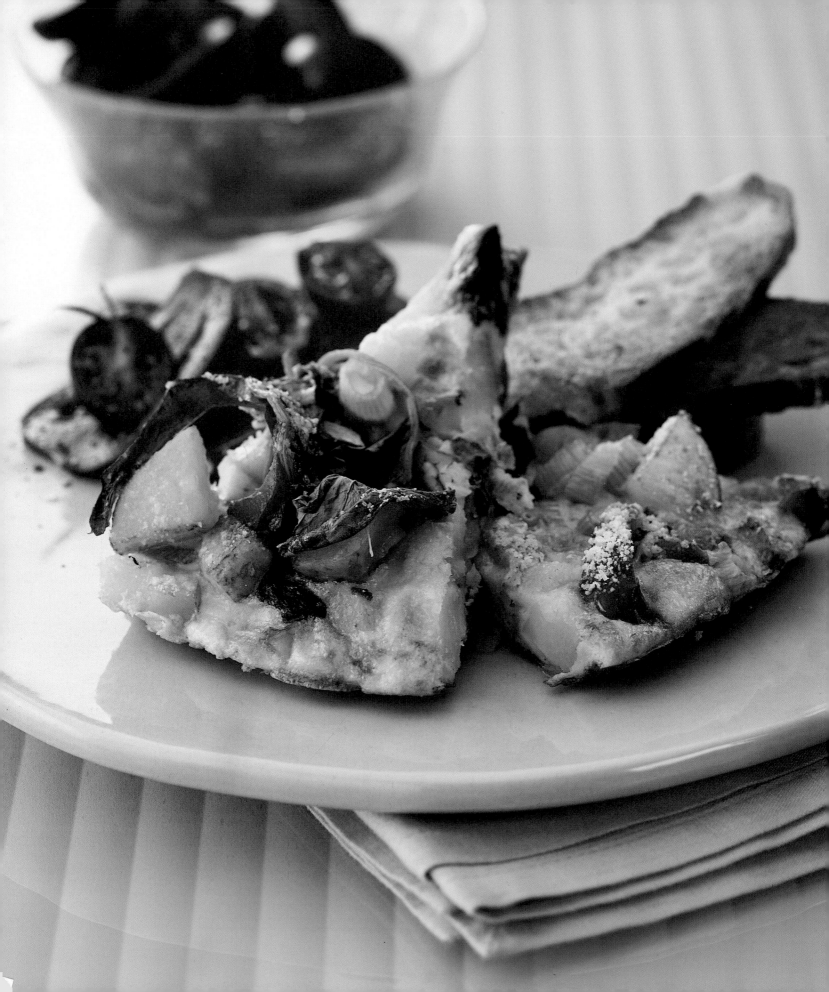

Spinach and potato frittata

This flat omelette makes a delicious vegetarian main course, and can be eaten hot or at room temperature. It is a very versatile recipe, as almost anything can be added to it – a handy way of using up leftovers. Serve with toasted ciabatta bread and sliced tomatoes and/or a mixed green salad for a quick supper.

Serves 4

500 g (1 lb 2 oz) potatoes, scrubbed and
    cut into 1 cm (½ in) cubes
225 g (8 oz) baby spinach leaves, trimmed
    of any large stalks
1 tbsp extra virgin olive oil
1 red pepper, quartered lengthways,
    seeded and thinly sliced
5–6 spring onions, thinly sliced
5 eggs
3 tbsp freshly grated Parmesan cheese
salt and pepper

Preparation and cooking time: 30 minutes

Each serving provides   ⓥ

kcal 320, protein 19 g, fat 15 g (of which
saturated fat 5 g), carbohydrate 26 g
(of which sugars 6 g), fibre 4 g

✓✓✓	A, B$_6$, B$_{12}$, C
✓✓	folate, calcium, iron
✓	B$_1$, B$_2$, E, potassium, zinc

1 Cook the potatoes in a saucepan of boiling water for 5–6 minutes or until almost tender. Put the spinach in a steamer or colander over the potatoes and cook for another 5 minutes or until the potatoes are tender and the spinach has wilted. Drain the potatoes. Press the spinach with the back of a spoon to extract excess moisture, then chop.

2 Heat the oil in a non-stick frying pan that is about 25 cm (10 in) in diameter. Add the pepper slices and sauté over a moderate heat for 2 minutes. Stir in the potatoes and spring onions and continue cooking for 2 minutes.

3 Beat the eggs in a large bowl, season with salt and pepper and mix in the spinach. With a draining spoon, remove about half of the vegetables from the pan and add to the egg mixture, leaving the oil in the pan. Stir the egg and vegetables briefly to mix, then pour into the frying pan. Cover and cook, without stirring, for about 6 minutes or until the omelette is almost set but still a little soft on top. Meanwhile, preheat the grill.

4 Dust the top of the frittata with the Parmesan cheese and place under the grill. Cook for 3–4 minutes or until browned and puffed around the edges. Cut into quarters or wedges and serve.

Some more ideas

• For a courgette and potato frittata, replace the spinach with 1 large or 2 small courgettes, quartered lengthways and sliced, and use 1 thinly sliced small leek instead of spring onions. Sauté the leek and courgette with the pepper slices for 3–4 minutes. Add the potatoes and stir. Mix a handful of torn fresh basil leaves with the beaten eggs, and cook the omelette as in the main recipe.

• Make a smoked salmon frittata. Omit the potatoes and red pepper, and sauté a courgette, quartered lengthways and sliced, with the spring onions. Add 75 g (2½ oz) slivered smoked salmon to the eggs with the spinach. Finish the frittata under the grill without the Parmesan.

Plus points

• Spinach is a good source of several antioxidants, including vitamin C and vitamin E, and it provides useful amounts of folate, niacin and B$_6$. Contrary to popular belief, it is not a particularly good source of iron.

• Although in the past people with a high risk of heart disease or stroke were advised to restrict the number of eggs they ate to 2 a week, a recent study suggests that unless you suffer from diabetes you can safely eat up to one egg a day.

Provençale roasted vegetable and feta slice

This colourful tart combines classic flavours of Provence – peppers, courgettes, tomatoes, garlic and fresh herbs – with piquant feta cheese in a crisp, olive oil pastry case. The tart can be served hot or cold, and would be lovely for a summer picnic or alfresco lunch in the garden.

Serves 4

170 g (6 oz) plain flour
pinch of salt
4 tbsp olive oil
1 egg, beaten with 1 tbsp tepid water
1 large red pepper, seeded and chopped
1 large yellow pepper, seeded and chopped
2 medium courgettes, thickly sliced
1½ tbsp extra virgin olive oil
2 garlic cloves, sliced
few sprigs of fresh thyme
4 plum tomatoes, quartered
150 g (5½ oz) feta cheese, roughly chopped
2 tsp semi-skimmed milk
1 tsp poppy seeds (optional)
salt and pepper

Preparation and cooking time: 1½ hours,
   plus 30 minutes resting

Each serving provides   Ⓥ

kcal 446, protein 14 g, fat 26 g (of which
saturated fat 8 g), carbohydrate 42 g
(of which sugars 9 g), fibre 4 g

✓✓✓	A, C
✓✓	B_{12}, E, calcium
✓	B_1, B_6, folate, niacin, copper, iron, potassium, zinc

1 Sift the flour and salt into a mixing bowl. Add the olive oil and beaten egg mixture and mix using a fork. Sprinkle with 3 tbsp cold water and mix in using a round-bladed knife. If the mixture does not clump together, add a drop or two more water, then gather together to make a firm but pliable dough. Wrap in cling film and leave to rest for at least 30 minutes.

2 Preheat the oven to 200°C (400°F, gas mark 6). Put the peppers and courgettes in a roasting tin, drizzle over the oil and turn the vegetables to coat. Sprinkle over the garlic and thyme sprigs, and roast for 15 minutes.

3 Add the tomatoes to the tin and roast for 10 minutes. Season with salt and pepper to taste, and set aside.

4 Roll out the pastry dough thinly on a lightly floured surface to make a rectangle about 30 x 40 cm (12 x 16 in). Use to line an 18 x 25 cm (7 x 10 in) non-stick baking tin that is 3 cm (1¼ in) deep. Reserve the pastry trimmings.

5 Prick the bottom of the pastry case using a fork. Bake it 'blind' for 10 minutes, then remove the paper and beans, and bake for a further 5 minutes or until golden.

6 Arrange the roasted vegetables evenly over the base of the pastry case and scatter the feta cheese on top.

7 Roll out the pastry trimmings and cut into thin strips. Lay the strips in a criss-cross pattern over the filling. Brush the pastry strips with milk and sprinkle with the poppy seeds, if using.

8 Bake for 15–20 minutes until the pastry lattice is golden. Serve hot or cold, cut into thin slices or squares.

Plus points

- Olive oil pastry is lower in saturated fat than shortcrust made with butter. Most of the fatty acids in olive oil are monounsaturated, which are thought to play a part in lowering high blood cholesterol levels.
- Feta cheese has a medium fat content. It is salty, so if you are watching your sodium intake soak the cheese in milk for 15–20 minutes before use (discard the milk).
- Peppers are an excellent source of vitamin C and beta-carotene. Their beta-carotene content depends on the colour of the pepper, with red peppers having the most and green peppers the least.

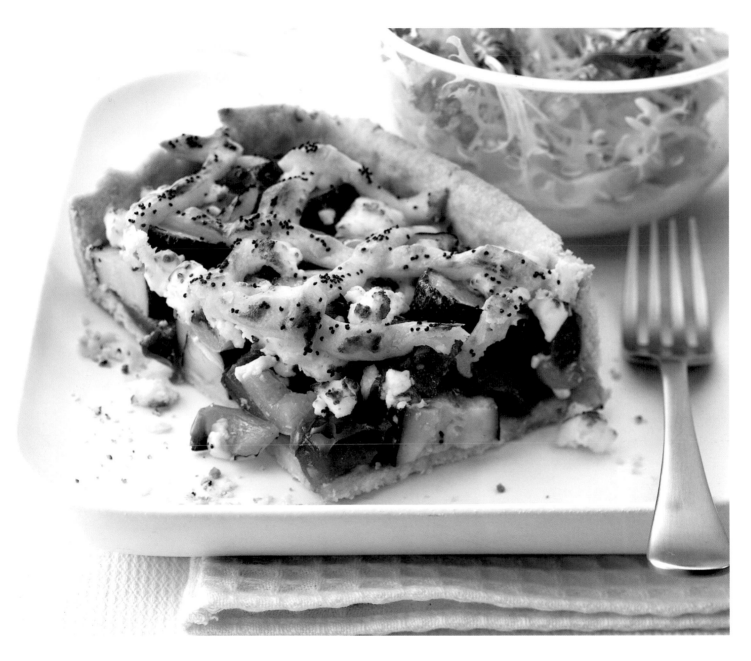

Some more ideas

● Instead of feta, use Caerphilly or Lancashire cheese.

● Make a Puy lentil and goat's cheese slice. For the filling, soften 1 chopped onion in 1 tbsp extra virgin olive oil with 1 crushed garlic clove and 2 tsp finely chopped, fresh root ginger. Add 200 g (7 oz) Puy lentils, 1 can of chopped tomatoes, about 400 g, with the juice, and 250 ml (8½ fl oz) vegetable stock. Bring to the boil, then reduce the heat and simmer for 10 minutes. Add 250 g (8½ oz) peeled and diced potatoes and cook for 10 minutes, then add 125 g (4½ oz) frozen peas. Bring back to the boil and cook for a further 5–10 minutes or until the potatoes and lentils are tender. Add a little more stock if needed. Stir in 50 g (1¾ oz) chopped watercress and season to taste. Spread evenly in the pastry case and scatter over 100 g (3½ oz) crumbled goat's cheese. Make a lattice top with the pastry trimmings, twisting the strips. Brush with milk and sprinkle with 1–2 tsp fennel seeds, if liked. Bake as in the main recipe.

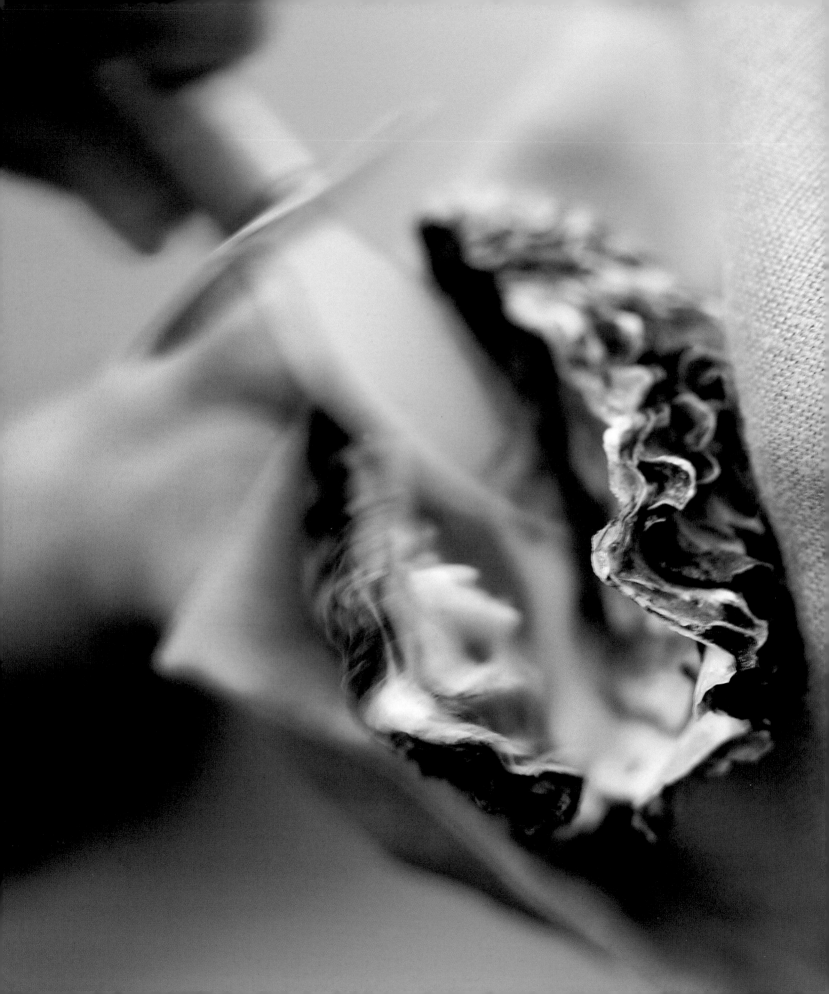

Fantastic Fish

Fish is an ideal food for our busy lives – quick and easy to cook and endlessly versatile. It makes the perfect healthy choice for all kinds of tempting meals, as it is a great source of protein and provides many vitamins and minerals. Oily fish also offer beneficial fats such as omega-3 which can help maintain a healthy heart. Shellfish, too, are packed with many essential nutrients, as are fat-free seaweeds and sea vegetables.

The wide variety of fish and shellfish – fresh or preserved – can be used to make delicious soups and starters, main-meal salads or family suppers, and is ideal for more elaborate dishes when entertaining.

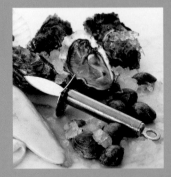

Fish in a healthy diet

Fish and other seafood are perfect for all kinds of meals. They are quick to cook, full of goodness and form an important part of a healthy, balanced diet.

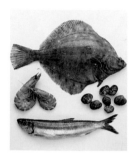

Why eat fish?

Fish and shellfish are very nutritious foods – full of first-class protein, low in saturated fat but often high in other beneficial fats, and packed with essential vitamins and minerals. Because of these benefits, nutrition experts agree that eating fish 2–3 times a week can be a positive aid to good health.

• Protein is essential to keep our bodies working efficiently and we need to eat protein-rich foods each day. A 140 g (5 oz) portion of cooked white or oily fish provides 55% RNI of protein for adult women and 45% RNI of protein for men.

• White fish offers many of the B-complex vitamins, in particular B_{12} which is vital for growth.

• Oily fish is a source of vitamin D, essential for healthy bones, and of vitamin A for healthy eyes and growth.

• Fish and other seafood supply many important minerals, including phosphorus for healthy bones and teeth; selenium, a powerful antioxidant that protects cells against damage by free radicals; and iodine, an important component of the thyroid hormones which control the rate food is converted into energy.

• Fish can be divided into two groups – white fish and oily fish. The principal difference between them is that in white fish the oil is found mainly in the liver; in oily fish, the oil is distributed throughout the flesh.

White fish for lean protein

White fish has very lean flesh and is low in fat and therefore in calories, making it an ideal food for helping to maintain a healthy weight. It is an important source of good-quality protein, providing similar amounts to lean meat but with lower amounts of fat. The deliciously delicate flavour makes white fish a popular choice with children who also like its texture – unlike meat, which has a fibrous texture, white fish has soft flesh containing little connective tissue, so it is easy to chew.

Oily fish for good fat

All fish is good for you, but oily fish can actually help to improve your health. These fish are a major source of polyunsaturated fatty acids such as omega-3, which can help to prevent arteries clogging and so minimise the risk of strokes and heart attacks. It is no coincidence that the Japanese, whose consumption of fish is the highest in the world, have the lowest incidence of heart disease. The old adage that fish is good for the brain is true, too – omega-3 fatty acids are vital for the development of the brain and can help to prevent cerebral haemorrhages by reducing the risk of blood clotting.

Nutritional differences between types of seafood
(typical values per 100 g/ 3½ oz raw edible fish)

	white fish	oily fish	shellfish
energy	80 kcals	180 kcals	76 kcals
protein	18.3 g	20.2 g	7.6 g
fat*	0.7 g	1.0 g	0.6 g
polyunsaturates	0.3 g	3.1 g	0.1 g
monounsaturates	0.1 g	4.4 g	0.2 g
saturates	0.1 g	1.9 g	0.1 g
carbohydrate	0.0 g	0.0 g	0.0 g
fibre	0.0 g	0.0 g	0.0 g
sodium	60.0 mg	45.0 mg	190 mg

* The total fat figure includes fatty compounds and other fatty acids in addition to mono and polyunsaturates.

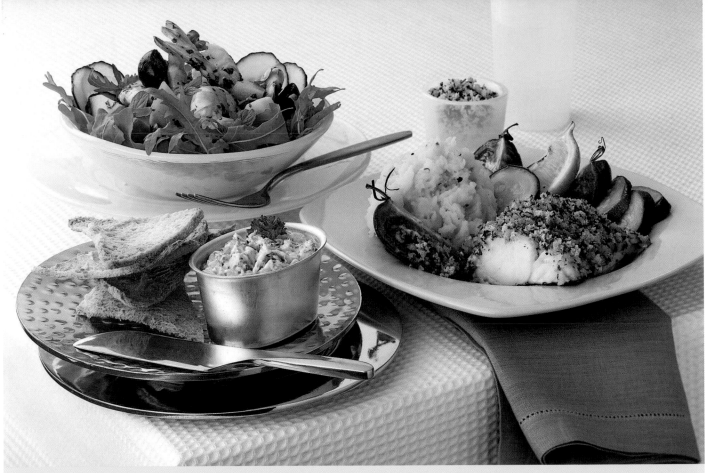

▲ Fish and shellfish can be turned into delicious and nutritious dishes, including simple starters, crunchy salads and satisfying main courses.

Put shellfish on the menu now and again

Like fish, shellfish are low in fat, although they contain a higher level of dietary cholesterol. They also contain a high level of sodium. But they offer many essential minerals such as iodine, potassium, iron and zinc. For example, oysters are an excellent source of zinc, and oysters and mussels contain more iron than red meat, when compared weight for weight of the edible part. And shellfish in general are the most reliable natural source of iodine in the normal diet.

An added bonus

Some seafood offers unexpected extra nutritional benefits.
• The canning process softens the bones of fish like sardines, pilchards and salmon and makes them palatable, and eating these bones boosts calcium intake.
• Fish roes provide vitamin C – some types of fish more than others. The fat content of fish fluctuates with the seasons and it is when the female fish are at their fattest, in late summer and early autumn, that they contain large quantities of roe.

• Seaweeds and sea vegetables, widely used in Japanese cookery, are virtually fat-free while offering protein, carbohydrate, and many essential vitamins and minerals.

The future of fish

Fish and shellfish are under constant threat from pollution and over-fishing. Industry effluents, careless sewage disposal and global warming have all played their part in harming the marine eco-system and polluting the world's seas, rivers and lakes. Whether you buy, catch or gather wild fish or shellfish, make sure that they come from unpolluted waters. Most farmed fish and seafood are carefully monitored to eliminate any harmful organisms, but sometimes careless farming can cause diseases in farmed fish. The trend nowadays is towards organic fish farming, which guarantees the fish are fed on only natural foods and are produced in clean, pollution-free waters.

Lean and versatile white fish

For family meals or special dinners, white fish is a great choice. Low in fat and high in protein, white fish is enhanced by subtle flavourings and textures.

Lean and lovely

Most white fish fall into two main categories: round and flat. Round fish, such as cod or haddock, have rounded bodies and eyes on either side of the head. They swim with the back fin uppermost. Flat fish, such as plaice or sole, have both eyes on their upper side and the skin there is usually marked as a form of camouflage. Flat fish lead an inactive life on the sea bed, so their flesh has little muscle tone. This makes it delicate and particularly easy to eat and digest.

White fish contain nutritious oils, mainly concentrated in the liver. Some of these – cod and halibut liver oils for example – have long been used as dietary supplements. Fish liver oils contain vitamin A which is essential for healthy vision; vitamin D, essential for growth and the absorption of calcium; vitamin E which works as an antioxidant; and omega-3 fatty acids.

Although fish is a very healthy food, some white fish are short on certain dietary essentials like iron and calcium, and most species contain no vitamin C. So it is a good idea to combine white fish with foods that do provide these nutrients, such as spinach and other iron-rich vegetables; calcium-rich dairy products such as yogurt and milk; and vitamin C-rich vegetables such as broccoli and tomatoes.

An ABC of white fish

The most common white fish are described below. An average portion is 140 g (5 oz), weighed before cooking, without skin and bones. All the healthy cooking methods, such as steaming, poaching and grilling, work well for white fish.

Bream

There are almost 200 different species of bream, of which the best to eat is the gilt-head or dorade – a beautiful fish with dense, juicy white flesh. Bream are usually sold whole or in fillets, and it is essential that their scales be removed before cooking. Sea bream are an excellent source of niacin, a B vitamin involved in the release of energy from food, and of vitamin B_{12}.

Cod

The firm, succulent white flesh of this popular fish becomes deliciously flaky when cooked. Most commonly sold cut into fillets or steaks, cod can also be bought whole and poached or baked. It is an excellent source of iodine, which plays a part in converting food into energy, and a useful source of potassium.

Haddock

This smaller relative of the cod has softer, more delicate flesh. At its best in winter and early spring, when the cold has firmed up the flesh, it is generally sold as fillets, and should be cooked with the skin on. It is an excellent source of iodine and provides useful amounts of potassium and vitamin B_6.

Hake

When very fresh this member of the cod family has firm, lean flesh. It contains few bones and must not be overcooked or it will fall apart. It is usually sold whole or as fillets or steaks. Hake is a good source of phosphorus, which is important for healthy teeth and bones, and a useful source of potassium.

Halibut

Largest of all the flat fish, halibut has dense, meaty flesh that can be dry if not carefully cooked. It is possible to buy whole small fish, known as chicken halibut, but larger fish are usually sold cut into steaks. Halibut is a good source of niacin, and the large roes provide vitamin C.

Hoki

A deep-sea relative of hake, hoki has lean flesh with a flaky texture and rather bland flavour, which is why it is often used in the manufacture of fish fingers. It is always sold as fillets. Hoki is an excellent source of selenium.

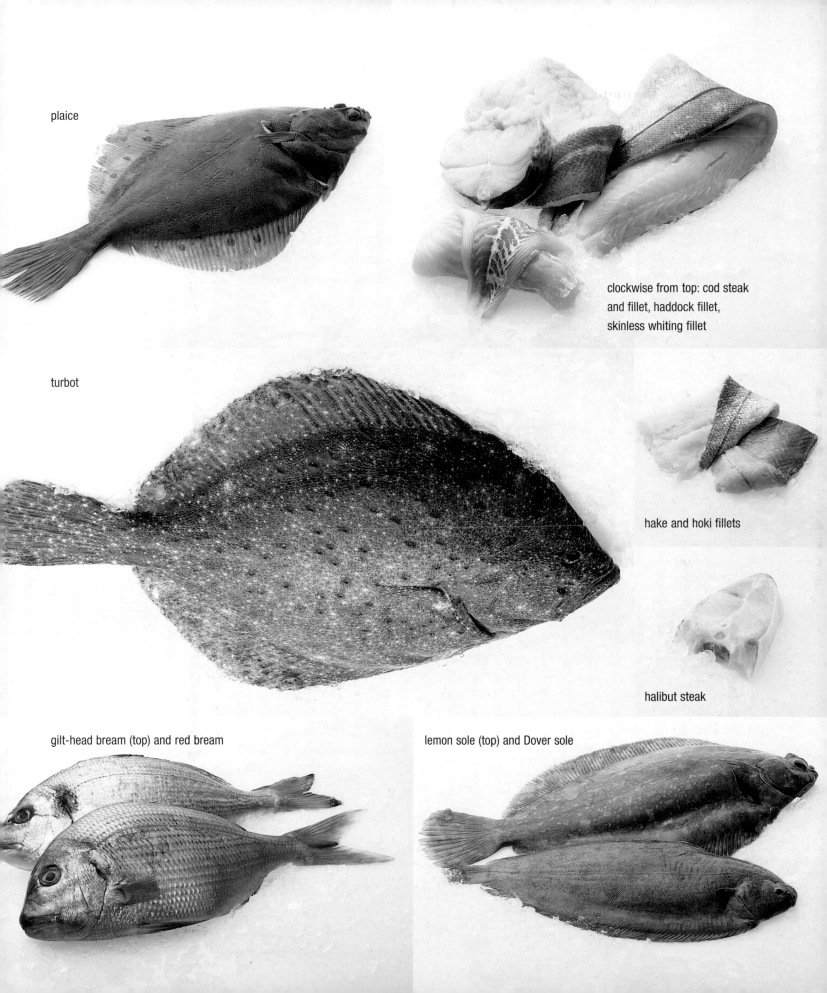

plaice

clockwise from top: cod steak
and fillet, haddock fillet,
skinless whiting fillet

turbot

hake and hoki fillets

halibut steak

gilt-head bream (top) and red bream

lemon sole (top) and Dover sole

John Dory

Although technically a round fish, the body of the John Dory is so slim that it looks almost like a flat fish swimming upright. Its flesh is firm and succulent. John Dory is a good source of phosphorus and a useful source of potassium, which is needed to regulate blood pressure.

Monkfish

This extraordinarily ugly fish has a huge head and a relatively small body. Only the tail is eaten, and it is sold whole or as fillets. The flesh is meaty and firm with a superb flavour. Monkfish is an excellent source of phosphorus and provides useful amounts of potassium.

Mullet

There are 2 types of mullet: red and grey. Red mullet has beautiful reddish-gold skin and lean, firm flesh that tastes a bit like lobster. Being a small fish, it is usually sold whole. The larger grey mullet is a dark silvery colour and has lean, well-flavoured flesh. Grey mullet is sold whole or as fillets, and must be scaled before cooking. The roes, which contain vitamin C, are a delicacy pan-fried and eaten fresh; when dried they are used to make taramasalata. Mullet are excellent sources of selenium and contain useful amounts of potassium.

Plaice

This flat fish has distinctive dark skin spotted with orange. The very soft white flesh can be bland, although it is easy to digest. Sold whole or as fillets, plaice must be very fresh or it will have a woolly texture, and it is best avoided in summer as it is in poor condition after spawning in the spring. Plaice provides many B vitamins – excellent B_{12} and good B_1, B_6 and niacin – and it is a useful source of potassium.

Sea bass

The delicate flesh of this sleek silvery fish has a superb flavour and holds its shape well during cooking. Sold whole or as fillets or steaks, it must be scaled before cooking. Bass is a good source of calcium.

Shark

Shark is a cartilaginous fish (like skate), which means that it has a skeleton composed entirely of cartilage rather than of bones. Its white or pale pink flesh is firm and meaty, and it is always sold skinned and in steaks or fillets. Mako and dogfish (sometimes called huss or rock salmon) are the species most widely available. Shark is an excellent source of selenium and

a good source of vitamin A, and unlike most other white fish it contains useful quantities of omega-3 fatty acids.

Skate

Only the 'wings' (actually large, flat pectoral fins) of this cartilaginous fish are generally sold, ready skinned. Skate is best in autumn and winter. Even when very fresh it has an ammoniac smell, but this disappears during cooking. The soft pinkish flesh, which is easily scraped off the cartilage after cooking, has a sweet flavour and its gelatinous quality makes it ideal for fish terrines and mousses. Skate contains excellent levels of vitamin B_{12}, which is vital for the maintenance of a healthy nervous system, and useful amounts of vitamins B_1, B_6 and niacin as well as potassium.

Sole

There are many varieties of these flat fish, including dabs, lemon sole and witch or Torbay sole, but the finest – and most expensive – is Dover sole. This superb fish has firm, juicy flesh with a delicious flavour. Depending on size, sole are sold whole or filleted. They provide useful amounts of vitamin B_{12} and potassium.

Swordfish

This huge game fish has no scales or teeth but a long sword-like nose. Its meaty flesh, usually sold as steaks, can easily dry out, so it is best marinated before cooking. Swordfish is very nutritious, providing excellent amounts of selenium, niacin and vitamin B_{12} as well as useful quantities of potassium.

Tilapia

Sold whole or as fillets, tilapia has lean, moist flesh that contains excellent levels of phosphorus, good amounts of calcium and useful quantities of potassium.

Turbot

The dark, warty skin of this large flat fish conceals dense, meaty flesh with a wonderful flavour. It is usually sold as fillets. Smaller 'chicken turbot' are sometimes available, and can be cooked whole to serve 4. Turbot is an excellent source of niacin and also offers good amounts of phosphorus and useful quantities of potassium.

Whiting

This fish resembles haddock in appearance. It has soft, bland flesh that can have a woolly texture if the fish is not very fresh. Whiting provides good quantities of selenium and is a useful source of potassium and phosphorus.

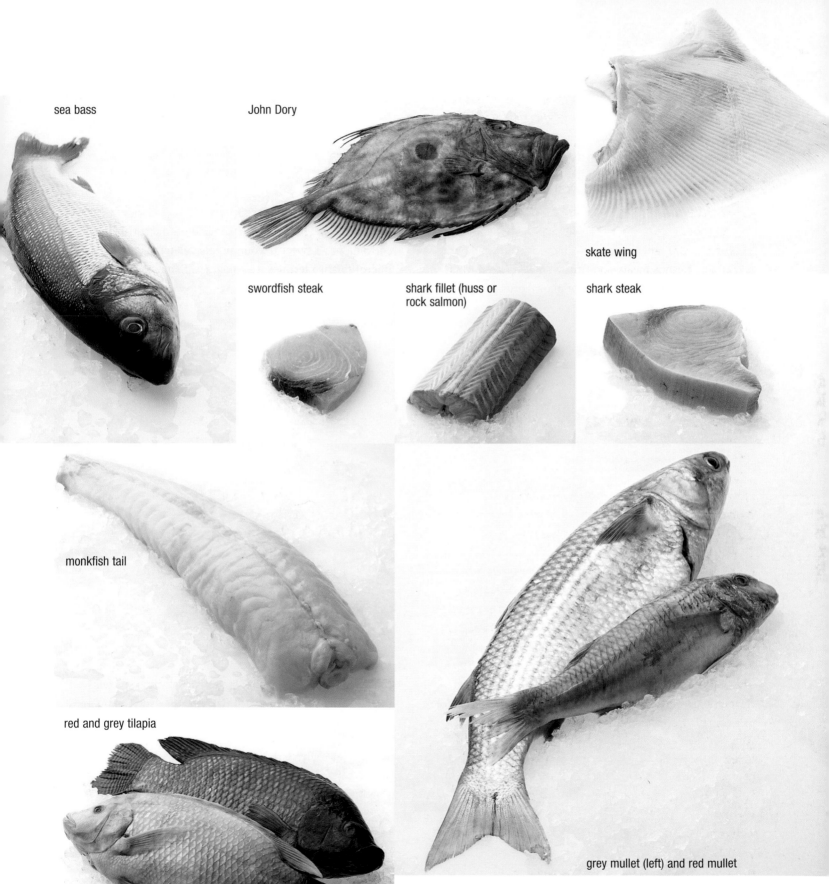

sea bass

John Dory

skate wing

swordfish steak

shark fillet (huss or
rock salmon)

shark steak

monkfish tail

red and grey tilapia

grey mullet (left) and red mullet

Heart-healthy oily fish

Oily fish offers many of the vitamins and minerals needed for good health. Eating it regularly is beneficial to your heart – and its delicious flavour is a bonus.

Rich and full of flavour

Most oily fish live in shoals near the surface of the sea. They contain more fat than white fish, but it is mainly mono or polyunsaturated fat. They also provide beneficial omega-3 fatty acids, which reduce the tendency of blood to clot, and

thus are helpful in the prevention and treatment of heart disease. These healthy fats are stored throughout the bodies of the fish, particularly in the head and muscle tissue. As a further bonus, oily fish offer vitamin A, important for healthy skin and vision; B vitamins, including vitamin B_{12} which is vital for growth; and vitamin D, needed for maintaining strong, healthy bones. Oily fish are rich in minerals too, such as iodine, phosphorus and selenium, as well as calcium if the bones of the fish are eaten.

All oily fish must be eaten when very fresh. They are quick and simple to cook and taste delicious. Their rich-tasting flesh is complemented by sharper flavours such as tart fruit (for example lemon, gooseberries and apple), mustard, pungent spices and herbs such as sorrel.

An ABC of oily fish

The most common oily fish are described below. An average portion is 140 g (5 oz), weighed before cooking, without skin and bones. The best methods for cooking oily fish are grilling, barbecuing and baking.

Anchovy

Usually canned or salted, this small silvery-blue fish is sometimes available fresh, when it can be grilled or pan-fried.

Maximising the healthy fats

Most oily fish do not feed when they are spawning, so during that time they draw their nutrients from the fats stored in their bodies. As a result, the level of fat falls during the spawning season and they are at their leanest just after spawning. For example, herrings have a fat content of about 20% in summer, dropping to only 3–4% in early spring. To benefit fully from the healthy fats contained in oil-rich fish, eat them when they are at their fattest and ready to spawn.

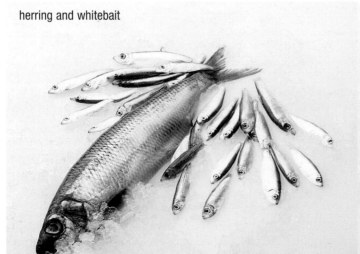

herring and whitebait

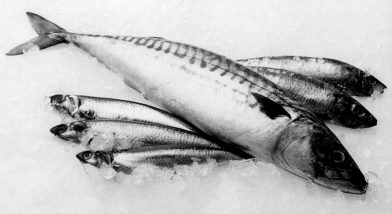

anchovies, mackerel and sardines

It may be under 10 cm (4 in) long, but its flesh is packed with flavour, and it provides phosphorus and calcium.

Herring

This sleek silvery fish is not popular with everyone as it contains numerous small bones, but it is very tasty and the nutritious pluses far outweigh this minus point – herring contain large quantities of polyunsaturated fat, excellent levels of vitamin D and useful amounts of vitamin A and potassium. Generally sold whole, herring are at their best when they are really plump and firm, just before spawning. At this stage they are full of roe: females have hard roes and males contain soft roes (milt). Herring roe is a useful source of vitamins A, E and B_1, and contains some vitamin C, so makes a delicious and nutritious snack when pan-fried and served on toast.

Mackerel

This beautiful fish has smooth, steel-blue skin and flesh with a distinctive, rich flavour. It is very nutritious, being an excellent source of iodine, vitamin D and niacin, a good source of vitamins B_2 and B_6, and a useful source of potassium. Mackerel are usually sold whole.

Salmon

Often called 'the king of fish', salmon migrate from the sea into freshwater rivers to spawn. Before spawning, they contain up to 13% unsaturated fat, but by the time they spawn, levels have fallen to about 5%. Wild salmon such as this is at its best in early summer. It contains excellent levels of vitamin B_{12} and useful amounts of potassium.

Salmon is also now raised extensively in fish farms, and this farmed salmon is much less expensive than its wild cousins. Both wild and farmed salmon are sold whole or cut into steaks or fillets.

Sardine

Fresh sardines are delicious, and ideal for grilling and barbecuing. This fish is best in summer, but it is available frozen so can be enjoyed year round. Sardines are an excellent source of selenium and a useful source of potassium.

Trout

There are several varieties of trout, including brown trout and sea trout (also called salmon trout), both of which have a wonderful flavour. The rainbow trout is easy to farm and so is widely available and inexpensive. Trout contain useful amounts of potassium and iodine.

Tuna

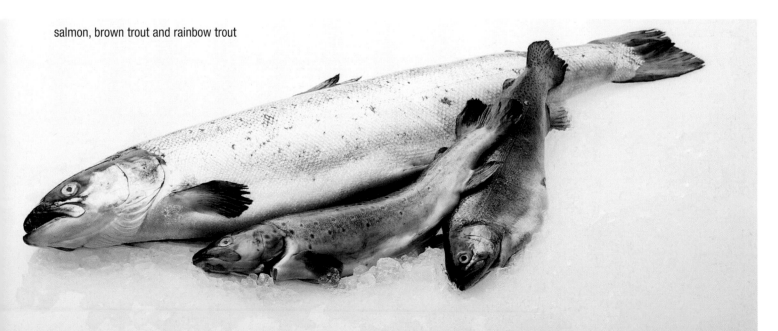

This fish can grow to a huge size, so is almost always sold cut into steaks. The dense, meaty flesh varies from pinky-beige to deep red, according to the variety of tuna. It can be dry if overcooked, so is best marinated first. Although lower in healthy fats than other oily fish, tuna is still very nutritious and also contains excellent levels of vitamins B_{12} and D and useful amounts of potassium.

Whitebait

A tiny silvery fish, whitebait is, in fact, young herring or sprats, and so offers the same nutritional benefits as herring. In addition, as it is eaten whole, bones and all, it is a useful source of calcium.

salmon, brown trout and rainbow trout

Fruits of the sea

For the true flavour of the sea, fresh shellfish is unbeatable. Not only is it quick and easy to cook, but it is low in fat and provides essential minerals.

Crustacean or mollusc?

The seas abound with curious creatures which we loosely call shellfish. There are two main categories of shellfish: 'crustaceans' which have shells and legs and 'molluscs' with shells but no legs.

Like fish, crustaceans and molluscs are low in fat, but unlike fish, they are high in dietary cholesterol. Cholesterol is an essential component of our body structure and a normal constituent of blood, but high levels of cholesterol in the blood are associated with increased risk of coronary heart disease. As a result, for some years shellfish were considered undesirable in a healthy diet. Now scientific research suggests that it is more important to reduce our intake of saturated fat and increase the quantity of foods containing soluble fibre than to avoid eating cholesterol-rich foods. For a small percentage of the population, reducing the amount of dietary cholesterol consumed can help to lower the level of cholesterol in the blood, but for the majority it is the level of saturated fats that is crucial, not the amount of dietary cholesterol.

So as long as shellfish are properly prepared and cooked, we can safely put them back on the menu. It is still important to eat shellfish in moderation, however, as they contain a high level of sodium. On the plus side, shellfish supply many essential minerals and a few vitamins too.

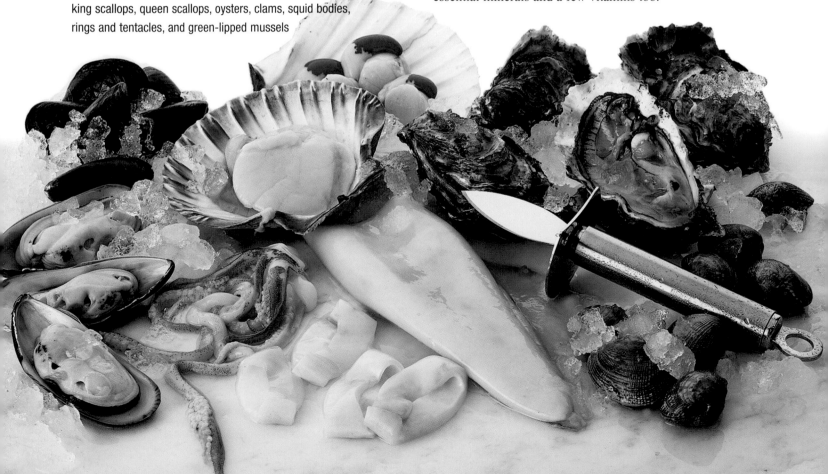

molluscs (clockwise from back left): blue mussels, large or king scallops, queen scallops, oysters, clams, squid bodies, rings and tentacles, and green-lipped mussels

An ABC of shellfish

Shellfish can be cooked in many healthy ways. An average portion (shelled weight of edible flesh) is 100 g (3½ oz).

Clam

This mollusc comes in myriad sizes, from tiny Venus clams to giant specimens. The flesh of most clams has a firm texture and sweet flavour. Clams can be eaten raw, but only if bought from a reputable source. They are an excellent source of phosphorus, which is important for healthy bones and teeth, and a good source of iron.

Crab

There are many different crabs, in all shapes and sizes, from tiny green swimming crabs to huge king crabs with long dangly legs like gigantic spiders. The most familiar in Britain is the common crab, which has brown meat in the body shell and white meat in the claws. The white meat is sweet and succulent with a flaky texture, while the brown meat is rich and creamy. The two can be eaten together or used separately – the brown meat is best mixed with other ingredients to make sauces, soups and so on. Crab is a good source of phosphorus.

Crabsticks are made from crab-flavoured white fish pulp. They are cheaper than fresh crab, but do not really taste like it.

Langoustine

Also known as scampi and Dublin Bay prawn, the langoustine looks like a pale pink miniature lobster. Once caught, the flesh deteriorates rapidly, so langoustines are often cooked and frozen at sea, then sold as frozen scampi tails. Langoustines are a rich source of vitamin E.

Lobster

The king of crustaceans, lobster has firm white meat with an exquisite sweet flavour. It is at its best in summer and autumn, and needs only brief cooking. Lobster contains excellent levels of the antioxidant selenium and useful amounts of iodine and zinc.

Mussel

The beautifully coloured, hinged shell of this mollusc conceals a nugget of sweet, juicy orange flesh. The simplest way to prepare mussels is to steam them open. Be sure to keep the delicious juices from the shells for soups and sauces. Mussels are mineral-rich, providing good quantities of iodine and iron

crustaceans (from left): langoustines, lobster, crab and dressed crab

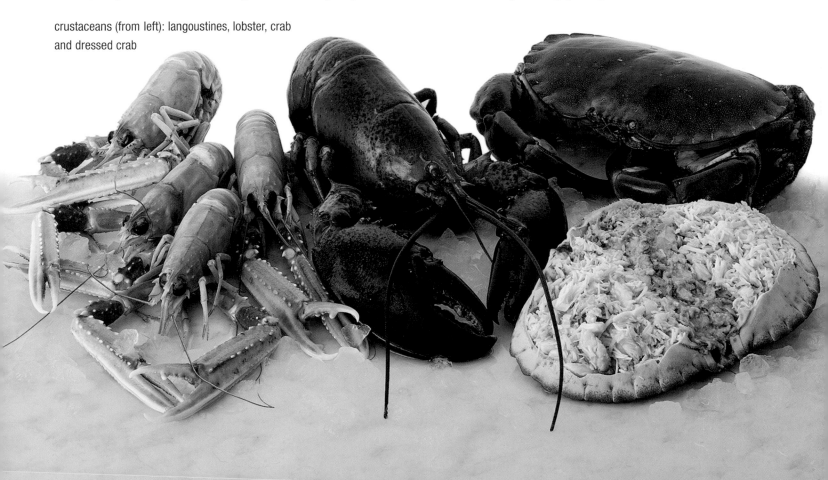

(more iron gram for gram than in red meat) and useful levels of calcium, phosphorus and zinc.

Oyster

Regarded as one of the ultimate luxury foods, oysters are traditionally eaten raw, with a few drops of lemon juice or Tabasco sauce to enhance their iodised flavour. They can also be lightly grilled, poached or steamed, but must not be overcooked or they will become rubbery. Oysters are one of the richest sources of zinc, a mineral needed for reproduction, which may be why they have a reputation for being an aphrodisiac. They also provide excellent amounts of iron and useful levels of potassium.

Prawn and shrimp

The different names given to these tasty crustaceans are only an indication of size – commercially, any prawn measuring less than about 5 cm (2 in) is known as a shrimp. Different species of prawns are found throughout the world and, generally speaking, those from cold waters have the best

flavour. If possible, buy prawns in the shell as they will taste better than those sold ready-shelled. Prawns are an excellent source of vitamin B_{12} and a useful source of calcium.

Scallop

For sheer beauty, the scallop is hard to beat, with its elegant fan-shaped shell. Inside, the thick disc of sweet white meat is attached to a vibrant orange, crescent-shaped roe or 'coral', which tastes as delicate and delicious as the white meat. Large or king scallops are sold both in and out of the shell. The small queen scallops are almost always sold shelled. Scallops are an excellent source of selenium and vitamin B_{12} and a useful source of phosphorus and potassium.

Squid

The squid is a cephalopod, a mollusc whose 'shell' has developed inside the body. Sold whole or as rings or tubes, squid requires either very brief or very long, slow cooking – anything in between makes it tough and rubbery. It is an excellent source of vitamin B_{12}.

prawns and shrimps (clockwise from back left): raw king prawns, cooked Mediterranean prawns (in shell and peeled), raw tiger prawns (in shell and peeled), peeled cooked brown shrimps, peeled cooked rose shrimps, and cooked Atlantic prawns (peeled and in shell)

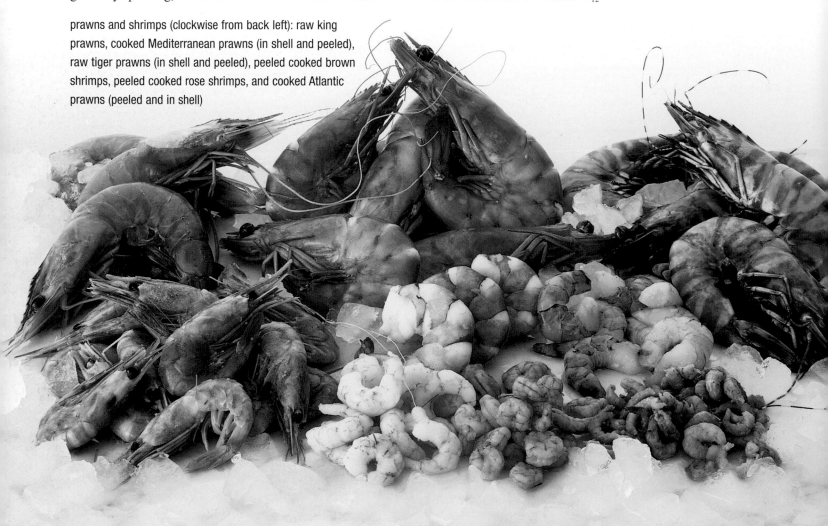

Vegetables from the sea

From a nutritional point of view, seaweeds and sea vegetables are superfoods as they contain protein, carbohydrate and essential vitamins and minerals and they are virtually fat-free.

Beside the seaside

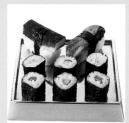

The Japanese have been eating seaweeds and sea vegetables (which grow near the salty shore) for thousands of years, and there has also been a long tradition of eating seaweed in Ireland and Wales. Elsewhere, the health-giving properties of these foods are just beginning to be appreciated. Edible seaweeds are sold in a variety of forms – fresh, dried, pickled in vinegar or flaked as a flavouring – and they can be found in large supermarkets, healthfood shops and speciality food shops. Some can be eaten raw or lightly blanched. All seaweeds are high in sodium, but they are also an excellent source of iodine, and the iodine flavour harmonises wonderfully well with fish and other seafood. Many seaweeds provide vitamin B_{12}.

Carrageen or Irish moss A fan-shaped seaweed from Ireland, this is reputed to be an excellent cure for coughs and colds when boiled and mixed with honey and lemon juice. In common with other seaweeds like agar-agar, carrageen has good gelling properties and is used as a vegetarian gelatine substitute to make jellies and mousses. Carrageen is a useful source of calcium.

Dulse Also called dillisk, this seaweed is popular in Ireland, where it is dried and chewed as a nutritious salty snack or added to soups to make a tasty sea-flavoured broth. Dulse can also be eaten fresh and is delicious cooked and spooned over buttered boiled new potatoes.

Nori and laver Anyone who has eaten sushi will be familiar with nori, the dark brownish seaweed that is dried and pressed into thin sheets to make sushi wrappers. Nori can also be eaten as it is, dipped in soy sauce, or toasted and shredded to be sprinkled over fish or vegetables as a garnish. Laver is the Welsh equivalent of nori. It is boiled to make a thick purée called laverbread, which is coated with oatmeal and fried, or spread on toast or oatcakes for breakfast. Both nori and laver are excellent sources of calcium, potassium and vitamin A.

Wakame Usually sold dried, this Japanese seaweed is an excellent source of calcium, phosphorus, magnesium and iodine. **Kombu** and **hijiki** are other seaweeds used in Japan.

Seashore feasts

Sea vegetables growing by the seashore contain all the goodness of seaweed. Steamed or quickly blanched and tossed in a little butter or lemon juice, they make the most delectable alternative to green vegetables.

Samphire, also called sea asparagus because of its appearance and texture, is at its best in spring and early summer, when its vibrant green shoots are young and tender. Samphire can also be bought pickled, but it has a completely different taste from fresh samphire and the pickling process changes it to greyish-green. Marsh samphire or glasswort is similar to rock samphire and can be eaten in a salad, cooked or pickled. It makes a good accompaniment for fish.

Seakale This cousin of the common cabbage can be tough, but if drifting sand covers the young shoots, shielding them from the light, the resulting yellowish stems will be pale and tender. They make a great alternative to asparagus and can be cooked in the same way. Seakale is a good source of vitamin C.

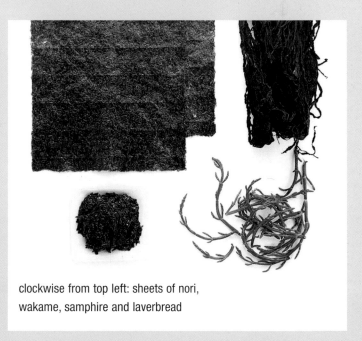

clockwise from top left: sheets of nori, wakame, samphire and laverbread

Preserved fish

Canning, smoking, drying, pickling and freezing are all healthy ways to preserve the goodness of fresh fish, for year-round enjoyment.

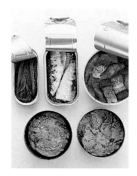

Canned goodness

Cans of fish are a very useful part of a well-stocked storecupboard. Oily fish like sardines, salmon and tuna are favourites and these fish retain their vitamin and mineral content when canned. Other ideal standbys are some of the more seasonal shellfish such as mussels, oysters and clams, all perfect for perking up fish pies and pasta sauces.

• Anchovy fillets have a high sodium content, but a little goes a long way and it takes only a small amount to add real flavour to fish dishes. Anchovies can also enhance the flavour of many non-fish dishes, including roast lamb, without making them taste fishy.

• Canned salmon comes in different grades, with the wild Alaskan red salmon having the best flavour. The canning process seals in all of salmon's natural beneficial oils and softens the bones to provide an extra source of calcium if they are eaten. Canned salmon makes a delicious healthy sandwich filling when partnered with watercress. It is also ideal for fish cakes and mousses.

• Sardines were the first fish ever to be canned and are among the most successful. Like salmon, if you eat the bones you will be adding valuable calcium to your diet. For one of the quickest and healthiest snacks possible, drain a can of sardines, mash them with a little lemon juice and serve on wholemeal toast.

• Pilchards are very similar to sardines although slightly larger. They have a coarser flavour but are equally nutritious.

• Tuna is a healthy fish that responds well to canning, and it is

Frozen for freshness

Many fish and shellfish are caught far out at sea, days or weeks away from land. To prevent deterioration, they are processed and frozen immediately on the fishing boats. This type of commercial freezing at very low temperatures preserves all the nutrients and ensures that the fish remains ultra-fresh. Frozen fillets and steaks are pre-packed and ready to cook, a wonderful convenience for busy cooks who may not have a fishmonger nearby but wish to include fish regularly in their diet. Other convenient frozen seafood includes shell-on or peeled prawns and mixtures that include mussels, prawns and squid.

preserved in oil, brine or spring water. Tuna is perfect for sandwiches and substantial salads.

The smoking story

There are two kinds of smoked fish: hot-smoked and cold-smoked. In hot-smoking, the fish is given an initial blast of hot air and then slowly cured in the smoke from a hot wood chip or sawdust fire. This cooks it too, so it is bought ready to eat. In cold-smoking, the fish is often salted or brined before curing over the smoke from a slow-burning wood fire. Some cold-smoked fish are eaten raw, while others need to be cooked further. Smoking, whether hot or cold, doesn't destroy the nutrients in the fish.

• Cod and haddock fillets are cold-smoked. When buying, look for the natural pale golden undyed fillets as they have a better flavour than the bright yellow fish which contains artificial colouring. Arbroath smokies are small whole hot-smoked haddock.

• Herrings are cold-smoked to become kippers and bloaters, or hot-smoked to become sprats and buckling. Like their fresh counterpart, they contain high levels of omega-3 fatty acids, which help to protect against stroke and heart disease.

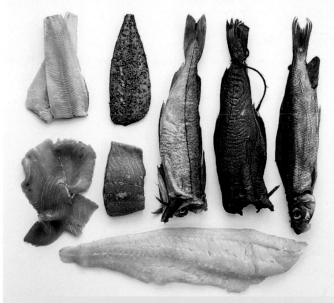

smoked fish (clockwise from top left): smoked trout, peppered smoked mackerel, smoked Finnan haddock, Arbroath smokie, kipper, smoked cod fillet, hot-smoked salmon and cold-smoked salmon

• Hot-smoking mackerel preserves all the nutritious oils and enhances its rich flavour. Smoked mackerel needs no cooking and can be eaten as part of a salad.

• Smoked salmon is usually produced by lightly salting the filleted fish and cold-smoking it, but it can also be hot-smoked which gives it a smoky, roasted flavour. Scottish smoked salmon is generally acknowledged to be the finest of all, but Irish salmon is also superb. Wild salmon has a gamier flavour and drier texture than farmed salmon. Smoked salmon from Canada and Norway is usually cheaper than British salmon and tends to be paler in colour with a lighter flavour.

• Hot-smoked rainbow trout is delicious in salads and sandwiches, or as a first course with bread and salad leaves.

In a pickle

Oily fish are well suited to pickling and can be preserved in flavoured vinegar or brine, or in a dry salt and spice mixture. Pickled fish are low in calories and high in flavour but may also be high in sodium, so should be eaten only occasionally.

• Gravad lax is fresh salmon 'dry' pickled with salt, crushed peppercorns and fresh dill. The process preserves all the goodness of salmon and the fish has a superb texture and flavour. Serve it sliced, with a dill and mustard sauce.

• Marinating herring fillets in vinegar with onions and spices preserves them in the same way that cooking does. Pickled

herrings are also available in a sour cream sauce. Rollmops are herring fillets rolled around peppercorns and onions and bottled with hot spiced vinegar.

Ancient methods of drying and salting

Air-drying is a natural process that removes moisture from food, preserving it and concentrating the flavour. Salting is another ancient way of extracting moisture. Both are well suited to fish and their roe. Dried and salted fish have been a staple food in many countries throughout the world for centuries, providing protein throughout the year.

• Dried, salted cod is known as stockfish in Scandinavia, bacalhau in Portugal and baccala in Italy. It looks like dried shoe leather, but after long soaking in many changes of water, it reverts to its original texture. The soaking process reduces the high sodium content. Poached or baked with tomatoes, onions and garlic, salt cod makes a tasty dish.

• Caviar is the salted roe of the sturgeon. It is available in grains or pressed and the grandest version is beluga. Caviar is low in fat with a moderate protein content, although as with other fish roes, it has high levels of cholesterol and sodium.

• Lumpfish roe, which can be black or orange, is a cheaper alternative to caviar as is the bright orange or red salmon roe.

• The hard roes of cod and grey mullet are salted, dried and pressed. They are often used for the Greek dip taramasalata.

▼ pickled, dried and salted fish (clockwise from left): dried salted cod, dried salted cod's roe, rollmops, marinated herring fillets, Bismarck herrings, salmon roe, gravad lax and black lumpfish roe

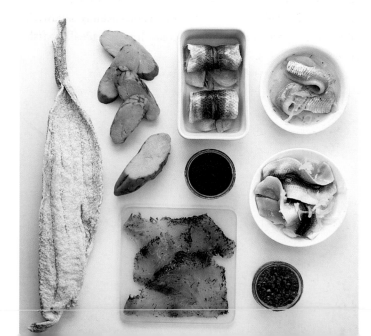

Cooking fish and shellfish

Healthy cooking methods like poaching, grilling, steaming and microwaving are perfect for the delicate flesh and subtle flavours of fish – and they are quick, too.

For fish, simplest is best

Fish does not need elaborate cooking. In fact, its delicate texture benefits from the fastest and simplest cooking methods to retain its natural juices and fresh clean taste. Some very fresh fish like salmon are sometimes simply marinated in citrus juice or other acidic liquid. This turns the flesh of the fish opaque and adds a tangy flavour, while retaining the valuable nutrients of the fish.

Unlike meat, fish has naturally tender flesh so it is always better to undercook rather than overcook it. Fish is ready if the flesh is still very slightly translucent when eased away from the bone, or flakes easily when tested with the point of a sharp knife or skewer. Alternatively, you can test by pressing the prongs of a fork into the thickest part of the fish; they should

▼ Baking fish in a parcel keeps it beautifully moist. Here a whole sea bass is baked with Oriental flavours.

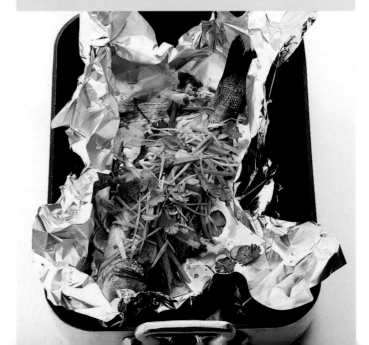

go in easily, just meeting a slight resistance near the bone.

Since most fish comes from the sea, it already has a natural salty taste so it needs little or no added salt.

Fish cooking know-how

● Cooking fish in parcels ensures the flesh stays moist and the fish cooks in its own juices. Whole fish can be stuffed with herbs or vegetables, then wrapped in foil or put in a baking dish and covered tightly, then baked in the oven at 180°C (350°F, gas mark 4). Allow about 10 minutes per 450 g (1 lb). Thick fillets or steaks can be parcelled up in baking parchment or foil with vegetables and herbs, moistened with wine or lemon juice and baked en papillote.

● Oily fish such as herrings, mackerel and trout are delicious grilled, and their own healthy oils can do all the basting. White fish should be marinated first or covered with a glaze or coating to protect its delicate flesh. Depending on size and thickness, fish will take 4–12 minutes to cook.

● Barbecuing is a tasty way to cook fish. Try whole oily fish like sardines, trout or mackerel and cook for 4–8 minutes on each side, depending on the size of the fish. If you use a special fish grill that holds whole fish, it will be easy to turn them over. White fish is best marinated if it is to be cooked straight on the barbecue, or it can be wrapped in foil parcels with herbs and lemon juice. Or cut chunky white fish into cubes and thread on skewers with vegetables to make wonderful kebabs. Be sure to oil the barbecue grid to ensure the fish doesn't stick to it.

● Fish can make a delicious and easy dish when braised with vegetables and a little fish stock or wine. As fish needs so little cooking, it is best to soften the chopped vegetables in a flameproof casserole first, then lay the fish on top and braise on the hob or in the oven. Allow 7–8 minutes for fillets and steaks or about 20 minutes for a whole 1 kg (2¼ lb) fish.

● Microwaving is an excellent way to cook fish, ensuring that it retains all its moistness, natural flavour and nutrients, and it

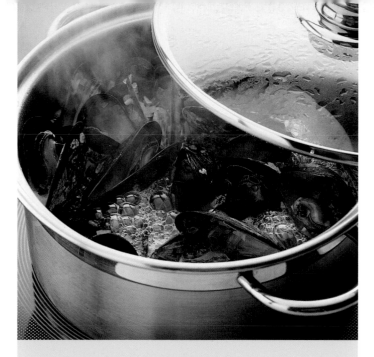

▲ Quick steaming is the traditional way to cook mussels.

Cooking crustaceans and molluscs

• When cooking a live crustacean, such as a lobster or crab, first wrap it in a damp tea towel and put it in the freezer for 1–2 hours to make it comatose. Then plunge it into a large saucepan of boiling water and quickly clamp on the lid. For crab, cook for 10–12 minutes, whatever its size; lobsters need about 15 minutes for the first 450 g (1 lb) and then 10 minutes for each subsequent 450 g (1 lb).

• Prawns and shrimps can be poached, pan-fried, grilled, barbecued or stir-fried. Raw prawns only take a few minutes to change to a bright pink colour, which indicates they are done. Keep the cooking of ready-cooked prawns very brief so that they are just heated through.

• Molluscs such as mussels and clams are usually steamed open, whereas oysters and scallops are more often prised open. Whether steamed, grilled, stir-fried or sautéed, cooking should be brief as overcooking will make the shellfish tough.

takes only a few minutes. When microwaving fish fillets or steaks, add a little stock or lemon juice and cover with kitchen paper. If you are microwaving whole fish, slash the skin a few times to prevent it from bursting.

• Poaching fish brings out its flavour and keeps it very moist. Fish stock, water and wine, or milk can all be used for poaching. The liquid will retain the water-soluble vitamins from the fish, so don't throw it away – use it to make a sauce or soup. When poaching fish, the liquid should never boil – it should be just under simmering point. For a whole fish (around 3.5 kg/6½ lb), put it into a pan with cold liquid to cover, put the lid on and bring to a simmer. Poach for 8–12 minutes, then remove from the heat and cool in the liquid.

• Steaming is one of the healthiest ways to cook fish as it uses no fat and, because the fish does not come into direct contact with liquid, most of the vital nutrients are retained. Use herbs and aromatics to add flavour, or steam fish on a bed of seaweed or samphire for an extra taste of the sea.

• Fish is delicious briefly pan-fried in a little oil or butter. If you use a non-stick frying pan or a ridged cast iron grill pan and heat the pan well, you'll need only a tiny amount of fat. Pan-fried fish takes only 2–3 minutes cooking on each side, depending on the thickness of the fish.

• Stir-frying is ideal for small pieces of fish, which take only moments to cook.

Beyond the fish finger

Fish is an ideal food for children but many are reluctant to try it. Encourage them to eat more fish by tempting them with colourful dishes like chunky kebabs with cherry tomatoes and courgettes, stir-fries or pasta dishes with fish, sweetcorn and peas. Form fish cakes into fishy shapes, or serve in burger buns with tomato ketchup. Or try sole goujons and chunky oven chips, shown below, served with a green vegetable. Skinless, boneless white fish makes a good addition to a toddler's diet as it has a delicate flavour and is easy to digest. Mash it with potato or carrot, stir tiny pieces into small pasta shapes or purée it into soup.

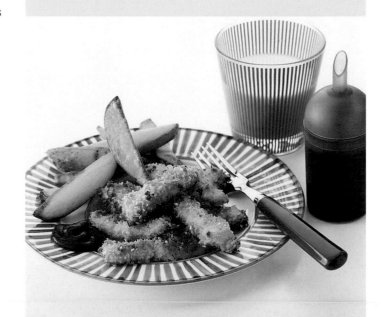

Back to basics

Nothing beats the flavour of fresh fish, but careful storage and preparation are essential. Always eat fresh shellfish and oily fish on the day they are bought.

Buying seafood

The best place to buy fresh fish and shellfish is from a trusted fishmonger, but they are becoming rare. Larger supermarkets now have excellent wet fish counters, and there are also mobile fish vans that travel around some parts of the country selling fresh seafood. Wherever you buy fish, always follow these guidelines.

• Really fresh fish do not smell fishy but give off an aroma of seaweed and the sea. When buying whole fish, check that the skin has a metallic shine and is covered in clear slime. The scales should be plentiful and firmly attached; stale fish shed their scales. The flesh should be firm and springy and the gills should be a vibrant red or deep pink; do not buy fish with brown or greyish gills. The eyes should be clear and slightly protruding; avoid fish with dull, sunken eyes.

• Testing pre-packed fish for freshness is more difficult, since you cannot smell it. For fish portions, check that the flesh is firm and moist, with a pearly translucency, and that any visible skin is shiny and bright. Buy from a reputable source that has a quick turnover.

• The flesh of all shellfish deteriorates rapidly and can become poisonous, so it is essential to buy only the very freshest. Seafood that is past its best has an unpleasant ammoniac or fishy odour. Crustaceans such as prawns and shrimps should have crisp, firm shells and should smell very fresh. On no account buy them if they smell of ammonia – a sure indication that they are stale.

• When buying molluscs, such as oysters, mussels or clams, always check with the fishmonger that they have come from 'clean' waters.

Freezing and thawing rules

When buying fresh fish, always ask the fishmonger if the fish has been previously frozen. Packaged fresh fish often has a label stating whether it has been frozen – if it has not, then ask. Basically, if the fish you are buying has been previously frozen then you must not re-freeze it as the texture will be ruined and harmful bacteria could cause food poisoning. However, it is fine to use this fish in cooked dishes like fish pies or lasagnes and then freeze the cooked dish. If absolutely necessary, you can freeze fresh (previously not frozen) white fish at home. To preserve the delicate texture, wrap the fish tightly in foil and freeze at the lowest possible temperature, preferably on fast-freeze. Once frozen, white fish can be stored for up to 3 months at -18ºC (-4ºF). Oily fish like herrings and mackerel do not freeze successfully as their oils cause them to spoil rapidly.

Fish should be thawed as slowly as possible to preserve the flavour and texture. Place in a dish, cover and leave overnight in the fridge, or thaw in the microwave on the defrost setting. Take care not to over-thaw it or it will dry out. Once thawed, pour off any liquid (you can use it in a nutritious soup or sauce), pat the fish dry with kitchen paper and cook it as soon as possible.

It is not advisable to freeze raw shellfish at home. Ready-frozen shellfish can be stored in a home freezer for 2 months.

• It is sometimes more convenient to buy frozen seafood. Obviously, you cannot apply the smell and feel tests, but do make sure the packaging is undamaged, and that there is no visible ice inside it and no sign of freezer burn or any discoloration. Frozen prawns and shrimps and seafood mixtures should still be solidly frozen in their bags; do not buy them if they have started to thaw.

Storing fresh seafood

• Ideally, fresh fish should be eaten on the day of purchase, but this is not always practical. As soon as you get it home, remove the packaging and wipe the fish with a clean damp

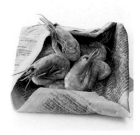

cloth. Place it on a plate, cover with cling film and store at the bottom of the fridge for no more than 24 hours.
• Live crustaceans, such as crabs or lobsters, should always be cooked on the day of purchase. If you cannot cook them immediately, wrap in wet newspaper or cover with a very damp tea towel and keep in the coldest part of the fridge.
• Live molluscs, such as mussels, clams, scallops and oysters, should also be eaten on the day you buy them. Put them in a large container, cover with a damp cloth and keep in the coldest part of the refrigerator until ready to cook. Oysters should be stored cupped side down to keep them fresh in the juices contained in the shell. Never store live molluscs in fresh unsalted water or they will die.

Safe handling

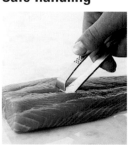

• Always use an immaculately clean, separate chopping board to prepare fresh fish and shellfish so that any harmful bacteria that might be present are not transferred to other foods. Wash your hands thoroughly before and after handling the fish.
• Make sure that fish fillets are free of small bones that might get stuck in the throat. Run your fingertips over the cut side of the fish to feel for bones and use clean tweezers to pluck out any that you find.
• The edible parts of a crab are the white meat in the claws and the creamy-brown meat in the body shell. When the crab's body has been separated from its hard shell, discard the greyish-white stomach sac and the feathery gills (dead men's fingers) as these are inedible.
• When taking lobster meat from the shell, discard the sac between the eyes in the head, the dark intestinal vein that runs down the tail and the grey spongy, feathery gills. The red coral or roe and the creamy greenish-grey liver (called the tomalley) can both be eaten.
• Before cooking mussels they should be well scrubbed and the wiry 'beards' removed. If any shells are slightly open, tap them sharply. If they do not close immediately, discard them.

Fish stock

A good home-made fish stock can enhance all kinds of fish dishes and it's very simple to make. Use fish trimmings – the head, skin and bones – from any white fish with a good flavour, such as sole, cod or plaice. (Oily fish are not suitable for making stock as they would give it a strong fatty flavour.) Once cooled, the stock will keep in the fridge for 1–2 days or it can be frozen for up to 1 month.

Makes about 1.2 litres (2 pints)
900 g (2 lb) trimmings from white fish, including skin, bones, and
     heads without gills
1 onion, thinly sliced
4 sprigs of parsley
2 bay leaves
2 carrots, thinly sliced
2 celery sticks, thinly sliced
4 black peppercorns
1.3 litres (2¼ pints) boiling water

Preparation time: 10 minutes, plus 10 minutes cooling
Cooking time: 35 minutes

1 Rinse the fish bones and heads well, then place in a large saucepan. Add the onion, parsley, bay leaves, carrots, celery and peppercorns, and pour in the boiling water. Bring back to the boil, then reduce the heat and simmer gently for about 30 minutes, skimming off the froth and sediment from the surface as it appears.

2 Remove from the heat and leave to cool for 10 minutes, then strain the stock through a fine sieve into a heatproof bowl. Discard the fish trimmings and vegetables. Use the stock at once or cool and chill.

Some more ideas
• For special-occasion fish dishes, use 300 ml (10 fl oz) white wine and 1 litre (1¾ pints) water.
• Use 400 g (14 oz) inexpensive white fish fillet, such as pollock, instead of the trimmings.
• Make a shellfish stock using prawn, crab, lobster or mussel shells instead of the white fish trimmings.

Piquant cod chowder

A variety of vegetables ensures that this wonderful soup is as healthy as it is delicious. The broth can be prepared a day in advance, ready for adding the fish at the last minute, which is useful when cooking mid-week meals. Planning ahead like this means a healthy dinner can be on the table in minutes.

Serves 4

2 sprigs of parsley

2 sprigs of fresh thyme

1 bay leaf

7.5 cm (3 in) piece of celery stick

1 can chopped tomatoes, about 400 g

750 ml (1¼ pints) fish stock, preferably home-made (see page 79)

4 tbsp medium cider

1 large onion, chopped

400 g (14 oz) waxy potatoes, cut into large chunks

225 g (8 oz) carrots, thickly sliced

225 g (8 oz) courgettes, thickly sliced

225 g (8 oz) green beans, cut into short lengths

1 yellow or red pepper, seeded and sliced

550 g (1¼ lb) cod fillet, skinned and cut into large pieces

salt and pepper

To garnish

2 tbsp finely chopped parsley

1 tbsp snipped fresh chives

finely shredded zest of 1 lemon

Preparation time: about 20 minutes

Cooking time: about 40 minutes

1 Tie the parsley, thyme and bay leaf with the celery to make a bouquet garni. Put the bouquet garni in a large saucepan. Add the tomatoes and their juice, the stock, cider and onion, stir and bring to the boil. Reduce the heat to low, half cover the pan and simmer for 15 minutes.

2 Add the potatoes and carrots. Increase the heat to moderate and cook, covered, for 15 minutes or until the vegetables are almost tender. Stir in the courgettes, green beans and yellow or red pepper and continue simmering, covered, for 5 minutes or until all the vegetables are tender. Discard the bouquet garni.

3 Season with salt and pepper to taste, then add the cod to the gently simmering broth. Cover and cook gently for 3–5 minutes or until the fish is opaque, just firm and flakes easily. Do not allow the broth to boil rapidly or the fish will overcook and start to break up.

4 For the garnish, mix the parsley, chives and lemon zest together. Ladle the fish and vegetables into warm bowls, then add the broth. Sprinkle the garnish over the top and serve at once.

Some more ideas

• Ring the changes by using different vegetables – broccoli florets, sliced leeks, sweetcorn, peas and green peppers are all suitable. Add them instead of the courgettes, green beans and yellow pepper in step 2.

• Smoked haddock is delicious in this dish, on its own or replacing half of the white fish.

Plus points

• Serving wholemeal rolls with the soup will add to the dietary fibre provided by all the vegetables.

• Green beans are a good source of fibre and they also provide valuable amounts of folate.

• Courgettes provide niacin and small amounts of vitamin B_6.

Each serving provides

kcal 290, protein 33 g, fat 2.5 g (of which saturated fat 0.5 g), carbohydrate 35 g (of which sugars 16 g), fibre 7 g

✓✓✓	B_6, B_{12}, C
✓✓	A, folate, iron, potassium
✓	B_1, niacin, calcium, selenium

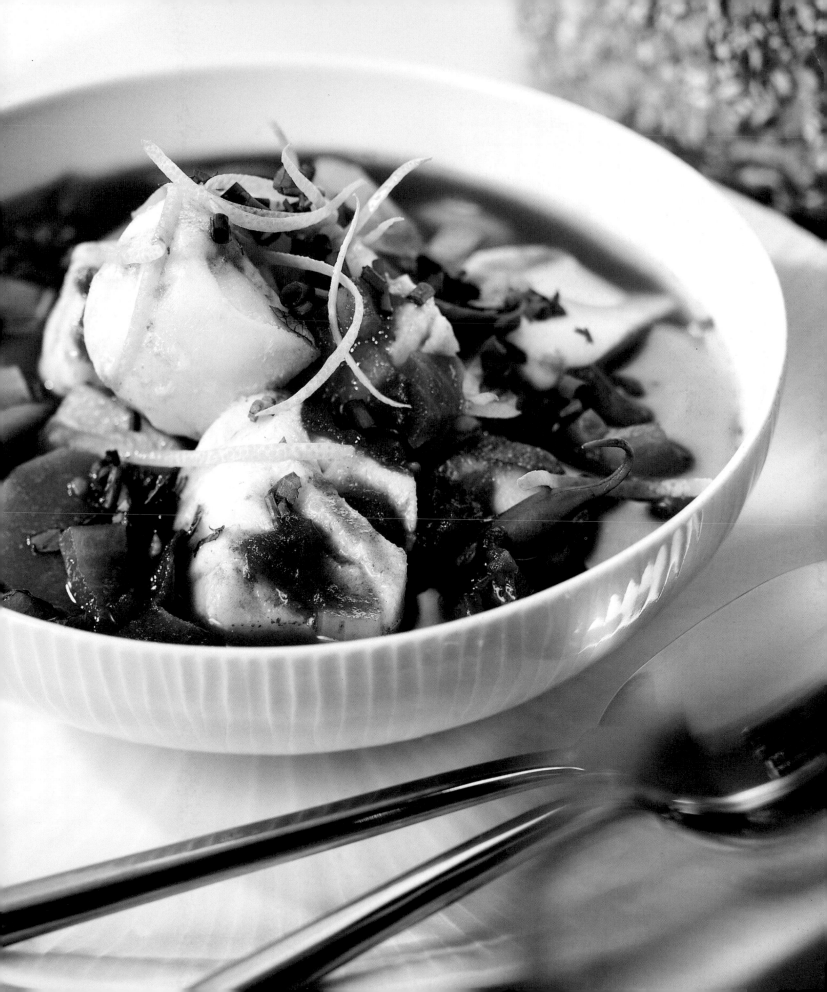

Monkfish and mussel sticks

To create these succulent mini kebabs, marinated cubes of monkfish fillet and fresh mussels are threaded onto skewers with a selection of colourful vegetables, then lightly grilled. They make an extra special hot nibble to hand round at a celebration party or present on a buffet table.

Makes 16 kebabs

finely grated zest and juice of 1 lemon

juice of 1 lime

1 tbsp extra virgin olive oil

2 tsp clear honey

1 garlic clove, crushed

1 tbsp chopped fresh oregano or marjoram

1 tbsp chopped parsley

200 g (7 oz) monkfish fillet, cut into
    16 small cubes

16 shelled fresh mussels, about 125 g
    (4½ oz) in total

1 small yellow pepper, seeded and
    cut into 16 small chunks

1 courgette, cut into 16 thin slices

16 cherry tomatoes

salt and pepper

lime or lemon wedges to garnish

Preparation time: 20 minutes,
    plus 1 hour marinating
Cooking time: 8–10 minutes

Each kebab provides

kcal 30, protein 3 g, fat 1 g (of which saturated fat 0.1 g), carbohydrate 2 g (of which sugars 2 g), fibre 0.5 g

✓✓	B$_{12}$
✓	C, E

1 Put the lemon zest and juice, lime juice, oil, honey, garlic, chopped oregano or marjoram, parsley, and salt and pepper to taste in a shallow non-metallic dish. Whisk together, then add the monkfish cubes and mussels. Turn the seafood to coat all over with the marinade. Cover and marinate in the fridge for 1 hour.

2 Meanwhile, put 16 wooden skewers in warm water and leave to soak for 10 minutes. Drain. Preheat the grill to moderately high.

3 Onto each skewer, thread 1 cube of monkfish, 1 mussel, 1 piece of yellow pepper, 1 slice of courgette and a cherry tomato. (Reserve the marinade.) Leave the ends of the skewers empty so they will be easy to hold.

4 Place the kebabs on a rack in the grill pan and grill for 8–10 minutes or until the monkfish is cooked and the vegetables are just tender, turning occasionally and brushing frequently with the marinade. Serve hot, garnished with lime or lemon wedges.

Some more ideas

• For scallop and prawn sticks, use 16 shelled fresh queen scallops and 16 raw peeled prawns in place of the monkfish and mussels.

• To make tuna or swordfish sticks, cut 300 g (10½ oz) fresh tuna or swordfish fillet into 16 small cubes and marinate in a mixture of the finely grated zest and juice of 1 lime, 1 small crushed garlic clove, 1 tbsp extra virgin olive oil, 1 tsp Cajun seasoning, and salt and pepper to taste. Seed 1 red pepper and cut into 16 small chunks, and quarter 4 shallots or baby onions. Thread the marinated fish onto skewers with the prepared vegetables and 16 very small button mushrooms. Grill as in the main recipe.

Plus points

• Monkfish has a huge, ugly head, and only the tail is eaten. The firm flesh tastes rather like lobster. Monkfish is an excellent source of phosphorus and a useful source of potassium, which is vital to help regulate blood pressure.

• Mussels provide several minerals, in particular iron, zinc, copper and iodine. Mussels are also an extremely good source of vitamin B$_{12}$, needed for the maintenance of a healthy nervous system.

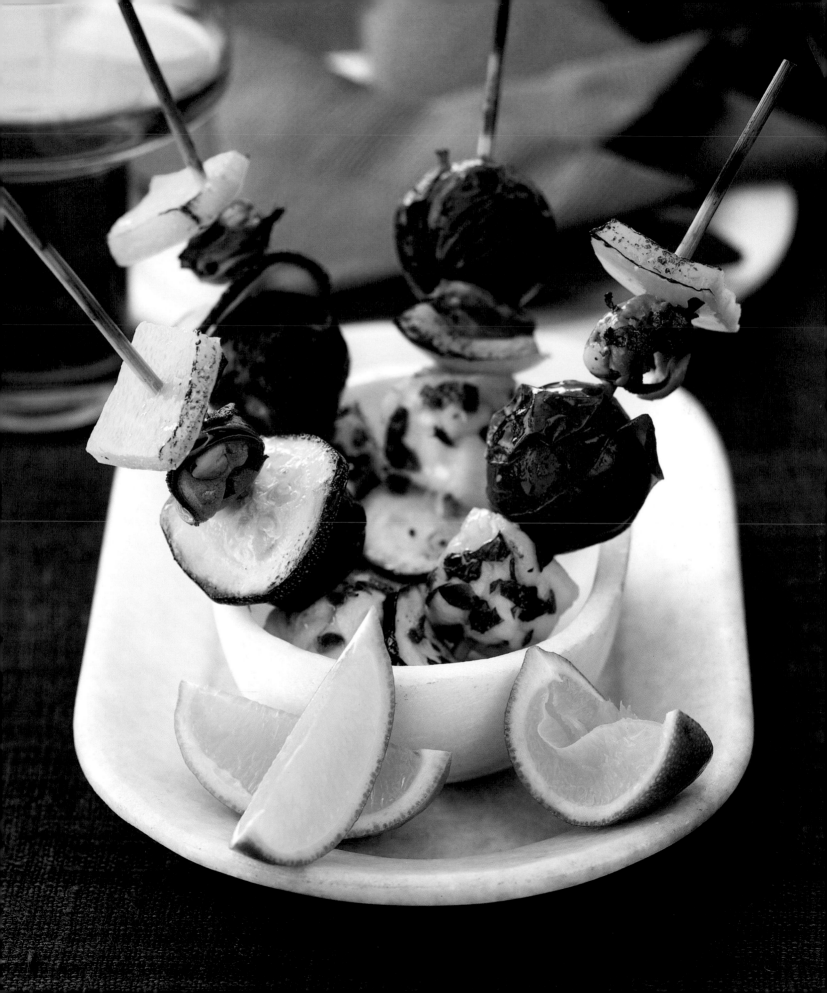

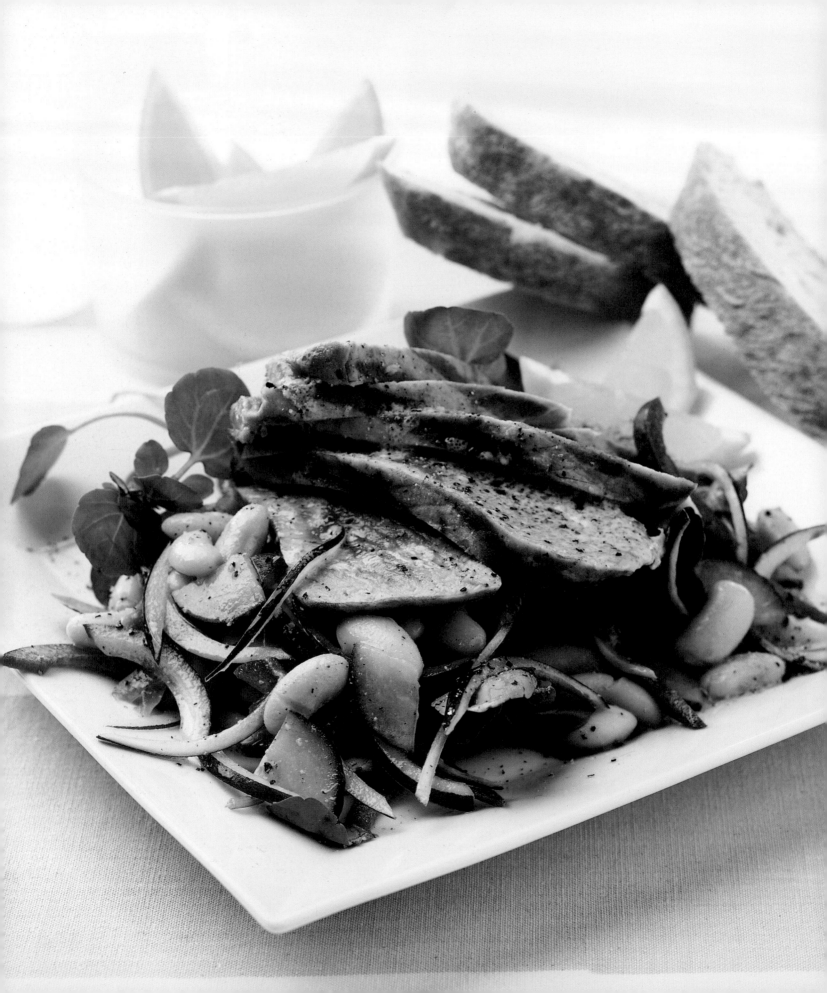

Seared tuna and bean salad

This healthy version of a classic salad is perfect for warm weather eating. Fresh tuna is quickly cooked in a hot pan so the outside is lightly browned, leaving the inside pink, moist and full of flavour, and then served on a cannellini bean and red pepper salad. Warm ciabatta bread, thickly sliced, is the best accompaniment.

Serves 4

400 g (14 oz) piece tuna steak, about 5 cm (2 in) thick
4 tbsp extra virgin olive oil
1 tbsp lemon juice, or to taste
1 garlic clove, crushed
1 tbsp Dijon mustard
1 can cannellini beans, about 410 g, drained and rinsed
1 small red onion, thinly sliced
2 red peppers, seeded and thinly sliced
½ cucumber, about 225 g (8 oz)
100 g (3½ oz) watercress
salt and pepper
lemon wedges to serve

Preparation and cooking time: 30 minutes

Each serving provides

kcal 380, protein 32 g, fat 17 g (of which saturated fat 3 g), carbohydrate 26 g (of which sugars 11 g), fibre 9 g

✓✓✓	A, B$_6$, B$_{12}$, C, selenium
✓✓	B$_1$, niacin, iron
✓	E, folate, copper, potassium, zinc

1 Brush a ridged cast-iron grill pan or heavy frying pan (preferably cast-iron) with a little oil and heat over a moderate heat. Season the tuna steak on both sides with coarsely ground black pepper.

2 Sear the fish in the hot pan over a moderately high heat for 4 minutes on each side – the outside should be browned and criss-crossed with dark lines from the grill pan, while the inside should be light pink in the centre. Take care not to overcook the tuna or it will become tough and dry. Remove from the pan and leave to rest while preparing the rest of the salad.

3 Mix together the oil, lemon juice, garlic and mustard in a salad bowl. Season with salt and pepper to taste and add more lemon juice, if needed. Add the cannellini beans, onion and peppers to the bowl. Cut the cucumber lengthways into quarters, then cut the quarters across into 1 cm (½ in) slices. Add them to the salad bowl together with the watercress. Toss the salad gently to mix.

4 Cut the tuna into slices about 1 cm (½ in) thick. Arrange the slices on top of the salad and spoon up a little of the dressing over the fish. Serve with lemon wedges.

Another idea

- For a warm chicken and bean salad, use 500 g (1 lb 2 oz) skinless boneless chicken breasts (fillets). Cook in the hot pan for 18–20 minutes, turning frequently, until the chicken is cooked through. Leave to cool while you make the salad. Instead of cannellini beans, watercress and cucumber, use 1 can borlotti beans, about 400 g, drained and rinsed, 100 g (3½ oz) baby leaf spinach or rocket, and 250 g (8½ oz) cherry tomatoes, halved, with the onion and peppers. Slice the chicken, arrange on the salad and spoon over the dressing.

Plus points

- The health benefits of eating watercress have been acknowledged for many centuries. Along with other dark green, leafy vegetables, it provides good amounts of several vitamins and minerals including vitamin C, vitamin E, carotenoid compounds and the B vitamins folate, niacin and vitamin B$_6$.
- Canned beans are a useful source of iron, and the vitamin C from the watercress and peppers will help enhance its absorption.

Soused fresh sardine salad

Cooking fish – traditionally by frying – and then submerging it in a 'souse' is a very tasty way to prepare it, and was once a means of preserving. Here sardines are grilled and marinated, then served on a Moroccan-spiced couscous, chickpea and pepper salad. It is a perfect prepare-ahead dish for summer entertaining.

Serves 4

8 fresh sardines, cleaned, scaled and
  heads removed
1 small lemon, cut into 8 thin slices and
  each slice halved
250 g (8½ oz) couscous
1½ tsp ground coriander
1 tsp turmeric
pinch of cayenne pepper
1½ tsp butter
600 ml (1 pint) boiling water
1 can chickpeas, about 410 g, drained
  and rinsed
4 spring onions, finely chopped
2 large peppers (1 red and 1 yellow),
  seeded and finely diced
1 large courgette, grated
140 g (5 oz) baby spinach leaves
fresh flat-leaf parsley to garnish
salt and pepper

Marinade

finely grated zest of 1 large lemon
4 tbsp lemon juice
1 tbsp garlic-flavoured olive oil
1 fresh red or green chilli, seeded and
  finely chopped
1 shallot, finely chopped
6 black peppercorns, lightly cracked
1 bay leaf

Preparation time: 25 minutes, plus at least
  30 minutes marinating

1 Preheat the grill to high. To make the marinade, put the lemon zest and juice in a bowl and whisk in the oil. Stir in the chilli, shallot, peppercorns and bay leaf.

2 Line the grill rack with foil and lightly brush with marinade. Tuck 2 lemon slice halves in each sardine cavity, then arrange the sardines on the foil. Brush with more marinade and grill for 2 minutes.

3 Carefully turn the sardines over, lightly brush with marinade again and grill for a further 2–3 minutes or until the skins are slightly crisp and the flesh flakes easily. Immediately transfer the sardines to a baking dish, arranging them in one layer, and pour over the marinade, including any remaining in the grill pan. Roll each sardine over so it is well coated. Leave to cool, then cover and chill for at least 30 minutes.

4 Meanwhile, put the couscous in a bowl and stir in the coriander, turmeric, cayenne pepper, butter and salt to taste. Pour over the boiling water and stir, then set aside to cool.

5 About 15 minutes before serving, remove the sardines from the fridge. Add the chickpeas, spring onions, peppers and courgette to the couscous, then stir to mix and fluff up the grains.

6 Divide the spinach leaves among 4 plates and spoon on the couscous. Remove the sardines from the marinade and place 2 fish on each plate. Sprinkle with the parsley and serve immediately.

Plus points

● Fresh sardines are an excellent source of vitamin B$_{12}$ and the antioxidant selenium, and also provide useful quantities of potassium.

● The vitamin C in the spinach leaves and the peppers helps with the absorption of iron from the sardines.

● As soon as vegetables are cut, their vitamin content starts to diminish, so if possible they should be prepared just before serving, as is done for this salad.

Each serving provides
kcal 586, protein 40 g, fat 18 g (of which saturated fat 5 g), carbohydrate 68 g (of which sugars 8 g), fibre 7 g

✓✓✓ A, B$_1$, B$_2$, B$_6$, B$_{12}$, C, E, folate, niacin, iron, selenium

✓✓ calcium, copper, potassium, zinc

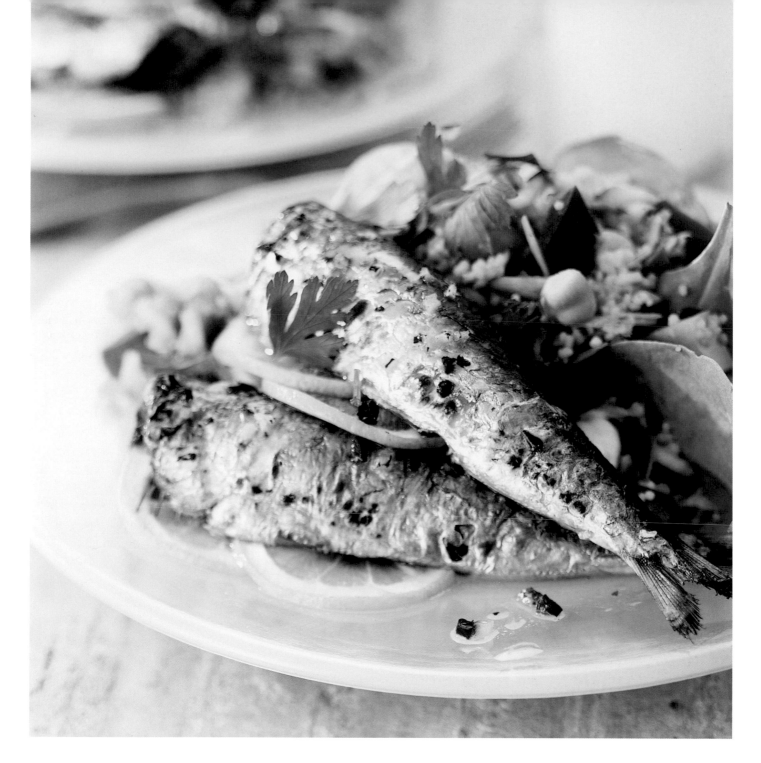

Another idea

• Make a soused trout salad with orzo, the small rice-shaped pasta. For the marinade, mix together the finely grated zest of 1 large lemon, 4 tbsp lemon juice, 1 tbsp orange juice, 100 g (3½ oz) thinly sliced shallots, 1 thinly sliced carrot, 1 bay leaf and 1 seeded and chopped fresh green chilli. Grill 4 skinless trout fillets, about 140 g (5 oz) each, for 6–7 minutes, turning once and brushing with the marinade. Transfer the fillets to a baking dish, pour over the marinade and leave to cool, then cover and chill. Meanwhile, cook 250 g (8½ oz) orzo in boiling water for 10–12 minutes, or according to the packet instructions, until al dente. Drain and leave to cool. About 15 minutes before serving, add 85 g (3 oz) baby spinach leaves, 55 g (2 oz) rocket and 1 red pepper, seeded and diced, to the orzo and fold together. Flake the trout and gently stir in, with the marinade, 4 tbsp chopped parsley and seasoning.

Grilled salmon in ciabatta

Here fresh salmon fillets are marinated, then lightly grilled and served in warm ciabatta rolls with mixed salad leaves and a basil mayonnaise, to create a very tempting and special lunch dish. Lightening the mayonnaise with yogurt reduces the fat without losing out on any of the creaminess.

Serves 4

juice of 1 lime

3 tbsp chopped fresh basil

4 pieces skinless salmon fillets, about 85 g
  (3 oz) each

2½ tbsp plain low-fat yogurt

2½ tbsp mayonnaise

½ tsp finely grated lime zest

4 part-baked ciabatta rolls, about 75 g
  (2½ oz) each

salt and pepper

mixed salad leaves, such as rocket,
  Oak Leaf lettuce, baby spinach, red chard
  and lamb's lettuce, to serve

Preparation time: 15 minutes,
  plus 30 minutes marinating
Cooking time: 10 minutes

Each serving provides

kcal 408, protein 26 g, fat 18 g (of which
saturated fat 3 g), carbohydrate 36 g
(of which sugars 4 g), fibre 2 g

✓✓✓	B$_{12}$, E
✓✓	B$_6$, niacin, selenium
✓	A, B$_1$, folate, calcium, potassium, zinc

1 Mix together the lime juice, 2 tbsp of the basil, and salt and pepper to taste in a shallow, non-metallic dish. Add the salmon fillets and turn them in the mixture to coat well all over. Cover and leave to marinate in a cool place for 30 minutes.

2 Meanwhile, mix together the yogurt, mayonnaise, lime zest and remaining 1 tbsp basil in a small bowl. Season with salt and pepper to taste. Cover and chill until required.

3 Preheat the grill to moderate, and preheat the oven to 220ºC (425ºF, gas mark 7). Lift the salmon fillets out of the marinade and place in the foil-lined grill pan. Brush with a little of the marinade, then grill for 4–5 minutes on each side or until the fish is just cooked and the flesh is beginning to flake, brushing again with the marinade after you have turned the fillets. While the fish is cooking, place the ciabatta rolls in the oven to bake for about 5 minutes, or according to the packet instructions, until crisp.

4 Split the ciabatta rolls in half and spread the cut sides with the basil mayonnaise. Put a cooked salmon fillet on the bottom half of each roll and scatter over a few mixed salad leaves. Place the top half of each roll in place and serve immediately.

Some more ideas

• Use other types of rolls, such as white baps, cheese-topped rolls or seeded rolls.

• For grilled tuna baps with tomato and ginger relish, use 4 fresh tuna steaks, about 85 g (3 oz) each, and marinate them in a mixture of 2 tsp finely chopped fresh rosemary, the juice of 1 orange, and salt and pepper to taste. Meanwhile, to make the relish, sauté 1 finely chopped small red onion, 1 crushed garlic clove and 1 tbsp finely chopped fresh root ginger in 1 tbsp extra virgin olive oil for 8–10 minutes or until softened. Remove from the heat and add 4 chopped plum tomatoes, 1–2 tbsp chopped fresh basil and salt and pepper to taste. Mix well. Grill the tuna for 3 minutes on each side or until cooked to your taste, then serve in wholemeal or Granary baps with salad leaves and the relish.

Plus points

• Combining mayonnaise with low-fat yogurt not only reduces total fat, it also increases the nutritional value of the dish, in particular adding calcium, phosphorus, and vitamins B$_2$ and B$_{12}$.

• Salad leaves such as rocket are useful sources of the B vitamin folate and of beta-carotene.

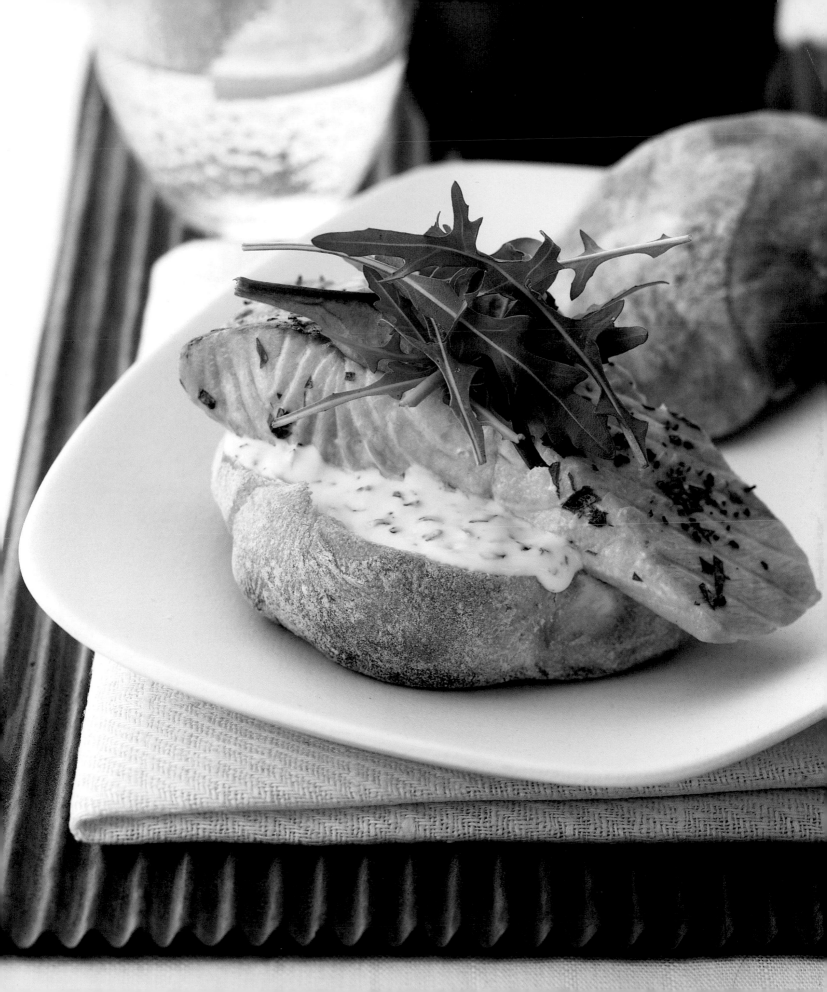

Steamed sea bass fillets with spring vegetables

Oriental steamer baskets are most handy for this dish – you can stack them so that everything can be steamed together. The moist heat from steaming ensures that the fish doesn't dry out. If using a liquid fish stock base or a cube, make up the stock half strength as it will get a lot of flavour from the marinade.

Serves 4

1 tsp grated fresh root ginger

1 tbsp light soy sauce

½ tsp toasted sesame oil

1 garlic clove, finely chopped

1 tbsp dry sherry, dry white wine or vermouth

4 sea bass fillets, 3.5 cm (1¼ in) thick, about 140 g (5 oz) each

700 ml (24 fl oz) fish stock

200 g (7 oz) couscous

1 strip of lemon zest

225 g (8 oz) baby carrots

12 spring onions, trimmed to about 10 cm (4 in) long

200 g (7 oz) asparagus tips

2 tbsp chopped parsley

salt and pepper

Preparation and cooking time: 30 minutes

Each serving provides

kcal 320, protein 34 g, fat 5 g (of which saturated fat 1 g), carbohydrate 35 g (of which sugars 8 g), fibre 3 g

✓✓✓	A, B₁₂
✓✓	C, folate, calcium, iron
✓	B₁, B₆

1 First make the marinade. Combine the ginger, soy sauce, sesame oil, garlic and sherry, wine or vermouth in a bowl. Add the fish and turn to coat in the marinade. Set aside.

2 Bring 250 ml (8½ fl oz) of the stock to the boil in a saucepan that will accommodate the steamer basket(s). Put the couscous in a bowl and pour over the boiling stock. Cover and leave to stand for about 15 minutes or until the couscous has swelled and absorbed the liquid.

3 Pour the remaining stock into the saucepan. Add the lemon zest and bring to the boil. Add the carrots. Reduce the heat so the stock simmers.

4 Place the fish, skin side down, in a single layer in a steamer basket. Add the spring onions and asparagus, or put them in a second stacking steamer basket. Place the steamer basket(s) over the gently boiling stock and cover. Steam for 10–12 minutes or until the fish is opaque throughout and begins to flake, and the vegetables are tender.

5 When the couscous is ready, add the parsley and fluff the grains with a fork to mix the couscous and parsley. Season with salt and pepper to taste.

6 Lift the steamer basket(s) off the pan. Drain the carrots, reserving the cooking liquid. Arrange the fish, carrots and steamed vegetables on warm plates with the couscous. Discard the lemon zest from the cooking liquid. Moisten the fish, vegetables and couscous with a little of the liquid, and serve with any remaining liquid as a sauce.

Plus points

• White fish such as sea bass are low in fat and calories and they offer many B-complex vitamins. Sea bass is also a good source of calcium, an essential mineral with many important functions in the body, including keeping bones and teeth strong.

• The active ingredient in asparagus, called asparagine, has a strong diuretic effect. Herbalists recommend eating asparagus as a treatment for rheumatism and arthritis, as well as for the bloating associated with PMT.

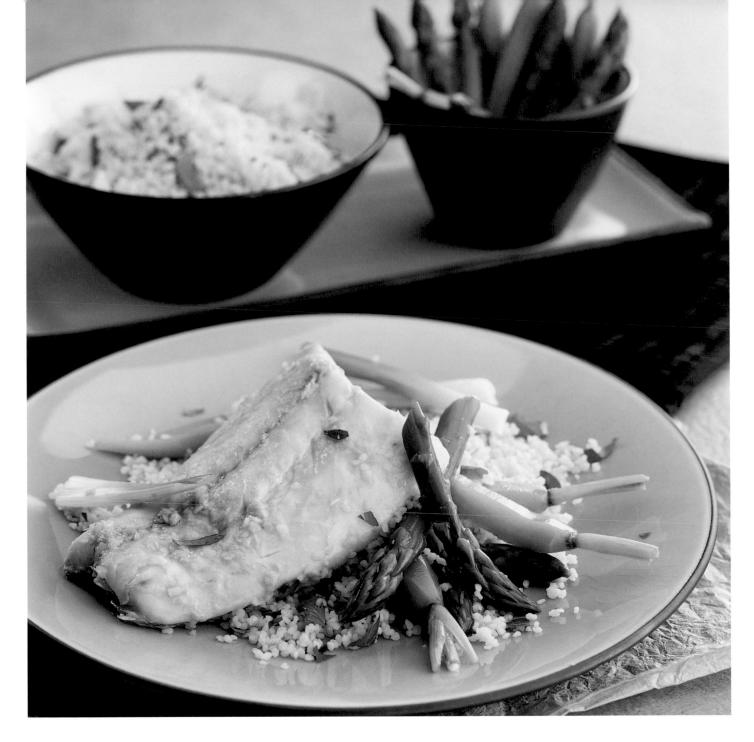

Some more ideas

- If you don't have a steamer, place the fish and vegetables in a colander, place inside a large pan and cover with a lid.
- Use salmon or cod fillets instead of sea bass. The cooking time may need to be reduced by a minute or 2 for thinner fish fillets; check for doneness after 8–9 minutes.

- For a simpler dish, omit the marinade and use water instead of fish stock. When the water comes to the boil, add 600 g (1 lb 5 oz) small new potatoes. Scatter 2 finely slivered small leeks and the finely grated zest of 1 lemon over the fish, then steam it over the potatoes. Meanwhile, cook 500 g (1 lb 2 oz) spinach until wilted; squeeze out excess water and chop.

Moisten with 4 tbsp single cream and season with salt and pepper to taste. Serve the fish on the creamed spinach, with the potatoes tossed with chopped fresh herbs.

- Instead of couscous, serve the fish with mashed potatoes. Use some of the fish cooking liquid instead of milk for mashing the potatoes and finish with a small knob of butter.

Red mullet parcels with orange

Whole red mullet are baked in the oven on a bed of aniseed-flavoured fennel and fresh orange segments. To save time, ask your fishmonger to scale and gut the fish for you. Serve one parcel per person and accompany it with new potatoes and some simply cooked green beans.

Serves 4

2 tbsp extra virgin olive oil

2 large bulbs of fennel, halved and very
   thinly sliced

2 garlic cloves, chopped

8 spring onions, cut into 2.5 cm (1 in) lengths

3 small oranges

4 red mullet, about 200 g (7 oz) each, scaled
   and gutted, and heads removed if liked

salt and pepper

Preparation time: 15 minutes
Cooking time: 12–15 minutes

Each serving provides

kcal 270, protein 32 g, fat 12 g (of which saturated fat 1 g), carbohydrate 10 g (of which sugars 9 g), fibre 3 g

✓✓✓	B_{12}, C, selenium
✓✓	B_6, potassium
✓	B_1, E, folate, niacin, calcium, copper, iron

1 Preheat the oven to 220°C (425°F, gas mark 7). Heat the oil in a saucepan, add the fennel, garlic and spring onions, and cook over a moderate heat for 5 minutes or until softened.

2 Meanwhile, squeeze the juice from one of the oranges. Cut the peel and pith from the remaining 2 oranges and, holding them over the orange juice container, cut between the membrane to release the segments.

3 Divide the fennel mixture and orange segments among 4 large sheets of baking parchment. Slash each fish 3–4 times on both sides, then place on top of the vegetables and orange. Sprinkle over the orange juice, and season with salt and pepper to taste.

4 Wrap the paper round the fish and fold over to seal each parcel. Place the parcels on a baking tray and bake for 12–15 minutes or until the fish is cooked. Set the parcels on individual serving plates still sealed, so they can be opened at the table.

Some more ideas

• To make haddock parcels with vegetable spaghetti, cut 2 parsnips and 2 carrots lengthways into thin strips using a swivel vegetable peeler. Thinly slice 2 leeks lengthways to make similar-sized strips. Heat 30 g (1 oz) butter in a frying pan, add the vegetables and

1 large garlic clove, crushed, and cook for 3–4 minutes or until softened. Season to taste and pile in the centre of the parchment sheets. Place a 140 g (5 oz) piece of skinned haddock fillet (a chunky piece from the top end) on top of each one and squeeze over the juice of ¼ lemon. Dot each piece of fish with 10 g (¼ oz) butter, then wrap up the parcels. Bake for 15 minutes or until tender.

• Use 4 pieces of salmon fillet, about 140 g (5 oz) each, instead of red mullet.

Plus points

• Red mullet has lean, firm flesh that tastes almost like shellfish. It is an excellent source of selenium and provides useful amounts of potassium.

• Oranges are an excellent source of vitamin C, with 1 large orange providing around double the recommended daily amount. They also contain phytochemicals that are believed to help thin the blood and lower cholesterol levels, thus helping to prevent strokes and heart attacks.

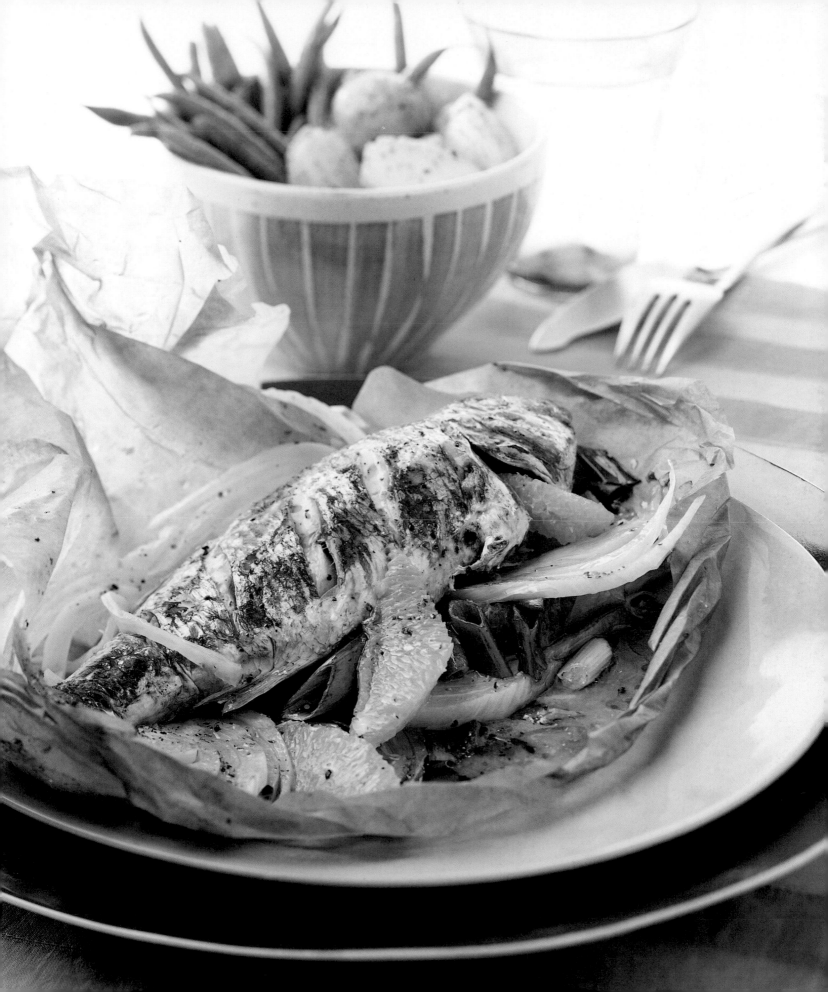

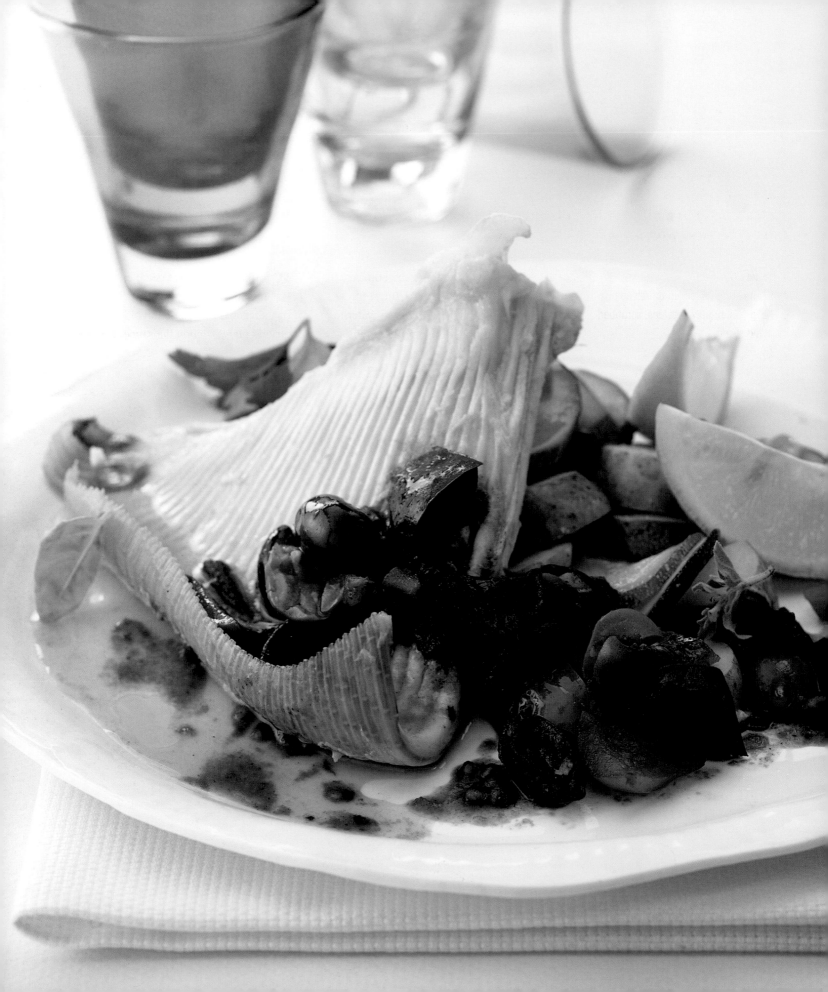

Poached skate with vegetables

Skate wings have a fine texture and flavour as well as an intriguing shape. Poaching them in stock with lots of vegetables is simple and quick, and lets each ingredient add its flavour to the others. A ladleful of the poaching stock turns sautéed peppers and tomatoes into a sauce to serve with the fish and vegetables.

Serves 4

600 ml (1 pint) chicken or fish stock
675 g (1½ lb) new potatoes, scrubbed
   and sliced
3 spring onions, thinly sliced
2–3 sprigs of fresh thyme
2 garlic cloves, chopped
4 medium or 2 large skate wings, 750 g
   (1 lb 10 oz) in total
2 courgettes, thinly sliced
juice of ½ lemon
2 tbsp extra virgin olive oil
1 red pepper, seeded and diced
1 green pepper, seeded and diced
3–4 large ripe tomatoes, diced
6 black olives, stoned and halved
6 green olives, stoned and halved
salt and pepper
chopped fresh herbs to garnish
lemon wedges to serve

Preparation and cooking time: 30 minutes

Each serving provides

kcal 350, protein 34 g, fat 9 g (of which
saturated fat 1 g), carbohydrate 37 g
(of which sugars 12 g), fibre 5 g

✓✓✓	A, B₆, B₁₂, C
✓✓	B₁, potassium
✓	B₂, E, folate, niacin, calcium, copper, zinc

1 Bring the stock to the boil in a large shallow saucepan. Add the potatoes and enough boiling water to cover them. Add the spring onions, thyme and half of the garlic. Bring back to the boil, then reduce the heat to moderate and cover. Simmer for about 5 minutes or until the potatoes are almost tender.

2 Add the skate wings to the pan and lay the courgette slices on top. Sprinkle over the lemon juice. The potatoes should be submerged in liquid, so add more boiling water if necessary. Cover again and cook over a moderately high heat for 5–7 minutes or until the potatoes are tender and the skate will flake when tested with a fork.

3 Meanwhile, heat 1½ tbsp of the olive oil in a frying pan and add the remaining garlic and the red and green peppers. Cook for 3–4 minutes or until the vegetables have softened. Add the tomatoes and cook over a high heat for 1–2 minutes, stirring.

4 Add a ladleful – about 120 ml (4 fl oz) – of the fish poaching liquid to the tomato mixture, and bubble over a high heat for 6–7 minutes or until the liquid has almost all evaporated. Add the olives and season with salt and pepper to taste. Remove the sauce from the heat and keep warm.

5 Lift the fish and vegetables from the pan with a draining spoon or fish slice and place on individual serving plates. Spoon the sauce over the fish. Garnish with chopped herbs and drizzle over the remaining ½ tbsp of olive oil. Serve with lemon wedges.

Another idea

• For saffron-scented fish with green beans, use 500 g (1 lb 2 oz) of skinless cod, haddock or monkfish fillet, cut into 4 pieces. Add 1 large pinch of saffron threads to the stock in step 1. In step 2, add the fish, which will need 7–10 minutes cooking. Instead of courgettes, use 250 g (8½ oz) fine green beans, adding them 3–4 minutes before the end of cooking.

Plus points

• Skate is an excellent source of vitamin B₁₂ and a useful source of potassium, vitamins B₁ and B₆ and niacin.
• Many people assume that olives are high in calories, but in fact both the black and green varieties provide relatively few – 30 g (1 oz) olives, which is about 10, contain about 30 kcals and just 3 g fat. Olives are a source of vitamin E, but are usually not eaten in large enough quantities to make a significant contribution to the diet.

Smoked haddock kedgeree

Kedgeree, a traditional Anglo-Indian dish of rice and smoked fish, is perfect for brunch, lunch or a light supper. It is also tasty cool as a salad. Serve with seeded wholegrain bread or warm naan bread.

Serves 4

280 g (10 oz) skinless smoked haddock fillet
1 bay leaf
1 sprig of fresh thyme
2 tsp extra virgin olive oil
300 g (10½ oz) basmati rice
1 onion, finely chopped
¼ tsp garam masala
¼ tsp ground coriander
½ tsp curry powder
225 g (8 oz) shelled fresh peas or frozen peas
4 tomatoes, halved
3 tbsp finely chopped parsley
2 spring onions, finely chopped
2 hard-boiled eggs, quartered
salt and pepper
sprigs of parsley to garnish

Preparation time: 10 minutes
Cooking time: 40 minutes

Each serving provides

kcal 462, protein 28 g, fat 7 g (of which saturated fat 1.5 g), carbohydrate 72 g (of which sugars 6 g), fibre 4 g

✓✓✓	B_1, B_6, B_{12}, niacin
✓✓	A, C, iron, selenium
✓	E, folate, calcium, potassium, zinc

1 Put the haddock in a saucepan, cutting into pieces to fit, if necessary. Cover with boiling water and add the bay leaf and thyme. Cook the fish, covered, over a low heat for 8–10 minutes or until it will flake easily (the water should just simmer). Remove the fish using a fish slice and set aside. Reserve the cooking liquid.

2 Heat the oil in a large saucepan over a moderate heat. Add the rice and stir to coat thoroughly, then cook, stirring frequently, for 2 minutes. Add the onion, garam masala, coriander and curry powder, and continue cooking for 2–3 minutes, stirring, until the onion starts to soften. Add 600 ml (1 pint) of the reserved cooking liquid together with the bay leaf and thyme. Reduce the heat to moderately low, cover and simmer for 12 minutes. Add the peas, cover again and continue cooking for 10–12 minutes or until the rice is tender.

3 Meanwhile, preheat the grill to high. Place the tomatoes, cut side up, on a baking sheet and grill for 2–3 minutes or until lightly coloured and heated through.

4 Flake the fish and gently fold it into the rice with the parsley and spring onions. Season with salt and pepper to taste and transfer to a warm serving dish. Add the egg quarters, garnish with parsley sprigs and serve with the grilled tomatoes.

Some more ideas

• For a fruity flavour, stir 55 g (2 oz) raisins or sultanas into the rice with the fish.

• Use brown basmati rice instead of white and cook for about 20 minutes before adding the peas.

• Add 100 g (3½ oz) sautéed sliced mushrooms with the flaked fish.

• Make a mixed seafood kedgeree. Use 150 g (5½ oz) smoked haddock and add 170 g (6 oz) cooked mussels or oysters. If using freshly cooked mussels, about 450 g (1 lb) in the shell, use the mussel cooking juices as part of the liquid to cook the rice. Canned and drained mussels or oysters can also be added. Another idea is to use 140 g (5 oz) each smoked

Plus points

• Peas, like other legumes such as lentils, soya beans and chickpeas, are a good source of protein. Peas are also rich in fibre, some of which is in the soluble form which can help to regulate blood sugar and cholesterol levels in our bodies.

• Eggs provide high-quality protein as well as zinc, vitamins A, D and E and B vitamins. Although eggs contain cholesterol, the health risks of eating eggs have often been exaggerated. Normally, dietary cholesterol has little effect on blood cholesterol levels. It is the intake of saturated fat that affects blood cholesterol.

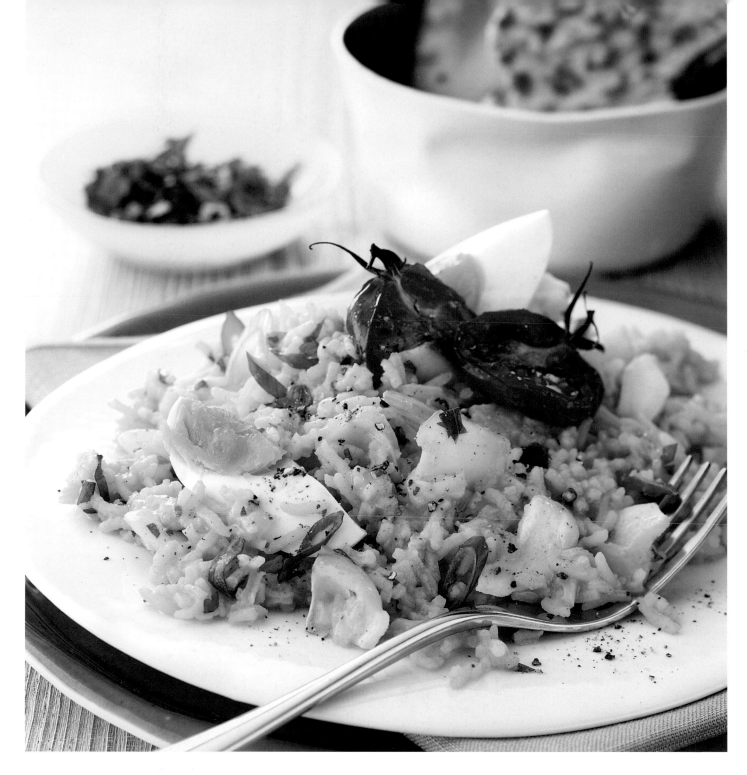

haddock and poached or steamed skinless fresh haddock or cod fillet.

• For a delicious herby salmon and rice dish, replace the smoked haddock with diced or flaked hot-smoked salmon fillet (no need to cook it first) or with poached salmon. Omit the spices and cook the rice in fish stock or water. Skin and chop the tomatoes instead of grilling them, and fold into the cooked rice with the salmon and parsley, plus 1 tbsp chopped fresh dill or tarragon and 1 tbsp snipped fresh chives. Instead of the hard-boiled eggs, fold in 1 peeled and diced avocado, if you wish. This dish is particularly good in the summer served at cool room temperature.

• Omit the grilled tomatoes and serve the kedgeree with a salad made from diced cucumber and halved cherry tomatoes.

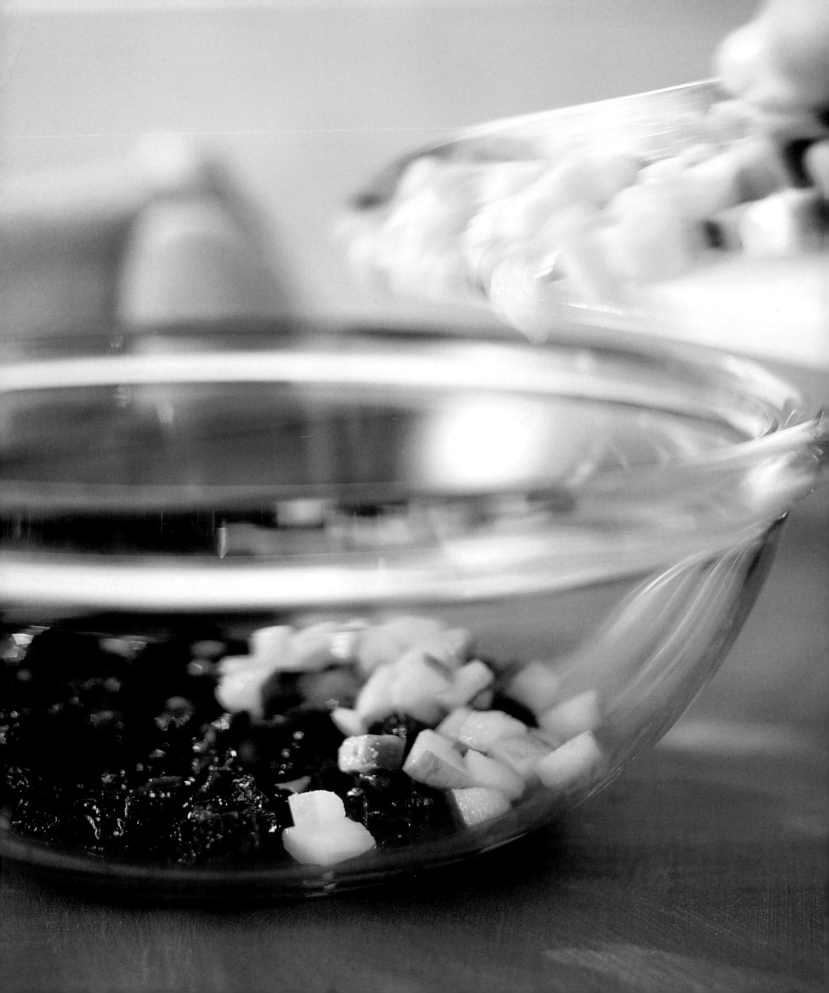

Perfect Poultry

It is no wonder that poultry today is so popular all over the world. It offers first-class protein, it provides many essential vitamins and minerals, and it is low in saturated fat – an unbeatable healthy profile. And the wonderful variety of poultry available – from well-loved chicken and turkey to duck, goose, guinea fowl, pigeon and quail – as well as game birds, such as pheasant, partridge and grouse, can be prepared in so many ways. Here, you'll find buying tips and guidelines on the preparation, storage and cooking of poultry and game birds. There are also ideas for flavourings and lower-fat preparations, and basic recipes for stock and stuffings.

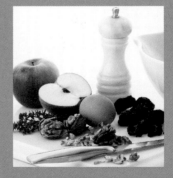

Poultry in a healthy diet

Protein repairs and maintains everything from muscle and bone to skin, hair and fingernails. It is essential to our good health and general well-being.

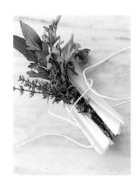

Essential for life

Protein is made up of amino acids, which are compounds containing the 4 elements that are necessary for life: carbon, hydrogen, oxygen and nitrogen. We need all of the 20 amino acids commonly found in plant and animal proteins. The human body can only make 12, so the remaining 8 have to be obtained from the food we eat. The proportions of amino acids in animal foods (meat, poultry, game and game birds, fish, milk, cheese and eggs) match human requirements more closely than the amino acids in vegetable foods, even though some vegetable foods, such as nuts and pulses, are very high in protein.

Protein foods should feature daily in the diet because amino acids cannot be stored in the body for later use. Any excess is used at the time as energy or stored as body fat.

Quality, not quantity

Despite protein foods being so vital, we do not need to eat them in great quantity – no more than 15% of our daily calorie intake should be from protein. The amount allocated to protein on the daily 'plate' in a well-balanced diet is, therefore, considerably smaller than accompanying starchy carbohydrate foods (such as pasta or rice), vegetables and fruit, which for some people may mean reducing the quantity of protein foods they eat.

In the UK, the average consumption of red meat – beef, lamb, pork and veal – is 8–10 portions a week, or 85 g (3 oz) a day. Current healthy eating guidelines suggest that this is sufficient, and that the rest of the protein requirement should come from other sources, such as poultry and game, fish, eggs, dairy foods, nuts and seeds, pulses and cereals.

Just 2 portions of protein food per day is thought adequate for most people, although the very active might need 3 or 4. With only a small quantity required, it is well worth choosing the best quality protein foods to eat. Lean poultry and game birds are far better nutritional value for money than high-fat products such as savoury pies, pâté, sausages and fatty meats, and can be low-fat alternatives to other protein foods such as red meat, eggs and full-fat cheeses.

Cutting the fat

Poultry and game birds are lower in saturated fat than most red meat – most of the fat they contain is unsaturated or

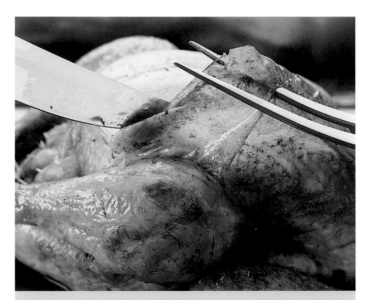

▲ Removing the skin from chicken reduces the fat content considerably, even if this is done after cooking – the fat in chicken skin does not transfer to the meat during cooking

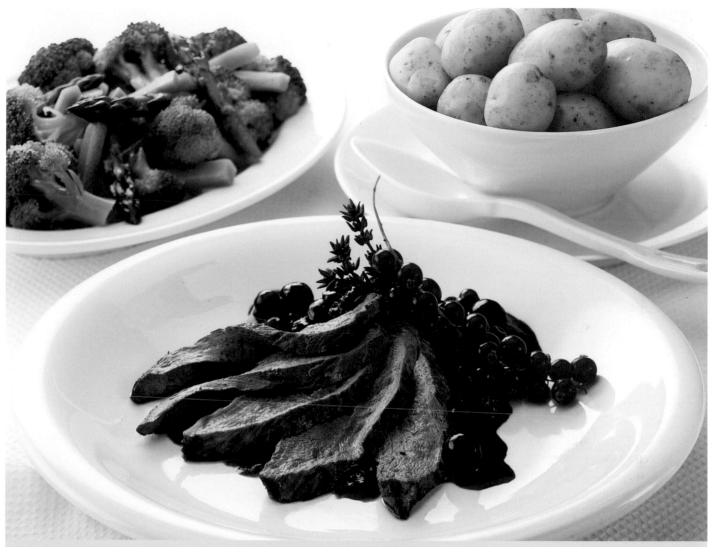

▲ In a well-balanced meal, protein foods make up the smallest portion. Here a tender duck breast with a redcurrant sauce is served with plenty of potatoes (starchy carbohydrate) and a selection of vitamin-rich vegetables

monounsaturated. Chicken and turkey are particularly lean birds, and most of their fat is in the skin, so if the visible fat and skin are removed, either before or after cooking, they are a good low-fat choice. Note, though, that if you eat both the meat and the skin of chicken and turkey, the fat content will be higher than an equivalent amount of beef or other red meat.

Duck, which is a fatty bird, can be enjoyed in a healthy diet too, if the skin and fat are removed before cooking. Once this is done, lean duck has about the same amount of fat as lamb.

Vitamins and minerals too

Poultry and game birds are an important source of B vitamins, including B_1 (thiamin), B_2 (riboflavin), niacin, B_6 and B_{12} – all essential for the body to run smoothly. They also provide many essential minerals such as zinc, iron, chromium, copper, selenium, phosphorus, potassium and magnesium. Eating lean poultry and game birds is one of the easiest ways to ensure you get enough iron, zinc and vitamin B_{12}. Chicken and turkey livers offer a lot of vitamin A too.

Popular poultry

Chicken and turkey are wonderfully versatile; they offer lean protein and essential vitamins. Duck, though fattier, is also a great source of protein.

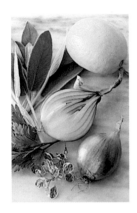

An ABC of poultry

Although to most people, the term poultry generally means just chicken and turkey, poultry is, in fact, the term for all domesticated birds reared for the table – even those that were wild until quite recently. Poultry, then, includes chicken, duck, goose, guinea fowl, quail, squab pigeon and turkey.

Chicken

Chicken – probably the world's most popular meat – is eaten in every country, and the range of preparations reflects this, using ingredients and flavours from all points of the globe. Today the choice of chicken to buy is wide – from fresh-chilled, intensively reared birds to organic chickens, free-range chickens and corn-fed chickens, as well as poulet de Bresse and other well-flavoured chickens from France.

Nutritionally, chicken is a very good source of protein: a 140 g (5 oz) portion of grilled breast (without skin) provides 88% RNI of protein for women and 71% RNI for men. Cooking chicken without too much additional fat and removing the skin, either before or after cooking, offers the lowest-fat option. Compare about 2g of fat per 100 g (3½ oz) in a grilled skinless boneless chicken breast (2% fat), with 12g of fat per 100 g (3½ oz) in a grilled chicken breast with skin (12% fat).

Although red meat is usually thought of as one of the best protein sources of vitamins and minerals, chicken compares very favourably. It is an excellent source of the B vitamin niacin: a 140 g (5 oz) portion provides more than the daily requirement for adults. It is also a useful source of vitamins B_2, B_6 and B_{12}, and the mineral zinc.

Corn-fed chickens are fed some corn (maize), but their attractive yellow-coloured flesh and fat is the result of an artificial dye in the food. A corn-fed chicken has very similar protein and fat levels to an ordinary chicken, and similar amounts of iron, zinc and B vitamins.

Chicken livers are a rich source of iron, zinc, vitamin A and many of the B vitamins, especially B_{12}. The iron present in liver is in a form that is easily absorbed by the body.

Whole chickens are best for roasting, and can also be poached, braised and pot-roasted. Young roasters are the most widely available, and one weighing 1.35–1.8 kg (3–4 lb) will serve 4–6 people.

Poussins are small, immature chickens. They are slightly lower in protein than older birds, and a little higher in fat. They do not have a lot of flavour, so need to be marinated and basted if being grilled or barbecued. Alternatively, cook them with flavourful ingredients. Allow one poussin per person.

Spring chickens, also called poulets, are a little older than poussins and thus a little bigger. One bird will feed 2 people.

Boilers, or boiling fowl, are old laying hens. Because of their age they are tougher than younger chickens, but they have much more flavour, and make delicious stock for soup. Unfortunately they are now hard to find.

Capons are neutered male birds, with a greater proportion of white meat to dark meat. Their meat is succulent as it is quite high in fat. Capons are available only from specialist outlets.

Joints are available on and off the bone, with skin or skinless. Common chicken joints are breasts (skinless boneless breasts are often called fillets), thighs, drumsticks, quarters and wings. Thigh and drumstick together are sometimes called a Maryland, and boneless breast and wing together a supreme.

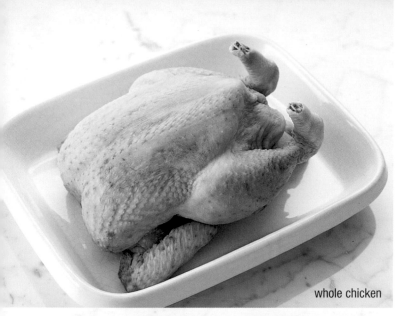

whole chicken

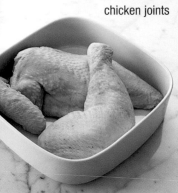

chicken joints

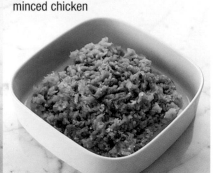

minced chicken

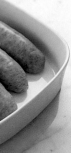

chicken sausages

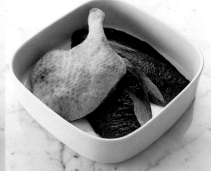

duck joints

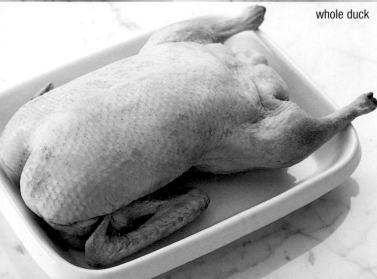

whole duck

Breast is the tenderest meat with the least fat; thigh is the fattiest and thus most moist.

Minced chicken can be used to make burgers, meat loaves, shepherd's pie and most other dishes that would traditionally use minced beef or other red meat.

Chicken products such as sausages can offer a lower-fat alternative to red meat products. They may not be as nutritious as chicken generally, however, because the meat will have been 'stretched' with bulking ingredients.

Duck

Duck has a similar protein content to chicken and turkey, but is higher in fat: roast meat contains 10% fat, even though no fat is visible, and duck meat, fat and skin together contain 29% fat. Most of the fat on a duck is found just below the skin. Although much of this fat is monounsaturated, from a health point of view it is still preferable to remove the skin and visible fat before cooking or, if roasting, to prick the skin all over before cooking to allow the fat to drain away.

Duck is rich in minerals, being an excellent source of zinc and a good source of iron, offering three times as much iron as chicken. It is also a very good source of B vitamins, and contains selenium and potassium.

The ducks we buy in butchers and supermarkets are bred for the table in sheds, in conditions almost identical to those for intensively reared chickens. They are very rarely kept free-range on ponds. The most common breed of duck in Britain is the Aylesbury. It is also possible to find Gressingham ducks (a cross between the domestic duck and the mallard) and two French breeds, the Barbary and Nantais.

Duckling was once the term for birds up to 2 months old, but it is now used until they reach 6 months. Although a duckling might be thought to have tenderer meat than a duck, this is not always the case, and being young it may not have a lot of meat on its bones. Ducklings can weigh as much as 3.2 kg (7 lb), according to the breed, although 1.5–2 kg (3 lb 3 oz–4½ lb) is more usual.

Ducks (like ducklings) do not have a lot of meat for their size, and the amount can vary according to the breed – for example, the Aylesbury is more fleshy than others. As a general guide, when buying allow about 750 g (1 lb 10 oz) per person.

Joints of duck widely available are legs and boneless breasts. The meat on duck legs is tough, so they are best used in soups and stews. The breasts can be pan-fried, grilled or barbecued – each breast will serve one – or cut up for stir-fries. The plump, meaty breasts (called magrets) from the French Moulard, the duck reared for foie gras, will each serve 2 people.

Goose

Being a waterfowl (like duck), the rich dark meat of a goose is a lot fattier than chicken and turkey. However, unlike duck, a greater proportion of goose fat is saturated, so it is particularly important to prick the skin before roasting so that the fat can run out, or to remove any visible fat and skin if cooking by other methods.

Goose has a similar protein content to other poultry. It provides as much zinc as duck and more iron – a 100 g (3½ oz) portion offers 31% RNI of iron for women and more than 50% for men. As for vitamins, goose is an excellent source of the B vitamins B_1, B_2, B_6, B_{12} and niacin.

Goslings are 6–8 months old. Being so young, they have very tender meat that is less fatty than that of older birds. Goslings weigh up to about 2.25 kg (5 lb) .

Goose, in its youthful prime, will weigh 3.2–5.4 kg (7–12 lb) . As the bird gets older and larger, the meat becomes tougher and more fatty. There is a lot less meat on a goose than on a chicken or turkey, so allow about 750 g (1 lb 10 oz) per person when calculating the size of bird to buy.

Guinea fowl

Semi-domesticated breeds of guinea fowl are not as lean as wild guinea fowl, which does not have a closed hunting season, but both are low in fat, particularly saturated fat. The meat of guinea fowl is like that of a slightly gamey chicken – darker than that of chicken, and with more leg meat and less breast meat. Guinea fowl is a good source of protein, and provides B vitamins and iron.

Pigeon

Pigeon, whether squab – the farmed bird – or the wild wood pigeon, is available all year, but is best between May and September. Despite being a small bird, pigeon is quite meaty, with very well-flavoured flesh. Like other poultry, it is a first-class source of protein and has a moderate fat content. Pigeon is an excellent source of iron, with a portion providing 100% RNI for both men and women, and a useful source of zinc.

Quail

Like guinea fowl and pigeon, quail is a game bird that is today bred for the table. It is very small, with delicately flavoured meat, and 2 birds are often served per person. The nutritional profile is similar to pheasant or partridge.

Turkey

While chicken has long been an everyday meat, turkey is traditionally reserved for special occasions such as Christmas and Thanksgiving. A large turkey, roasted to perfection, is the ideal bird for a festive dish – it can feed a large gathering and still leave plenty of meat for sandwiches and other meals. Smaller turkeys and turkey joints are now widely available and are well worth enjoying throughout the year.

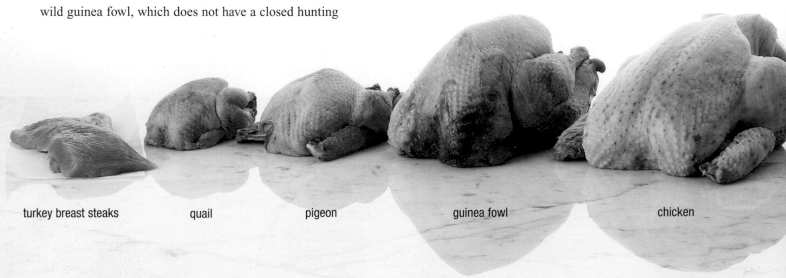

turkey breast steaks   quail   pigeon   guinea fowl   chicken

Sizing up turkey

Judging how big a turkey to buy depends on how many people you want to serve – and the leftovers you want to enjoy over the following few days. Here is a rough guide:

2.25–3.2 kg (5–7 lb)	bird serves	6–9
3.6–4 kg (8–9 lb)	bird serves	10–11
4.5–5 kg (10–11 lb)	bird serves	12–14
5.4–6 kg (12–13 lb)	bird serves	16–18
6.2–7.6 kg (14–17 lb)	bird serves	20–24
8–9 kg (18–20 lb)	bird serves	26–30

Nutritionally, turkey is very similar to chicken, although it contains slightly more vitamin B_{12} and niacin and more zinc. The dark leg meat offers three times as much zinc as the light breast meat and twice as much iron.

There are free-range and organic turkeys available, but most are reared under intensive conditions. On a much smaller scale, some schemes exist to produce 'traditional' turkeys, which are special breeds, such as the Norfolk Black and the Cambridge Bronze. These turkeys are hung to develop flavour, and do not have water added during processing.

Whole turkeys range in size from young birds at 2.25–3.6 kg (5–8 lb) up to huge birds weighing 11.25–13.5 kg (25–30 lb). See the chart, left, for judging the size of turkey to buy.

Joints on the bone are drumsticks, thighs and breasts. They can be quite large, and one joint will probably serve 2 people. There are also boneless breast steaks, escalopes and fillets for single servings. The whole breast on the bone, without the legs and wings, is often called a crown roast.

Minced turkey makes a lower-fat alternative to red meat minces for burgers and in meat sauces for dishes such as lasagne.

Turkey products such as sausages can be a good lower-fat choice, although many are breaded and deep-fried, which makes them high in fat. Turkey 'rolls' and 'roasts' can contain a lot of additives as well as water, so check the labels.

A buyer's guide to poultry

When choosing poultry, look for fresh, unblemished skin and meat. Avoid birds with dry or discoloured skin, or skin with bruises or tears, and especially birds that have an 'off' odour. Be sure that the wrapping on pre-packaged birds isn't torn and that the package isn't leaking. If the bird is frozen, check carefully that there is no freezer burn (brown or greyish-white patches on the skin).

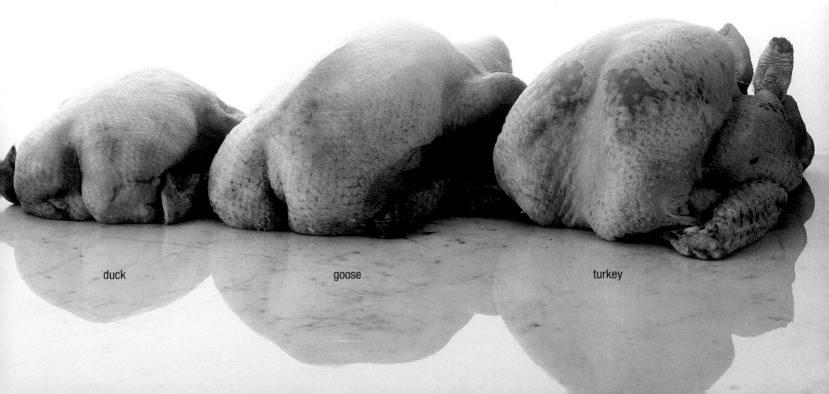

duck   goose   turkey

Glorious game

British native game birds offer a healthy lower-fat form of protein. Their popularity is growing steadily and many are now available in supermarkets.

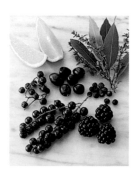

An ABC of game birds

Some game birds that once lived in the wild, such as quail and guinea fowl, are now reared for the table and, as such, are classed as poultry. Pheasant and partridge are often intensively reared, and then released into the 'wild' for the shooting season. Other birds remain truly wild, feeding on their traditional forage rather than on processed feed, with all the physical activity that entails. As a result, the meat of wild game birds tastes quite different from that of their farmed or 'semi-wild' counterparts, and it is more lean. It is also free of growth hormones and antibiotics.

Small young game birds – whether farmed or wild – are best roasted, or they can be grilled or barbecued. Older birds, particularly wild ones, can be tough and their meat tends to be dry, so they benefit from marinating before cooking, or a moist method of cooking such as braising or pot-roasting. Alternatively, use them in pies, soups and so on.

Duck

The wild members of the duck family are much tougher and lower in fat than the duck bred for the table, but like supermarket duck the meat has a very rich flavour. Mallard is the most common and largest wild duck – one bird will serve 2–3 people. Widgeon, thought to be superior in flavour to mallard, will serve 2 at a stretch. Teal, the smallest wild duck, will serve one. The season is 1 September to 31 January.

Grouse

This small, ground-scratching game bird is hunted on moors in northern England and Scotland – the 'Glorious Twelfth' (12 August) marks the start of the shooting season, which ends on 10 December. The birds feed on heather shoots, berries and small insects, and their dark red meat is richly gamey in flavour. A young grouse weighs about 750 g (1 lb 10 oz) and will serve one person.

Grouse contains marginally more protein than poultry, and is extremely low in fat – only 5 g per 100 g (3½ oz) – most of which is unsaturated. It is an excellent source of B vitamins, with a typical 140 g (5 oz) portion providing all an adult's daily B_2 and niacin needs, as well as over half the B_1 requirements. When roasted, grouse is an excellent source of iron and a good source of zinc.

Partridge

A small game bird, the same size as grouse, partridge is perhaps best known for its appearance in a pear tree in the traditional Christmas song. In fact, Christmas is in the middle of the shooting season for partridge, which is from 1 September to 1 February. Partridge has pale meat with a delicate flavour – it is usually hung for 3–4 days before being

---

Hanging poultry and game birds

In the past, most meat and poultry – even fish – was 'hung', to allow the enzymes and spoilage bacteria that are naturally present to break down and tenderise the muscle, in the process contributing distinctive flavour changes. Modern methods of farming produce poultry and game birds that do not need to be hung, probably because the muscles are not as 'tough' as they are in wild birds or in some free-range produce. Traditional poulterers and game dealers still hang pheasant and wild duck, and organic and specialist chicken and turkey producers often hang poultry before it is 'dressed' (i.e. plucked and gutted).

plucked and gutted. A bird will make one serving.

Partridge has one of the highest meat protein contents, equalled only by venison, and a fat content of 7% in its meat. It is also an excellent source of both iron and phosphorus.

Pheasant

Slightly larger than most other game birds, pheasant is quite tame, and as a result is now intensively reared. The shooting season lasts from 1 October to 1 February. The meat of a pheasant has quite a gamey flavour, and modern tastes prefer unhung birds, although older birds benefit from being hung for several days to tenderise them before cooking. A pheasant weighing about 1.5 kg (3 lb 3 oz) will serve 2–3 people.

Pheasant is an excellent source of protein. It is relatively high in fat for a game bird, at 10–12%, although this is mainly monounsaturated. Generally, the plump hen (female) birds contain more fat than the cocks (males). Pheasant is lower in iron than some other game birds, but is still an excellent source, as it is for B vitamins.

Other game birds

Black game, related to grouse and similar in flavour, is about the size of a pheasant. It is native to the hills and moors of Scotland and northern England. The shooting season is 20 August to 10 December. Other game birds similar to grouse include capercailzie, or capercaillie, a large bird which is in season 1 October to 31 January, and ptarmigan, in season 12 August to 10 December.

Two of the smallest game birds are snipe (12 August to 31 January) and woodcock (1 October to 31 January). Traditionally these birds are not gutted before cooking.

Free-range vs intensive farming

Free-range poultry, in theory, contains less saturated fat and more unsaturated fat than intensively reared birds that are unable to exercise. Physical activity alters the fat profile of a bird or animal in a way that is beneficial both for its own health and for the people who eat it. However, some of the older/rarer breeds favoured by organic and free-range poultry producers are less lean than breeds used in intensive farming. Also, some systems are more free-range than others.

Chickens were originally jungle fowl, and they are not always happy roaming in a field under the open sky, which is often the only type of 'range' available, so many free-range birds in fact remain quite sedentary. In contrast, some free-range farms offer wooded areas in which the chickens are happy to roam and forage for worms and insects to supplement their feed.

Because free-range birds are less intensively fed and are slaughtered when they are older, they tend to have a better flavour than intensively reared birds.

Is organic poultry any healthier?

While all poultry and meat are monitored and controlled by government regulatory bodies (in the same way that fruit and vegetables are monitored for pesticide and other agrochemical residues), there are concerns that antibiotic residues, in particular in intensively farmed meat and poultry, may transfer drug resistance problems to humans. Organic poultry is not given antibiotics and other routine veterinary drugs, nor artificial growth-promoting hormones in its feed, and so should be free from drug residues.

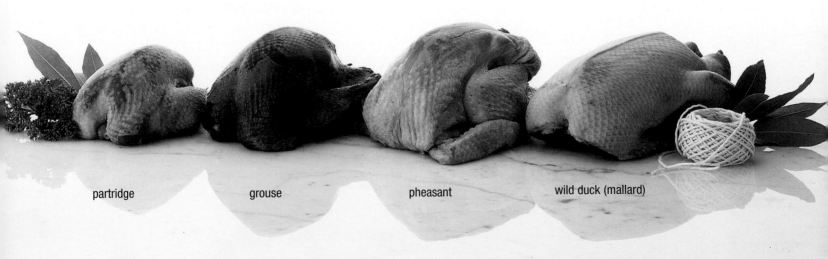

partridge   grouse   pheasant   wild duck (mallard)

Handle with care

Poultry and game birds must be handled carefully, stored properly and cooked thoroughly. Follow a few simple rules to safely enjoy these versatile birds.

Safe handling

Food poisoning comes from eating food contaminated with large numbers of bacteria or the toxins that some of them produce. Bacteria are naturally present in the air, water and soil and on our bodies. Because of modern intensive farming techniques, they are also widespread in meat, and particularly in poultry. The most common bacteria found in poultry are salmonella and campylobacter. Food poisoning can be caused by eating undercooked poultry or by eating lightly cooked food or raw food such as salad that has been in contact with raw poultry or its juices.

All poultry is extremely perishable, and bacteria multiply rapidly in warm conditions, so the first golden rule after buying your bird is to get it home and into the fridge as soon as possible. On a warm day, put the bird into an insulated container for the journey.

Storing in the fridge

If you are going to cook the bird within a few hours, you can put it into the fridge in its original wrapping. Otherwise, unwrap the bird (take any giblets out of the body cavity), put it on a plate and cover lightly with greaseproof paper or foil, or put it into a loosely covered container. Then put it into the fridge, ideally at the bottom – it is important that juices from poultry do not drip onto other food, particularly if that food will not be cooked before eating. Don't overcrowd the fridge – make sure there is room for cold air to circulate; the temperature inside should be no higher than 5°C (41°F).

In general, poultry must be cooked within 2 days of purchase – stick to the use-by date on the package, or ask your supplier for guidance.

Freezing and thawing

Poultry can be stored for up to 6 months in a freezer. Before cooking, a frozen bird must be thoroughly thawed – if it is still partially frozen, its centre will not reach a high enough temperature during cooking to destroy any food poisoning bacteria that might be present (salmonella survives freezing). Thawing should be done slowly – rapid thawing will spoil the texture of the meat, and warm conditions will encourage the growth of any bacteria.

The best way to thaw poultry is in the fridge: set the bird, still in its freezer wrapping, in a deep dish and put it in the fridge. Leave it until the wrapping is loose, then remove this and pour off any liquid that has collected in the dish. Cover the bird loosely with greaseproof paper and put it back in the fridge to continue thawing slowly. Remove any giblets as soon as they are loose, and thaw them in a separate, covered basin. Once the bird is completely thawed, it

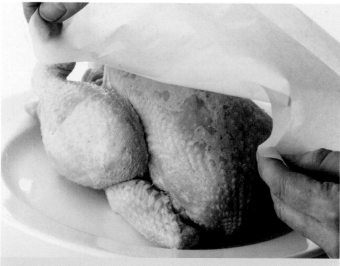
▲ Store poultry in the fridge, loosely covered so air can circulate

A guide to thawing times in the fridge

Frozen weight range	Thawing time
1.35–2.25 kg (3–5 lb)	20 hours
2.7–3.2 kg (6–7 lb)	30 hours
3.6–4 kg (8–9 lb)	36 hours
4.5–5 kg (10–11 lb)	45 hour
5.4–9 kg (12–20 lb)	60 hours

should be cooked very soon afterwards.

An alternative, slightly faster method of thawing is in cold water: immerse the bird in a large basin or sink of cold water (not warm), and change the water every 30 minutes or so as the bird thaws to keep it cold.

Keeping tools clean

Use a separate chopping board for raw poultry, meat and fish. This prevents bacteria that might be present in the raw food from transferring to cooked food or to other foods that are to be eaten raw. If you have to use the same board (or work surface), wash it well with hot soapy water or use an antibacterial spray between uses.

Before you start

Wash your hands thoroughly with hot soapy water both before and after handling raw poultry, and between handling raw and cooked poultry. (It is also essential to wash your hands after visiting the bathroom, after coughing, blowing your nose, or touching your face or hair, or after using cleaning products.)

A final rinse?

Current advice is that raw poultry should not be rinsed before cooking as this is thought to encourage the spread of any bacteria that might be present. If your bird seems too moist, wipe it over, inside and out, with kitchen paper.

Safe cooking

To be sure any food poisoning bacteria that might be present is killed, poultry such as chicken and turkey must be cooked thoroughly. It must never be cooked partially – if there is bacteria in the uncooked portions, it will flourish.

Stuffing

Although it was once common to stuff the body cavity of poultry – particularly turkey – before roasting, this is now not recommended, because the stuffing can prevent heat penetrating to the centre of the bird. Also, the stuffing itself can harbour bacteria, which will not be destroyed unless the stuffing reaches a safe temperature inside the bird. If you do want to stuff the cavity, fill it only two-thirds full, and weigh the bird again after stuffing to calculate cooking time. Then, after cooking, test the temperature of the stuffing with an instant-read thermometer; it should be at least 75°C (170°F). Alternatively, stuff the neck end only, or cook the stuffing separately. Do not stuff a bird more than 3 hours before cooking. If the stuffing is warm, cook the bird straightaway.

Trussing

Just tucking the wing tips under the bird's back and tying the ends of the legs loosely together is sufficient – a tight trussing may keep the bird in a neat compact shape, but it can also prevent the leg meat from cooking through as rapidly as the drier breast meat.

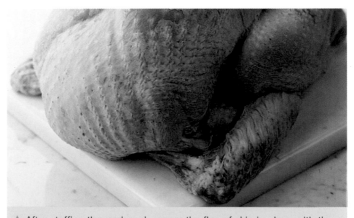

▲ After stuffing the neck end, secure the flap of skin in place with the wing tips rather than trussing the bird

Testing for doneness

The traditional way of testing poultry and game birds to see if they are cooked is to pierce the thickest part of the meat with a skewer or the point of a sharp knife, and then to note the colour of the juices that run out. An alternative method for a roasted bird is to lift it up with a two-pronged fork and tip it so that the juices run out of the cavity. For chicken, turkey and goose, the juices should be completely clear and not at all pink; however, for duck and many game birds served rare, the juices that run out will still be pink.

Another, more precise way to check if poultry is thoroughly cooked is to use an instant-read thermometer. At the end of the recommended cooking time, insert the thermometer probe into the thickest part of the meat. For chicken and turkey, the internal temperature of the dark thigh meat should be at least 75°C (170°F); the white meat of the breast should have reached 71°C (160°F).

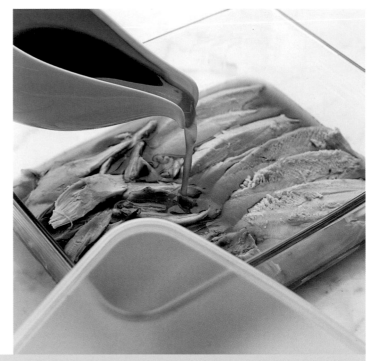

▲ To freeze cooked poultry, take the meat off the bone, then pack in a rigid container, with gravy to cover completely

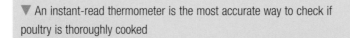

▼ An instant-read thermometer is the most accurate way to check if poultry is thoroughly cooked

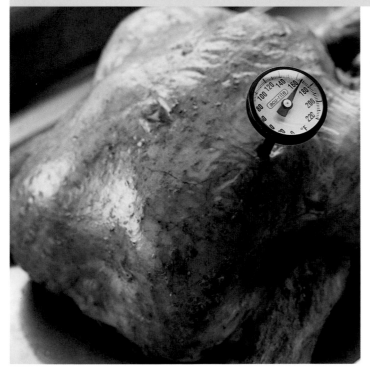

If not eating immediately

As soon as chicken and turkey are cooked, they should be served and not kept warm. For leftovers, cool them as quickly as possible (2 hours maximum at room temperature). When cold, remove any stuffing, wrap the bird in foil and store in the fridge. It can be kept for 3–5 days.

Reheat cooked poultry only once. To reheat in gravy or a sauce, bring to the boil and cook for 5 minutes. Or reheat in the microwave, stirring during cooking to avoid cold spots and to ensure that the food is piping hot throughout.

For longer storage, remove the meat from the bones, put it in a freezer bag and label, then freeze. The meat can also be frozen in gravy: pack the meat in a rigid container and pour over the gravy to immerse the meat completely, then cover, leaving 2.5 cm (1 in) headroom for expansion of the frozen gravy. Or freeze in a freezer bag inside a casserole or dish, and remove the bag when frozen. Cook from frozen, thawing gently and then reheating as above.

A world of flavours

Poultry and game birds are wonderfully versatile, being suitable for many preparations and complemented by an almost endless range of flavourings. Cooks in every country have favourite flavour partnerships – chicken with saffron in a Spanish paella, hotly spiced for an Indian curry or in a stew with peanuts in the West Indies; turkey with a chilli and chocolate mole sauce in Mexico or with cranberry sauce in the USA; roast goose with apples in Germany or prunes in Scandinavia, or stuffed with potatoes in Ireland; duck with star anise in China, with pomegranates and walnuts in the Middle East or with horseradish sauce in Sweden; juniper-scented quail wrapped in vine leaves in France; guinea fowl with ginger and chestnuts in Poland; and pheasant with spiced cabbage in Eastern Europe or with bread sauce in the UK.

Here are some popular flavourings for poultry and game birds. All go well with the mild meat of chicken and turkey and most will also complement stronger-flavoured birds.

Pungent flavourings such as onions, shallots, garlic, fresh root ginger and chives.

Delicate herbs such as tarragon, basil, parsley (both curly and flat-leaf), coriander and chervil.

Robust herbs such as thyme, rosemary, lemon grass, bay leaf, marjoram, oregano and sage.

Warm spices such as juniper berries, allspice berries, star anise, cumin (seeds and ground) and caraway seeds.

Hot spices such as chillies (fresh, dried and ground), peppercorns (black, white, green and pink) and mustard (seeds and ground).

Fruit and nuts such as citrus (oranges, lemons and limes), mangoes, cranberries, cashews and chestnuts.

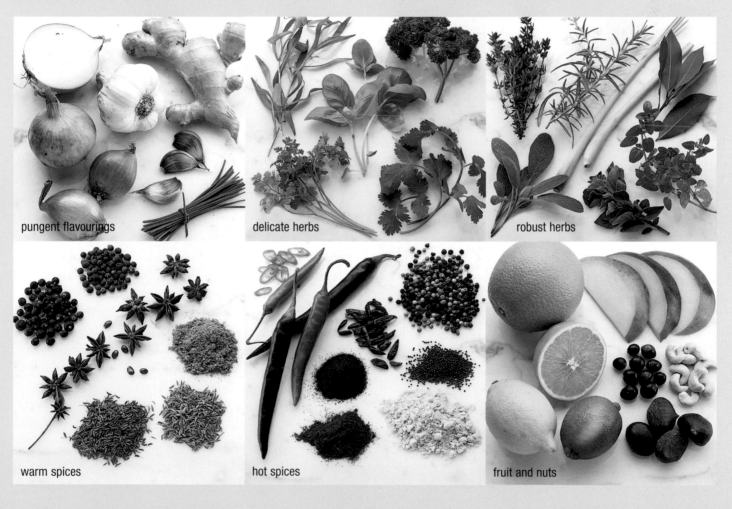

pungent flavourings

delicate herbs

robust herbs

warm spices

hot spices

fruit and nuts

Back to basics

Poultry and game birds are ideal for healthy, lower-fat cooking methods. Using the bones and giblets to make flavoursome stock means there is no waste, either.

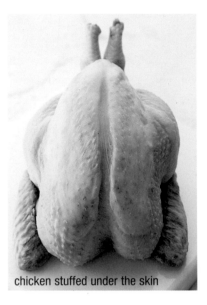

chicken stuffed under the skin

Taking off the fat

Because most of the fat in many birds is in the skin, removing this before or after cooking is a good way to reduce the total fat content of a dish. When roasting, grilling or barbecuing, you can leave the skin on to keep the juices in during cooking, and then remove it before serving. If removing the skin before roasting or grilling, a steep in a marinade will help to keep a bird moist, as will regular basting.

Marinades

A marinade is a seasoned liquid used to flavour and tenderise as well as to add moisture. Game birds, particularly older ones that tend to be a bit tough and dry, benefit from a steep in a marinade for several hours, or even longer. Poultry, on the other hand, is more likely to be marinated briefly in a thicker mixture, often based on oil, vinegar, lemon juice, yogurt, herbs and spices.

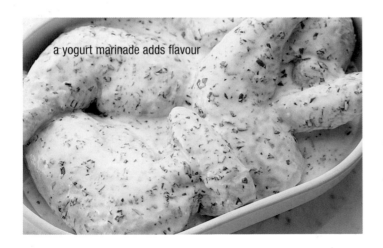

a yogurt marinade adds flavour

Tips for lower-fat cooking

● Softened butter is often spread over the breast meat of poultry, under the skin, to add moisture. Fromage frais can be used in the same way, simply seasoned or mixed with herbs, citrus zest or other flavourings.

● Game birds are traditionally barded – the breast is covered with pork fat or streaky bacon – to compensate for the natural leanness of the breast meat. Back bacon rashers, stretched very thin, or Parma ham are good lower-fat substitutes for streaky bacon, but barding isn't necessary for game birds that are now intensively reared.

● If you put chicken or other poultry on a trivet in the roasting tin, it will prevent the bird from sitting in its own fat during roasting. It also allows fat to be poured away easily, before the meat juices are used to make a gravy or sauce.

● Placing a bird upside-down for the first half of the roasting time helps to keep the breast meat moist, and there is no need to baste with extra fat.

● Basting can be done with lemon juice or a small amount of oil rather than butter or other saturated fats, or you can use the juices released by the bird during cooking.

● After skimming most of the surface fat from the roasting juices, pour them into a gravy strainer, also called a gravy separator, which is a jug with a spout rising from the bottom. This allows you to pour off the juices, leaving behind the fat that is floating on the top.

Fresh chicken stock

A home-made stock is a far cry from over-seasoned cubes and pastes, and cheaper than the chilled stocks many supermarkets sell these days. This version, made with the leftovers from a roast chicken, can be used as a base for soups, casseroles, sauces and gravies.

Makes about 1 litre (1¾ pints)

1 chicken carcass or the bones from 4 chicken pieces

1 onion, quartered

1 large carrot, cut into large chunks

1 celery stick, cut into large chunks

1 fresh or 2 dried bay leaves

8 black peppercorns

½ tsp salt

Preparation time: 10 minutes
Cooking time: 2 hours

1 Break up the chicken carcass or bones and put into a large pan. Add the vegetables, bay leaves, peppercorns and salt. Pour over 2 litres (3½ pints) of water.

2 Bring to the boil over a high heat, then turn the heat down so the liquid is simmering gently. Cover the pan and leave to bubble for 2 hours.

3 Strain the stock through a sieve into a bowl, discarding the bones and vegetables. Skim the fat from the surface with a spoon, if using the stock straightaway. Alternatively, chill the stock first, which will make it easier to remove the fat.

Some more ideas

● If you don't have a chicken carcass or bones to hand, use 450 g (1 lb) chicken wings, which are extremely economical. Heat 1 tbsp of sunflower oil in a large pan and brown the wings (this will give a richer flavour and colour to the stock). Add the rest of the ingredients and cook as above.

● You can make the stock from a raw chicken carcass or bones. When bringing to the boil, skim off all the scum that rises to the surface, then leave to simmer.

● For a stronger flavour, boil the strained stock rapidly, without a lid, to reduce the quantity.

● For a giblet stock, put the giblets (gizzard, heart and neck, but not the liver, which can give a bitter flavour) in a pan with 1 quartered unpeeled onion, 1 roughly chopped carrot and 1 chopped celery stick. Add a bouquet garni of 1 bay leaf, a few parsley stalks and a sprig of fresh thyme, tied together, and a few black peppercorns. Cover with cold water and bring to the boil, skimming off any scum. Then reduce the heat and simmer for 1 hour. Strain, cool quickly and refrigerate.

● Use the carcass of a turkey or other bird, rather than chicken.

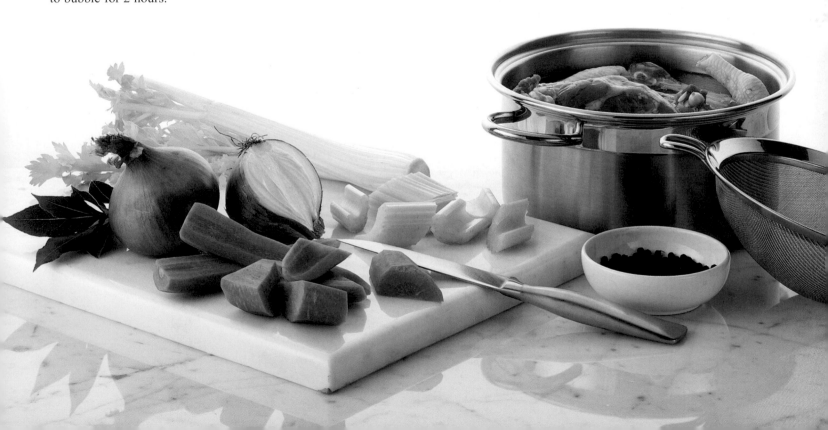

Stuffings for poultry

Packed with flavour and texture, these stuffings are also low in fat and high in fibre and carbohydrate. Stuffed into a bird, or baked alongside, they enable you to serve smaller portions of meat – with lots of vegetables – which means your meal will be in the right, healthy proportions. If you have a large bird, just increase the quantities for all these stuffings.

Apple, walnut and prune stuffing

Serves 6

100 g (3½ oz) pitted Agen prunes

3 tbsp port or fresh orange juice

1 small dessert apple, cored and finely chopped

2 shallots, finely chopped

30 g (1 oz) walnut pieces, coarsely chopped

75 g (2½ oz) fresh Granary breadcrumbs

1–2 tbsp fresh thyme leaves

1 egg, beaten

salt and pepper

Preparation time: 15 minutes

Cooking time: 20 or 40 minutes,
   depending upon method used

1 Snip the prunes into small chunks using scissors. Place in a small saucepan and add the port or orange juice. Set over a low heat and bring almost to the boil, by which time the prunes will have absorbed the liquid and become plump. Spoon into a mixing bowl.

2 Add the apple and shallots and stir. Add the walnuts, breadcrumbs, thyme, egg and seasoning, and mix.

3 Stuff into the neck end of a chicken or turkey, shaping any leftover stuffing into walnut-sized balls to cook separately. If you have made stuffing balls, arrange them on a lightly oiled baking tray and put into the oven for the last 20 minutes of the bird's cooking time.

4 Alternatively, put all of the stuffing into a lightly greased ovenproof dish, about 17.5 cm (7 in) in diameter, spreading it out evenly and packing it down. Bake in a preheated oven at 200°C (400°F, gas mark 6) for 40 minutes.

Another idea

• Instead of prunes, soak chopped ready-to-eat dried apricots in Armagnac and mix with almonds in place of walnuts, and 2 celery sticks, finely chopped, instead of apple. Season with 1 tsp ground cinnamon and ½ tsp freshly grated nutmeg.

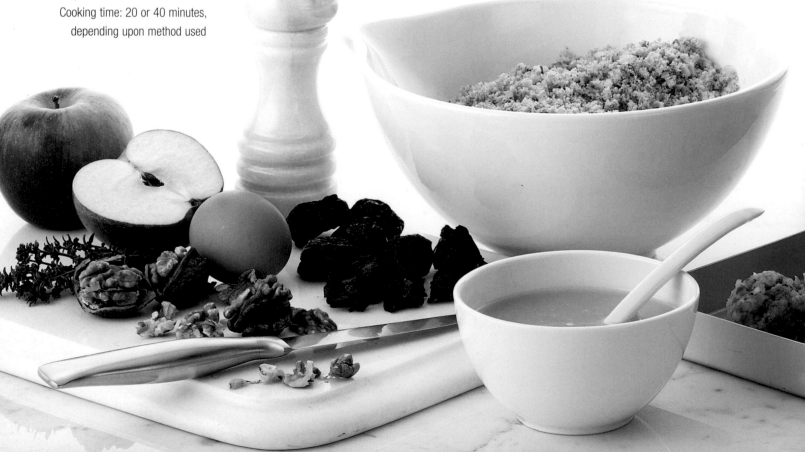

Sausage and chestnut stuffing

Serves 6

100 g (3½ oz) premium high-meat-content pork sausages

100 g (3½ oz) cooked or vacuum-packed chestnuts, finely chopped

2 shallots, finely chopped

75 g (2½ oz) fresh breadcrumbs

1½ tbsp chopped fresh sage

1 egg, beaten

salt and pepper

Preparation time: 10 minutes

Cooking time: 30 or 40 minutes, depending upon method used

1 Remove the sausage meat from the skins and put into a bowl. Add the chopped chestnuts and shallots and mix into the sausage meat. Add the breadcrumbs, sage, egg and some seasoning and mix thoroughly.

2 Stuff into the neck end of a chicken or turkey, shaping any leftover stuffing into walnut-sized balls to cook separately. If you have made stuffing balls, arrange them on a lightly oiled baking tray and put into the oven for the last 30 minutes of the bird's cooking time.

3 Alternatively, put all of the stuffing into a lightly greased ovenproof dish, about 17.5 cm (7 in) in diameter, spreading it out evenly and packing it down. Bake in a preheated oven at 200°C (400°F, gas mark 6) for 40 minutes.

Some more ideas

• Substitute canned unsweetened chestnut purée for the chopped chestnuts.

• Use wholemeal breadcrumbs to boost the fibre content.

• For a simple sage and onion stuffing, chop 3 medium-sized onions and cook in 30 g (1 oz) butter until soft and golden. Transfer to a bowl and add 170 g (6 oz) fresh breadcrumbs, 2 tbsp chopped fresh sage or 2 tsp crumbled dried sage, 1 beaten egg and seasoning to taste.

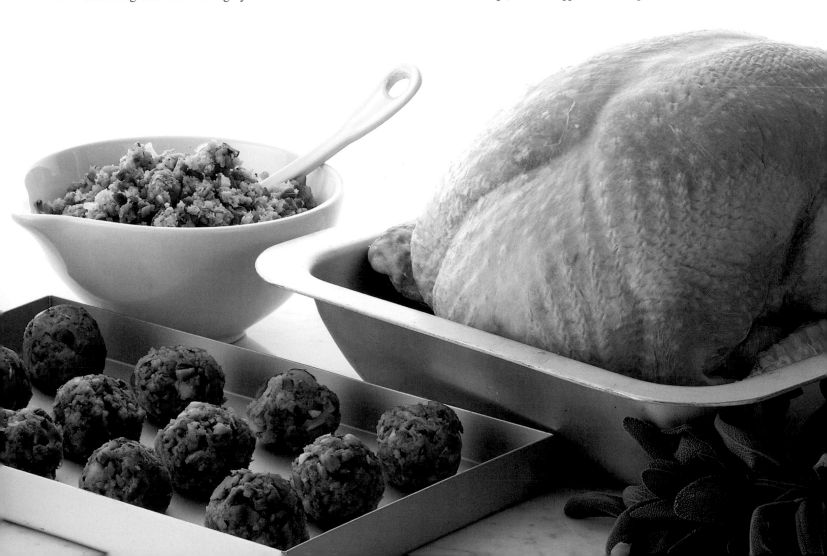

Braised duck with crunchy Oriental salad

Braising boneless duck breasts in red wine with garlic and ginger, plus a little redcurrant jelly for sweetness, produces moist, tender and flavoursome meat. The duck is cut into strips and served on a colourful mixture of crisp raw vegetables and fruit. Rice cakes would be an interesting Oriental-style accompaniment.

Serves 4

3 boneless duck breasts, about 525 g
    (1 lb 3 oz) in total
120 ml (4 fl oz) red wine
1 tbsp redcurrant jelly
1 tsp bottled chopped garlic in oil, drained
1 tsp bottled chopped root ginger in oil,
    drained
2 tbsp extra virgin olive oil
2 tsp balsamic or sherry vinegar
2 oranges
225 g (8 oz) red cabbage, finely shredded
¼ head of Chinese leaves, shredded
150 g (5½ oz) beansprouts
85 g (3 oz) watercress
1 can water chestnuts, about 220 g,
    drained and sliced
salt and pepper

Preparation and cooking time: 30 minutes

1 Preheat the oven to 220°C (425°F, gas mark 7). Remove all the skin and fat from the duck breasts. Place them in an ovenproof dish, pour over the wine and add the redcurrant jelly, garlic and ginger. Place the dish in the oven and cook the duck for 20–25 minutes or until tender.

2 Meanwhile, mix together the oil, vinegar and salt and pepper to taste in a large salad bowl. Cut the peel and pith from the oranges with a sharp knife and, holding each orange over the bowl to catch the juice, cut between the membrane to release the segments. Add them to the bowl. Add the red cabbage, Chinese leaves, beansprouts, watercress (reserving a few sprigs for garnishing) and water chestnuts. Toss well to coat everything with the dressing.

3 Remove the duck from the oven and transfer it to a warm plate. Pour the cooking liquid into a saucepan. Boil the liquid rapidly for 1–2 minutes to reduce slightly, while cutting the duck diagonally across the grain into neat slices. Pour the wine sauce over the salad and toss together. Pile the slices of duck on top, garnish with the reserved sprigs of watercress and serve.

Plus points
- All types of cabbage are rich in a range of vitamins, minerals and cancer-fighting phytochemicals.
- Duck is higher in fat than other poultry; however, removing the skin and all visible fat reduces the fat content considerably. The meat is rich in minerals, providing iron and zinc, as well as B vitamins.
- This salad contains a wide selection of different vegetables served raw, which preserves their vitamin value.
- Red wine is a rich source of flavonols, which are powerful antioxidants.

Each serving provides
kcal 334, protein 31 g, fat 12 g (of which saturated fat 3 g), carbohydrate 20 g

(of which sugars 16 g), fibre 4 g	
✓✓✓	B₆, B₁₂, C
✓✓	B₁, B₂, folate, niacin, copper, iron, potassium, zinc
✓	A, calcium

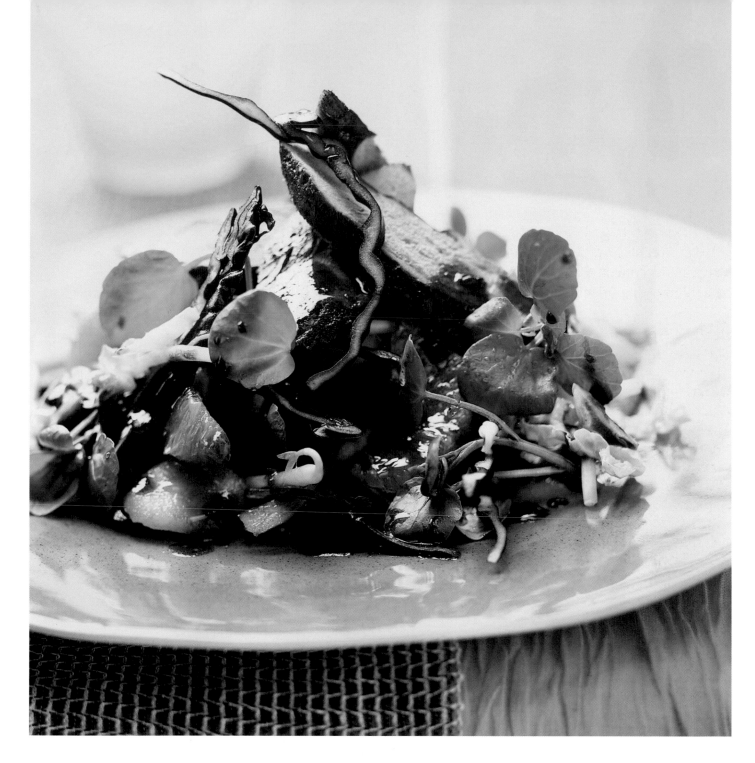

Some more ideas

• If fresh redcurrants are available, add a handful to the salad for extra vitamins and flavour.

• For a sesame roast pork salad, use 450 g (1 lb) pork fillet (tenderloin). Mix together 1 tbsp groundnut oil, 2 tbsp hoisin sauce and 1 tsp five-spice powder, and spoon the mixture over the pork. Sprinkle with 1 tsp sesame seeds. Roast in a preheated 180ºC (350ºF, gas mark 4) oven for 20–25 minutes. Make the salad using 1 cos lettuce, shredded, 1 orange pepper, seeded and chopped, 125 g (4½ oz) sliced mushrooms, 125 g (4½ oz) mange-tout, and the sliced water chestnuts. Toss the salad with 1 tbsp each olive oil and toasted sesame oil. Serve with the sliced pork on top.

• Other vegetables that could be added to the salad are lightly cooked baby corn, sliced raw courgettes or steamed asparagus spears.

• Sprinkle the salad with toasted cashew nuts.

Mango chicken salad

Here is a very special salad – new potatoes, slices of tender grilled chicken and asparagus tossed in a mellow fresh orange dressing while still warm and then gently mixed with juicy mango slices and baby salad leaves. It makes a delicious and well-balanced meal all on its own.

Serves 4

1 garlic clove, crushed
1 tsp grated fresh root ginger
1 tbsp light soy sauce
2 tsp sunflower oil
2 skinless boneless chicken breasts (fillets), about 170 g (6 oz) each
800 g (1¾ lb) new potatoes, scrubbed
2 large sprigs of fresh mint
125 g (4½ oz) asparagus spears
1 ripe mango, peeled and sliced
150 g (5½ oz) mixed baby salad leaves, such as spinach, red chard, and cos and Lollo Rosso lettuces

Fresh orange dressing

½ tsp finely grated orange zest
1 tbsp orange juice
1 tsp Dijon mustard
2 tbsp sunflower oil
1 tbsp walnut oil
salt and pepper

Preparation and cooking time: 50 minutes, plus 15 minutes marinating

Each serving provides

kcal 361, protein 24 g, fat 13 g (of which saturated fat 2 g), carbohydrate 40 g (of which sugars 9 g), fibre 4 g

✓✓✓	B₁, B₆, C, E, folate, niacin
✓✓	A, potassium, zinc
✓	B₂, iron

1 Put the garlic, ginger, soy sauce and sunflower oil in a bowl and whisk together. Add the chicken breasts and turn to coat both sides, then leave to marinate for 15 minutes.

2 Put the potatoes in a saucepan, pour over boiling water to cover and add the mint sprigs. Cook for 15–20 minutes or until tender. At the same time, put the asparagus in a steamer basket or metal colander, cover and set over the pan of potatoes to steam. Cook thin spears for 4–5 minutes, thick spears 8–10 minutes, or until just tender. Drain the potatoes (discard the mint) and leave until cool enough to handle, then cut into thick slices. Cut the asparagus diagonally into 6 cm (2½ in) lengths.

3 Preheat the grill to moderate. Remove the chicken from the marinade and place it on the grill rack. Grill for about 15 minutes, brushing frequently with the marinade and turning once, until cooked through and the juices run clear when the chicken is pierced with the tip of a knife. Leave to rest for 3–4 minutes, then slice.

4 To make the dressing, put the orange zest and juice, mustard and sunflower and walnut oils in a large serving bowl, and whisk together until slightly thickened. Season with salt and pepper to taste.

5 Transfer the warm sliced chicken, potatoes and asparagus to the serving bowl and gently toss together to coat with the dressing. Add the mango and salad leaves and toss gently again. Serve immediately, while still warm.

Plus points

• Mango is an excellent source of vitamin C and beta-carotene, both antioxidants that help to protect against damage by free radicals. Due to the beta-carotene content, mango is also one of the best fruit sources of vitamin A, providing more than 50% of the daily needs in half a large fruit.

• Chicken is an excellent source of protein, and by removing the skin, the fat content is kept low. It also contains B vitamins.

• Although potatoes contain much less vitamin C than fruit and other vegetables, they are an important source of this vitamin in the diet because they are eaten in such large quantities.

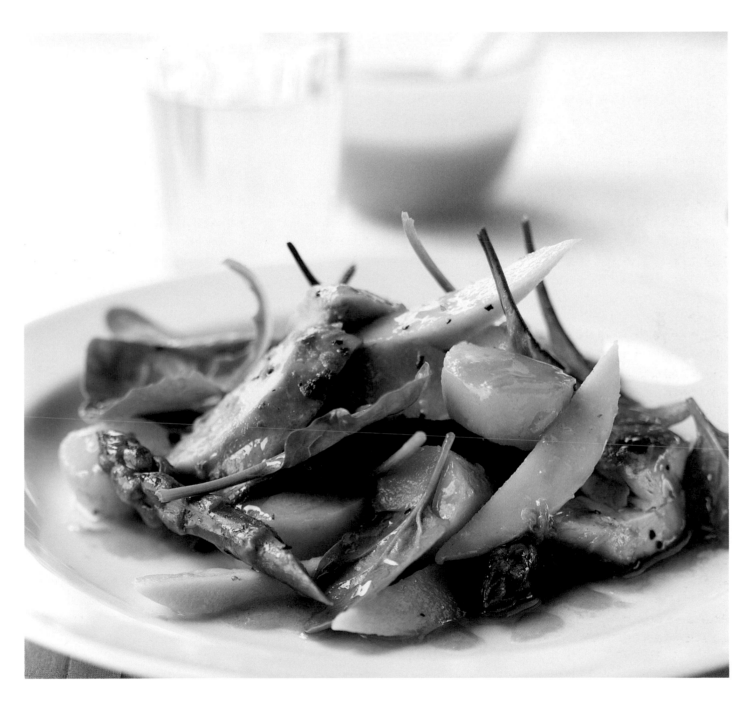

Some more ideas

- To save time, buy cooked or smoked chicken breasts. Remove the skin and slice.
- For a sharper citrus dressing, use lime zest and juice instead of orange.
- Make a turkey salad with fresh blueberries. Use turkey breast fillets, and marinate and grill as for the chicken in the main recipe. Cut 900 g (2 lb) new potatoes into 2 cm (¾ in) dice and cook in boiling salted water for 10 minutes or until just tender. Drain well and toss with the warm turkey slices in the fresh orange dressing. Put 150 g (5½ oz) blueberries in a small pan with 1 tbsp balsamic vinegar and 2 tsp clear honey. Gently bubble for 3–4 minutes or until the blueberries are tender. Add the salad leaves to the turkey and potato mixture and gently toss together, then drizzle over the warm blueberries.

Chicken and vegetable filo rolls

These filo pastry rolls make an excellent starter, or you could serve two rolls each for a light meal. The filling is a colourful mixture of low-fat minced chicken and plenty of vegetables, with a little smoked ham and fresh herbs to add to the flavour. The rolls are served with a piquant cranberry relish.

Serves 8 (makes 8)

1 large carrot, about 100 g (3½ oz), cut into
 very fine matchsticks

75 g (2½ oz) savoy cabbage, finely shredded

2 spring onions, cut into fine shreds

225 g (8 oz) minced chicken

55 g (2 oz) lean smoked ham, finely chopped

½ small onion, finely chopped

2 tbsp fresh white breadcrumbs

2 tsp chopped fresh sage

2 tsp chopped fresh thyme

4 large sheets filo pastry, each about
 46 x 28 cm (18 x 11 in)

2 tbsp extra virgin olive oil

15 g (½ oz) butter, melted

1 tsp sesame seeds

salt and pepper

Cranberry relish

3 tbsp cranberry sauce

1 tbsp extra virgin olive oil

1 tbsp red wine vinegar

1 tsp made English mustard

To serve

115 g (4 oz) mixed salad leaves

Preparation time: 40 minutes
Cooking time: 30 minutes

1 Blanch the carrot, cabbage and spring onions in boiling water for 1 minute. Drain, then plunge into a bowl of cold water to refresh. Drain again and pat dry with kitchen paper. Put the vegetables in a large mixing bowl with the chicken, ham, onion, breadcrumbs, herbs and seasoning. Mix together well, then set aside.

2 Preheat the oven to 190°C (375°F, gas mark 5). Halve each filo pastry sheet lengthways and then trim to a strip measuring 36 x 12 cm (15 x 5 in). Mix the oil and butter together.

3 Brush one pastry strip lightly with the butter mixture. Place an eighth of the filling at one end, shaping it into a sausage. Roll up the filling inside the pastry, folding in the long sides as you go, to make a spring roll-shaped parcel. Place on a baking sheet and brush with a little of the butter and oil mixture. Repeat to make another 7 parcels.

4 Score 3 diagonal slashes on top of each parcel. Sprinkle over the sesame seeds. Bake for 30 minutes or until the pastry is golden.

5 Meanwhile, put all the relish ingredients in a screw-top jar, season to taste and shake well.

6 Arrange the mixed salad leaves on serving plates, place a filo roll on each and drizzle around the relish.

Plus points

● Unlike most other types of pastry, filo contains very little fat – in 100 g (3½ oz) filo there are 2 g fat and 300 kcal. The same weight of shortcrust pastry contains 29 g fat and 449 kcal.

● Using a mixture of oil and butter to brush the sheets of filo reduces the amount of saturated fat, and brushing it on sparingly keeps the overall fat content down.

● By bulking out the poultry with plenty of vegetables you reduce the amount of fat in the dish as well as providing extra vitamins and dietary fibre.

Each roll provides
kcal 130, protein 8.5 g, fat 7.5 g (of which saturated fat 2 g), carbohydrate 7 g (of which sugars 4 g), fibre 1 g

✓ A, B$_6$

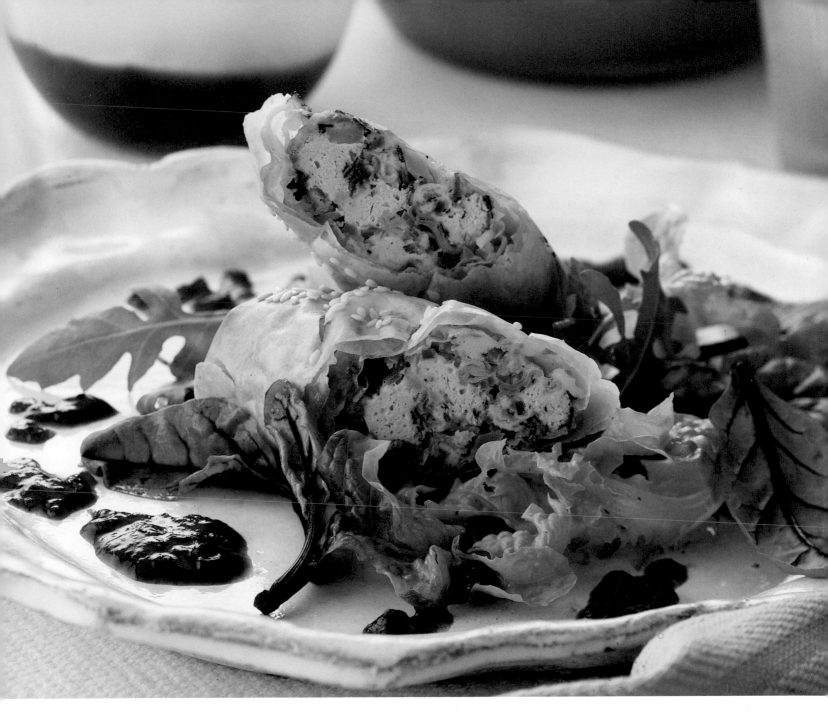

Some more ideas

- Use minced turkey instead of chicken.
- For Greek-style chicken parcels, cook 30 g (1 oz) long-grain rice in boiling water for 12 minutes or until just tender; drain and rinse with cold water. Meanwhile, soften 1 finely chopped onion in 1 tsp extra virgin olive oil for 5 minutes, then set aside to cool. Put the rice and onion in a bowl with 225 g (8 oz) minced chicken or turkey, 2 tbsp toasted pine nuts, 2 tbsp raisins, 2 tbsp chopped fresh mint and 2 tbsp chopped fresh dill. Season to taste. Mix together well and divide into 8 equal portions. Cut the sheets of filo pastry into 8 strips as before. Brush each pastry strip lightly with the olive oil and butter mixture, and put one portion of the filling at one end. Fold the pastry over the filling into a triangle. Continue folding down the pastry strip to make a triangular-shaped parcel. Brush all the parcels with the butter and oil mixture, and scatter over 1 tsp poppy seeds. Bake for 30 minutes. Serve the filo triangles on a tomato and onion salad: thickly slice 3 beef tomatoes and scatter over 1 sliced red onion, 15 small black olives and 1 tbsp chopped fresh dill. Season with salt and pepper and drizzle over 1 tbsp extra virgin olive oil.

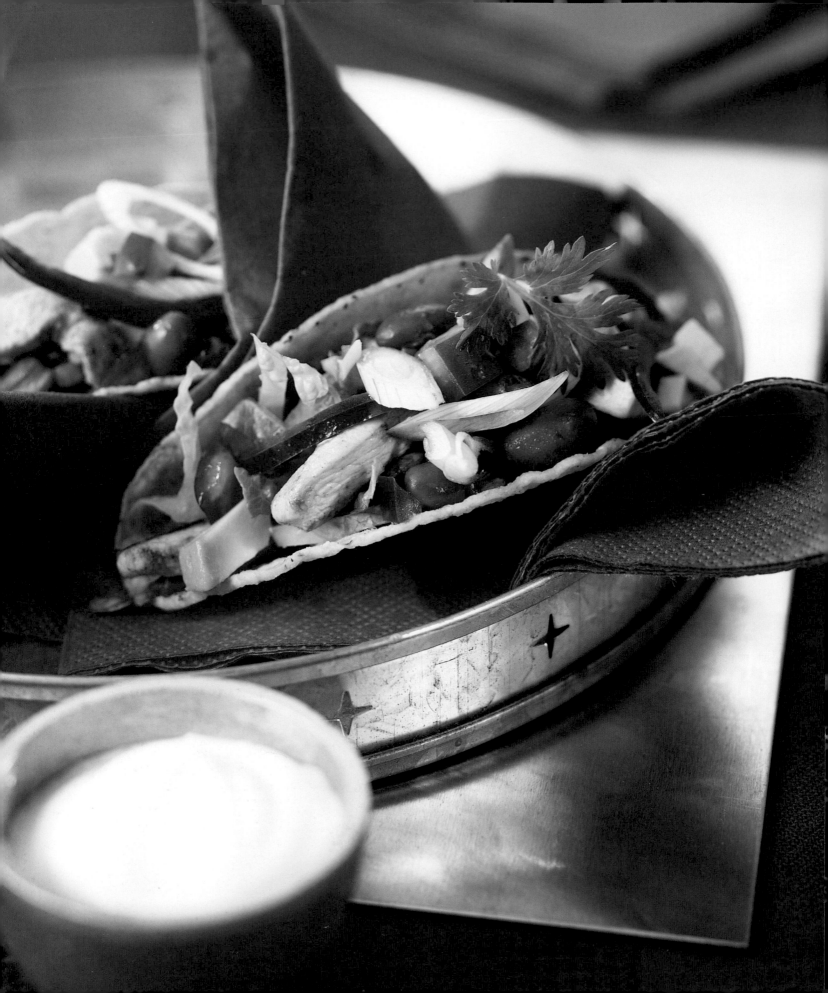

Chicken and pinto bean tacos

Here, tender chicken in a spicy mixture is quickly cooked to make a succulent filling for crisp taco shells. Sliced peppers and pinto or borlotti beans add to the mix, as does a scattering of shredded lettuce, spring onions and avocado. A dash of Tabasco sauce or other bottled hot sauce gives a piquant kick.

Serves 4

350 g (12½ oz) skinless boneless chicken
   breasts (fillets), cut into strips
3 garlic cloves, chopped
juice of 1 lime
¾–1 tsp Mexican seasoning mix
1 tbsp extra virgin olive oil
2 red, green or yellow peppers, seeded and
   thinly sliced
1 can pinto or borlotti beans, about 400 g,
   drained and rinsed
8 taco shells (crisp corn tortilla shells)
1 avocado
85 g (3 oz) crisp lettuce leaves, torn or
   shredded
3 spring onions, thinly sliced
3 tbsp fresh coriander leaves
1 tomato, diced or sliced
Tabasco or other hot sauce to taste
4 tbsp fromage frais
salt and pepper

Preparation and cooking time: 25 minutes

Each serving provides

kcal 490, protein 32 g, fat 21 g (of which
saturated fat 3 g), carbohydrate 45 g
(of which sugars 4 g), fibre 3 g

✓✓✓	C, B$_6$
✓✓	B$_1$, E, folate, niacin, copper, iron, zinc
✓	A, B$_2$, selenium

1 Preheat the oven to 180°C (350°F, gas mark 4). Put the chicken, garlic, lime juice and Mexican seasoning mix in a bowl and season to taste with salt and pepper. Mix well.

2 Heat the oil in a heavy non-stick frying pan or wok. Add the chicken mixture and cook for 1 minute without stirring. Add the peppers and stir-fry over a high heat for 3–5 minutes or until the chicken is lightly browned. Add the beans and heat them through, stirring occasionally.

3 Meanwhile, arrange the taco shells, open end down, on a baking tray and warm in the oven for 2–3 minutes. Peel and dice the avocado.

4 Spoon the chicken and pepper mixture into the taco shells, dividing it equally among them. Add the avocado, lettuce, spring onions, tomato, coriander and Tabasco or other hot sauce to taste. Serve at once, with the fromage frais to be spooned on top of the tacos.

Some more ideas

● Use 1 red or green pepper and replace the other pepper with 150 g (5½ oz) baby corn or sweetcorn kernels (frozen or canned). Add to the pan with the chicken mixture.
● For lamb and hummus wraps, trim any fat from 250 g (8½ oz) lean boneless lamb, such

as leg, and slice thinly. Heat 1 tbsp extra virgin olive oil in a frying pan, add the lamb with 1 red pepper, seeded and cut into thin strips, 3 chopped garlic cloves, the juice of 1 lemon, ½ tsp ground cumin, and salt and pepper to taste, and fry for 7–10 minutes. Meanwhile, heat 4 large plain or tomato-flavoured flour tortillas in the oven or microwave, according to the packet instructions. Spread each tortilla with about 45 g (1½ oz) hummus, top with a portion of the lamb mixture and add some sliced or diced cucumber, sliced or diced tomatoes and chopped fresh mint and coriander. Sprinkle with 2–3 chopped spring onions and a little Tabasco or other hot sauce, if desired, then roll up. Serve hot.

Plus points

● Avocados are a rich source of mono-unsaturated fat and vitamin B$_6$ – one small avocado provides over half the daily requirement for B$_6$. They also contribute useful amounts of vitamin E and several important phytochemicals.
● Herbs, spices and mixtures such as the Mexican seasoning used in this recipe are a good way of adding flavour to food rather than using lots of salt.

Chicken jamboree

This healthy chicken and vegetable casserole makes an easy mid-week meal. To make it even quicker, you could use supermarket washed-and-cut carrots and broccoli, ready to go from packet to pan. Mixed wild and long-grain rice goes well with the casserole, and adds sustaining and nourishing carbohydrate.

Serves 4

2 tbsp extra virgin olive oil

350 g (12½ oz) skinless boneless chicken
   breasts (fillets), cut into small cubes

1 small onion, chopped

225 g (8 oz) button mushrooms

1 bay leaf

2 large sprigs of fresh thyme or ½ tsp
   dried thyme

3 large sprigs of fresh tarragon or ½ tsp
   dried tarragon (optional)

grated zest of 1 small lemon or
   ½ large lemon

150 ml (5 fl oz) dry sherry

300 ml (10 fl oz) boiling water

225 g (8 oz) baby carrots

225 g (8 oz) broccoli florets

1 tbsp cornflour

3 tbsp chopped parsley

salt and pepper

Preparation time: 10 minutes
Cooking time: about 20 minutes

Each serving provides

kcal 260, protein 23 g, fat 10 g (of which
saturated fat 2 g), carbohydrate 11 g
(of which sugars 6 g), fibre 4 g

✓✓	B₆, C
✓	folate, niacin, selenium

1 Heat the oil in a large sauté pan with a lid or fairly deep frying pan. Add the chicken and brown the pieces over a high heat for 3 minutes, stirring constantly. Reduce the heat to moderate. Stir in the onion, mushrooms, bay leaf, thyme, tarragon if used and lemon zest. Cook for 4 minutes or until the onion and mushrooms are beginning to soften.

2 Pour in the sherry and water. Add the carrots and seasoning to taste, and stir to mix all the ingredients. Bring to the boil, then reduce the heat and cover the pan. Simmer for 5 minutes.

3 Stir in the broccoli florets. Increase the heat to bring the liquid back to a steady simmer. Cover the pan and cook for 5 minutes or until the pieces of chicken are tender and the vegetables are just cooked. Remove and discard the bay leaf, and the sprigs of thyme and tarragon, if used.

4 Blend the cornflour to a smooth paste with 2 tbsp cold water. Stir the cornflour paste into the casserole and simmer for 2 minutes, stirring constantly, until thickened and smooth. Check the seasoning, then stir in the parsley and serve.

Plus points

• Broccoli and related cruciferous vegetables (such as cabbage and cauliflower) contain several potent phytochemicals that help to protect against cancer. Broccoli is also an excellent source of the antioxidants vitamins C and E and beta-carotene. It provides good amounts of the B vitamins B₆ and niacin, and useful amounts of folate.

• This recipe uses vegetables to extend a modest amount of chicken. Served with a starchy (complex) carbohydrate, such as rice, it makes a well-balanced meal, especially if followed by fresh fruit for a vitamin boost.

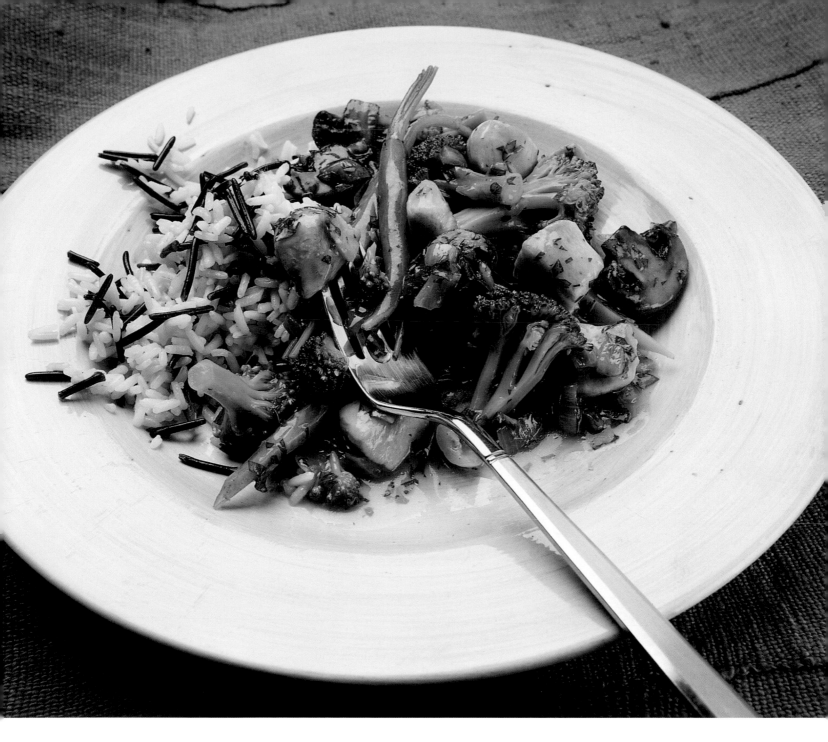

Some more ideas

● Semolina or fine oatmeal can be used to thicken the casserole instead of cornflour. Use 1 tbsp of either ingredient. Blend the oatmeal to a smooth paste with cold water and add as for the cornflour; sprinkle the semolina into the casserole, stirring, and continue stirring until the sauce boils and thickens.

● Small patty pan squash are good in this casserole. Trim off and discard the stalk ends from 225 g (8 oz) squash and slice them horizontally in half. Add them to the pan with the broccoli. When cooked, the patty pan should be tender but still slightly crunchy.

● For a creamy chicken and mushroom casserole, increase the quantity of button

mushrooms to 340 g (12 oz) and leave out the broccoli. Simmer for 5 minutes longer in step 2. Stir in 4 tbsp single cream after thickening the casserole with the cornflour, then heat for a few more seconds.

● Ready-prepared stir-fry strips of turkey, pork or chicken are ideal for this casserole. They reduce preparation time and cook quickly.

Turkey kebabs with fennel and red pepper relish

Here lean little bites of turkey are marinated with wine and herbs to add juiciness and flavour, and then threaded onto skewers to be grilled or barbecued. A colourful raw-vegetable relish provides a nice splash of vitamin C as well as a delightful taste contrast. Serve with a complex carbohydrate such as couscous.

Serves 4

450 g (1 lb) skinless turkey breast steak

3 garlic cloves, chopped

1½ tbsp lemon juice

2 tbsp dry white wine

1 tbsp chopped fresh sage or 2 tsp
    dried sage, crumbled

1 tbsp chopped fresh rosemary

1½ tsp fresh thyme leaves or ½ tsp
    dried thyme

1 tsp fennel seeds, lightly crushed

2½ tbsp extra virgin olive oil

1 red pepper, seeded and finely diced

1 bulb of fennel, finely diced

1 tbsp black olive paste (tapenade) or
    10 black Kalamata olives, finely diced

8 stalks of fresh rosemary (optional)

8 shallots or button onions

salt and pepper

Preparation time: 20 minutes, plus at least
    10 minutes marinating
Cooking time: 15 minutes

1 Cut the turkey into 24 pieces, each about 5 x 2 cm (2 x ¾ in). Combine the turkey pieces with 2 of the chopped garlic cloves, 1 tbsp lemon juice, the wine, sage, rosemary, thyme, fennel seeds, 2 tbsp of the olive oil and seasoning. Toss so that all the turkey pieces are covered with the herb mixture. Leave to marinate for at least 10 minutes, or up to 1 hour if you have the time.

2 Meanwhile, make the relish. Put the red pepper, diced fennel and olive paste or diced olives in a bowl together with the remaining garlic, ½ tbsp lemon juice and ½ tbsp olive oil. Season to taste. Mix well, then set aside.

3 Preheat the grill to high, or prepare a charcoal fire in the barbecue. Thread the marinated turkey pieces onto the rosemary stalks if using, or onto skewers, and top each one with a shallot or button onion.

4 Grill or barbecue the kebabs for about 15 minutes or until cooked through and the turkey pieces are lightly browned in spots. Turn the kebabs and baste with the remaining marinade frequently. Serve the kebabs hot, with the red pepper relish.

Plus points

- Red peppers are an excellent source of vitamin C and they are rich in beta-carotene. Both of these nutrients are powerful antioxidants that can help to counteract the damaging effects of free radicals and protect against many diseases including cancer and heart disease.
- Fennel provides useful amounts of potassium and the B vitamin folate. Another of fennel's advantages is that it is low in calories – 100 g (3½ oz) contains 12 kcal.

Each serving provides

kcal 224, protein 28 g, fat 9.5 g (of which saturated fat 1.5 g), carbohydrate 7 g (of which sugars 6 g), fibre 2.5 g

✓✓✓	B_6, B_{12}, C
✓✓	A, niacin
✓	E, folate, copper, iron, potassium, zinc

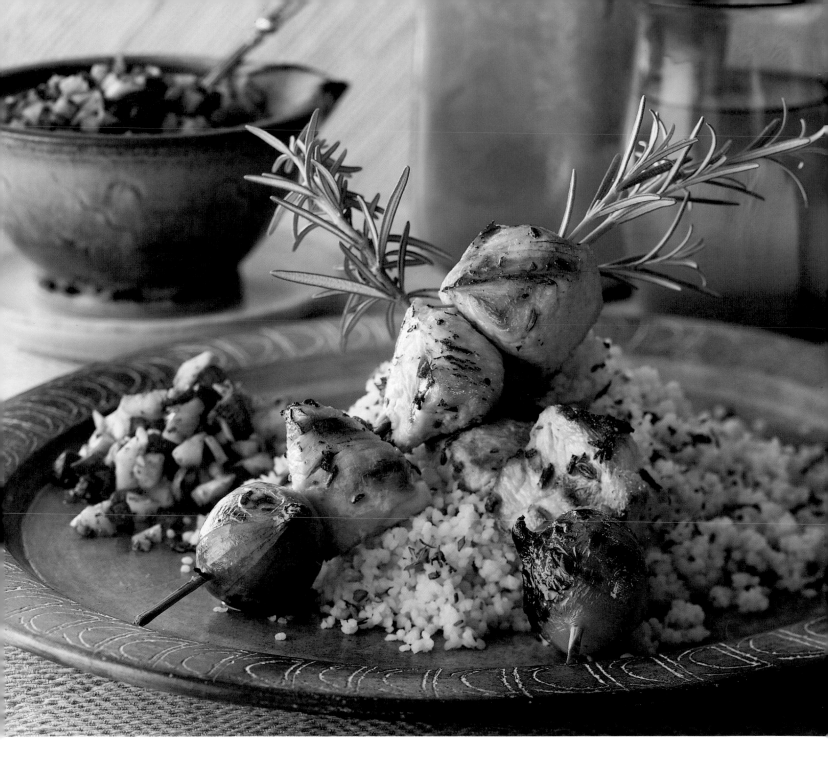

Some more ideas

• Instead of making a vegetable relish, add the red pepper and fennel to the kebabs. Cut the pepper and fennel into 2.5 cm (1 in) chunks. Alternate the vegetable chunks with pieces of turkey on the skewers, and brush all over with the turkey marinade. Grill or barbecue as above, then serve the turkey and vegetable kebabs drizzled with the remaining extra virgin olive oil and lemon juice.

• Another delicious relish, containing no oil, can be made with roasted red pepper and tomatoes. Cut a large red pepper in half and grill the skin side until it is blistered and charred. Put into a polythene bag and leave until cool enough to handle, then peel off the skin. Finely dice the flesh and mix with 1 diced tomato, 1 finely chopped shallot, 2 chopped garlic cloves, 2 tbsp chopped fresh basil or parsley, a splash of balsamic vinegar, and salt and pepper to taste.

Stuffed turkey rolls with lentils

Tender turkey rolls filled with an apricot stuffing are delicious served on a bed of orange-scented Puy lentils, chestnuts and vegetables. The only accompaniment needed is a crisp leafy salad.

Serves 4

4 skinless turkey breast steaks, about
  500 g (1 lb 2 oz) in total

1 tbsp extra virgin olive oil

1 onion, finely chopped

1 parsnip, cut into 1 cm (½ in) cubes

2 carrots, cut into 1 cm (½ in) cubes

1 tbsp plain flour

600 ml (1 pint) chicken stock, preferably
  home-made (see page 113)

2 tsp Dijon mustard

1 can whole peeled chestnuts, about
  240 g, drained

200 g (7 oz) Puy lentils

2 tsp balsamic vinegar

salt and pepper

sprigs of fresh flat-leaf parsley to garnish

Apricot stuffing

1 onion, finely chopped

75 g (2½ oz) ready-to-eat dried apricots,
  finely chopped

2 garlic cloves, crushed

75 g (2½ oz) fresh breadcrumbs

3 tbsp chopped parsley

1 egg yolk

grated zest and juice of 1 orange

Preparation time: 40 minutes

Cooking time: 1¼ hours

1 Preheat the oven to 180°C (350°F, gas mark 4). One at a time, lay the turkey steaks between 2 pieces of cling film and bat out with a rolling pin into a rectangle measuring about 15 x 12 cm (6 x 5 in).

2 For the stuffing, put the onion, apricots, garlic, breadcrumbs, parsley, egg yolk, a third of the orange zest and 1 tbsp of the orange juice in a bowl (set the remaining orange zest and juice aside to add to the lentils later). Season the stuffing ingredients to taste and mix well together. Divide this stuffing among the turkey slices and use a fork to spread it over them, pressing it down evenly. Roll up each slice from a narrow edge and secure with wooden cocktail sticks in 2–3 places to keep the roll in shape during cooking.

3 Heat the oil in a flameproof casserole. Add the turkey rolls and fry over a moderate heat for 5 minutes, turning occasionally to brown them evenly. Use a draining spoon to transfer the rolls from the casserole to a plate.

4 Add the onion to the casserole and cook for about 5 minutes or until it is softened. Stir in the parsnip and carrots, then sprinkle in the flour and stir until it is evenly distributed. Pour in the stock and stir in the mustard. Add the chestnuts, and bring to the boil, stirring. Replace the turkey rolls in the casserole, cover and transfer to the oven to cook for 1¼ hours or until the turkey is tender.

5 About 30 minutes before the turkey rolls finish cooking, place the lentils in a large saucepan with plenty of cold water to cover. Bring to the boil and cook for about 20 minutes or until the lentils are tender. Drain the lentils and return them to the pan. Add the reserved orange zest and juice, and the vinegar.

6 Use a draining spoon to transfer the turkey rolls to a board and the vegetables to the pan of lentils. Lightly mix the vegetables into the lentils. Remove the cocktail sticks from the turkey rolls and slice them neatly.

7 Spoon the lentil mixture and some of the cooking liquid onto warm plates. Arrange the turkey slices on top. Garnish with parsley and serve.

Plus points

- Puy lentils are a good source of soluble fibre and a useful source of iron. Vitamin C in the orange juice helps the body to absorb the iron.
- Parsnips provide potassium and some of the B vitamins, including B_1 and folate.

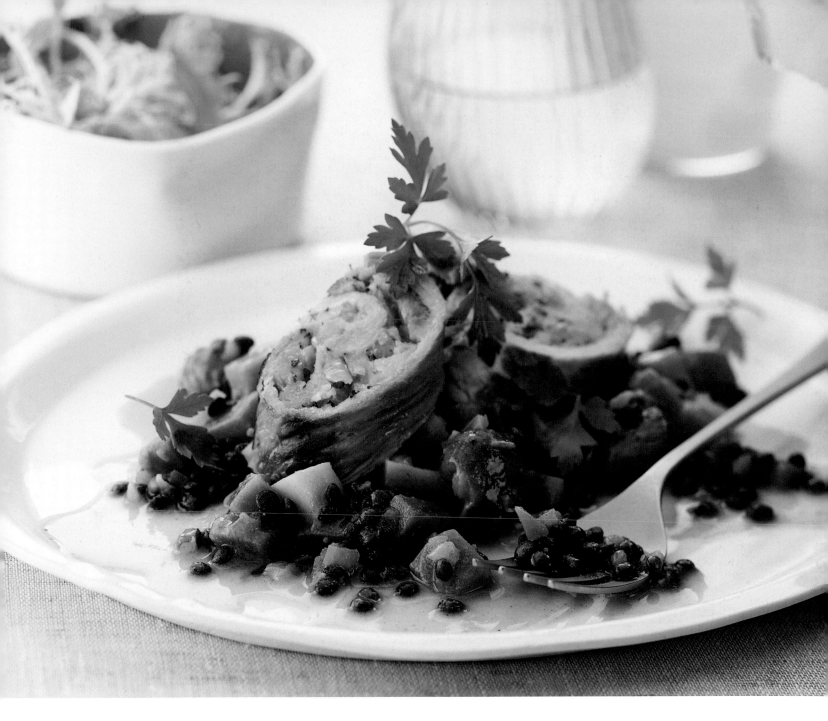

Some more ideas

● Try ready-to-eat pitted prunes instead of apricots and use quartered baby turnips instead of parsnips. Reduce the stock to 450 ml (15 fl oz) and add 150 ml (5 fl oz) red wine. Omit the lentils and serve the turkey rolls and vegetables with mashed potato.

● For an Italian-style stuffing, use chopped sun-dried tomatoes instead of apricots, and 3 tbsp chopped fresh basil or 1 tsp pesto instead of parsley. Use a whole egg, beaten, rather than an egg yolk. After stuffing and shaping the turkey rolls, wrap 1 slice of pancetta or Parma ham around each before browning as in the main recipe. Omit the parsnips and carrots and instead add 1 seeded and finely chopped red pepper and 3 chopped celery sticks.

Each serving provides

kcal 600, protein 47 g, fat 11 g (of which saturated fat 2 g), carbohydrate 83 g (of which sugars 21 g), fibre 12 g

✓✓✓	B_6, B_{12}, copper, iron, phosphorus
✓✓	A, B_1, C, folate, niacin, potassium, zinc
✓	B_2, calcium

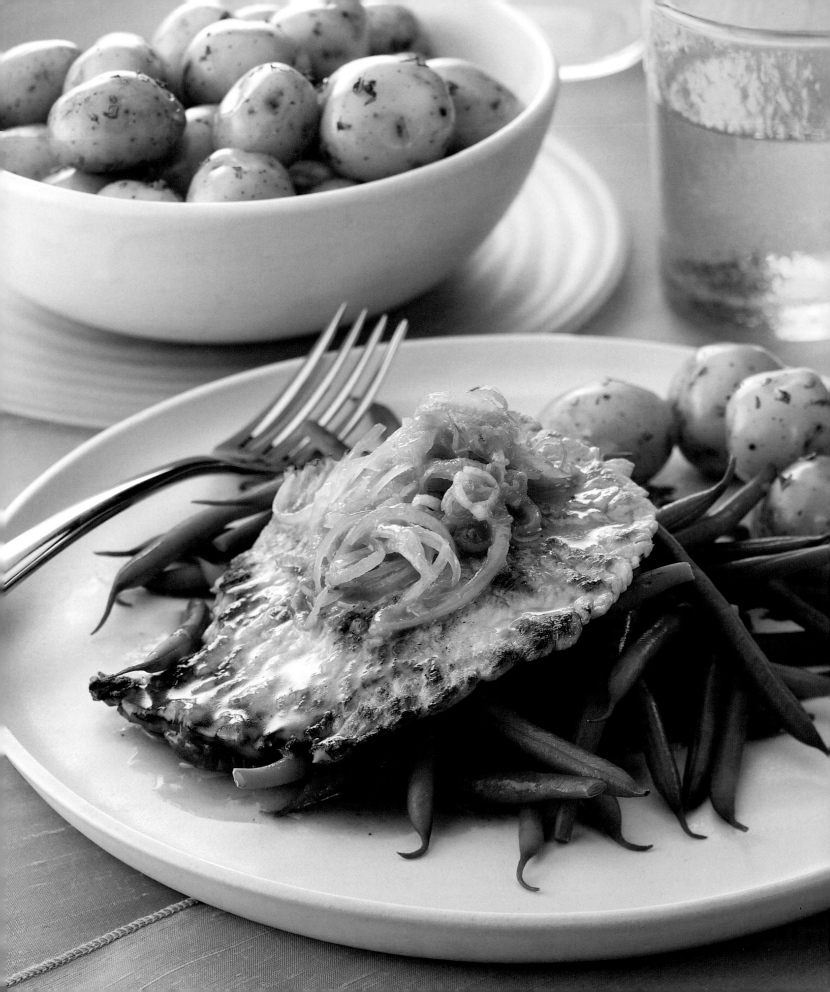

Pan-fried turkey escalopes with citrus honey sauce

The tanginess of citrus fruit marries extremely well with poultry, especially turkey which can sometimes be a little light on flavour. Here, orange and lemon, together with honey and shallots, create a tasty sauce for turkey escalopes, served on a stack of green beans. For a simple accompaniment, steam some new potatoes.

Serves 4

4 small skinless turkey breast steaks, about 115 g (4 oz) each

30 g (1 oz) butter

4 large shallots, thinly sliced

1 garlic clove, crushed

400 g (14 oz) fine French beans, trimmed

2 tbsp clear honey

grated zest and juice of 1 orange

grated zest and juice of 1 lemon

salt and pepper

Preparation time: 15 minutes
Cooking time: about 15 minutes

Each serving provides

kcal 245, protein 27 g, fat 9 g (of which saturated fat 5 g), carbohydrate 14 g (of which sugars 13 g), fibre 2.5 g

✓✓✓	B$_{12}$
✓✓	B$_6$, C, folate, niacin, iron, zinc
✓	A, copper, potassium

1 Put the turkey steaks between sheets of cling film and pound them to flatten to about 5 mm (¼ in) thickness. Set these escalopes aside.

2 Melt the butter in a large frying pan, add the shallots and garlic, and cook, stirring, for 2–3 minutes or until softened but not brown. Remove the shallots from the pan with a draining spoon and set aside.

3 Put the turkey escalopes in the pan, in one layer, and fry them for 2–3 minutes on each side.

4 Meanwhile, cook the beans in a saucepan of boiling salted water for 3–4 minutes or until just tender. Drain and rinse briefly in cold water to stop the cooking. Keep the beans warm.

5 Mix the honey with the zest and juice of the orange and lemon. Remove the turkey escalopes from the pan and keep hot. Pour the honey mixture into the pan, return the shallots and garlic, and add seasoning to taste. Bring to the boil and bubble for about 2 minutes, stirring constantly.

6 Make a pile of beans on 4 plates and place a turkey escalope on top of each pile. Spoon over the sliced shallots and pan juices, and serve.

Some more ideas

• Use 4 skinless boneless turkey breast fillets, about 125 g (4½ oz) each. Being a bit thicker than escalopes, they will need to be cooked for 5 minutes on each side.

• Replace the turkey steaks with 4 small boneless duck breasts, about 550 g (1¼ lb) in total. Remove the skin and all fat from the breasts. Pan-fry for 3 minutes on each side, if you like duck a little pink, or a little longer for well-done duck. For the sauce, use the zest and juice from a pink grapefruit instead of the orange and lemon. Also add a piece of stem ginger, cut into fine slivers, and 1 tbsp of the stem ginger syrup.

• Replace the beans with 3 finely shredded leeks, stir-fried in 1 tbsp sunflower oil.

Plus points

• Turkey contains even less fat than chicken, making it one of the lowest fat meats available.

• All citrus fruits are an excellent source of vitamin C. Studies have shown a correlation between a regular intake of vitamin C and the maintenance of intellectual function in elderly people.

Pheasant casseroled with ginger

Casseroling is an excellent way to cook pheasant, as it produces succulent meat and a rich sauce. Cutting the bird into 8 pieces will allow each person to get a piece of breast as well as dark meat. Herby mashed potatoes, baby carrots and broccoli are good accompaniments for this aromatic dish.

Serves 4

1 large bulb of fennel, about 300 g (10½ oz)

1 tbsp sunflower oil

1 pheasant, about 1 kg (2¼ lb), jointed into 4 or 8 pieces

100 g (3½ oz) shallots or button onions, halved

4 pieces stem ginger, about 115 g (4 oz) in total, cut into thin strips

4 tbsp ginger wine

300 ml (10 fl oz) chicken stock, preferably home-made (see page 113)

salt and pepper

Preparation time: 15 minutes
Cooking time: about 1½ hours

Each serving provides

kcal 235, protein 30 g, fat 11 g (of which saturated fat 3 g), carbohydrate 3.5 g (of which sugars 3 g), fibre 2 g

✓✓✓	B_6, B_{12}, niacin, iron
✓✓	B_2, potassium, zinc
✓	E, folate, calcium, copper

1 Preheat the oven to 190°C (375°F, gas mark 5). Trim the fennel, retaining any feathery leaves for the garnish, then cut the bulb lengthways into 8 wedges. Set aside.

2 Heat the oil in a large flameproof casserole over a moderately high heat. Add the pheasant joints and shallots or button onions and fry to brown on all sides.

3 Add the fennel wedges. Turn the pheasant joints skin side up and sprinkle over the strips of ginger. Add the ginger wine and enough stock to come halfway up the pheasant joints but not cover them. Season to taste.

4 Bring to the boil, then cover the casserole and transfer to the oven. Cook for 1–1¼ hours or until the pheasant is tender. Serve garnished with the reserved fennel leaves.

Some more ideas

• Try a pheasant casserole with chestnuts and cabbage. Brown the pheasant joints and shallots, then add 200 g (7 oz) vacuum-packed chestnuts and 200 g (7 oz) red cabbage, cut into 4 wedges, instead of the fennel wedges. Replace the stem ginger with 2 tbsp marmalade and use red wine instead of ginger wine.

• Other game birds can be jointed and cooked in the same way.

• When game is out of season, use duck or chicken joints.

Plus points

• Ginger is a useful alternative remedy for travel sickness or morning sickness. In herbal medicine it is used to aid digestion, to protect against respiratory and digestive infections, and to relieve flatulence.

• Pheasant is an excellent source of protein as well as iron and B vitamins. Although it is higher in fat than other game birds, most of this fat is monounsaturated.

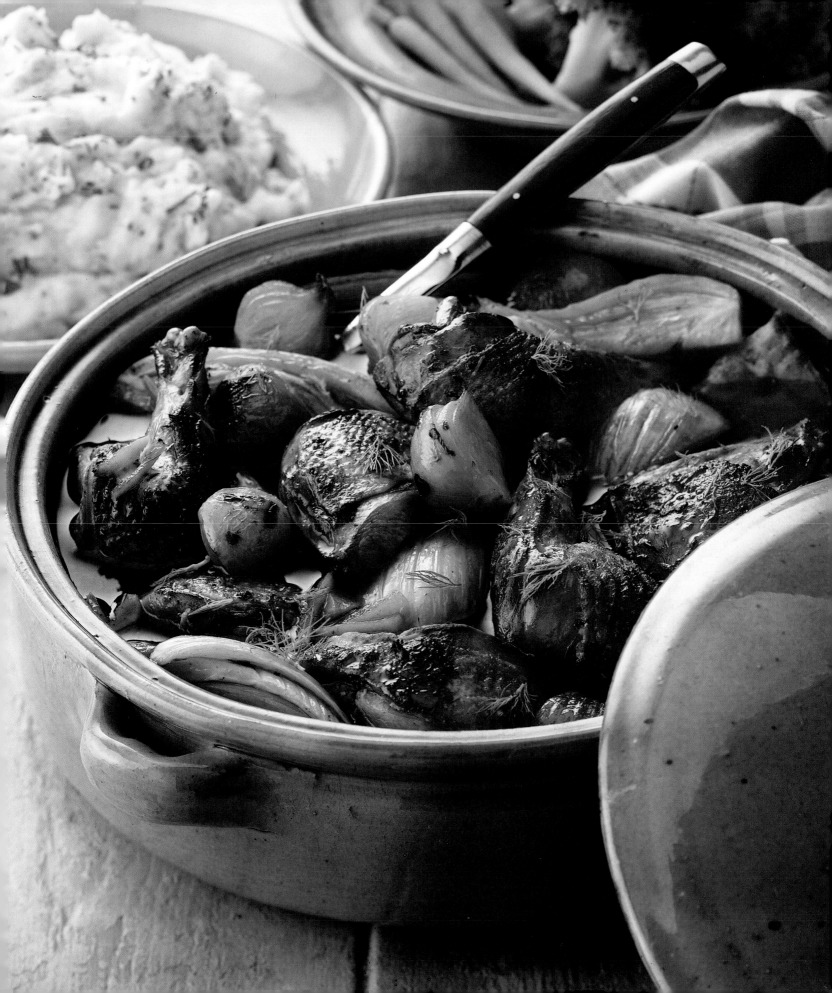

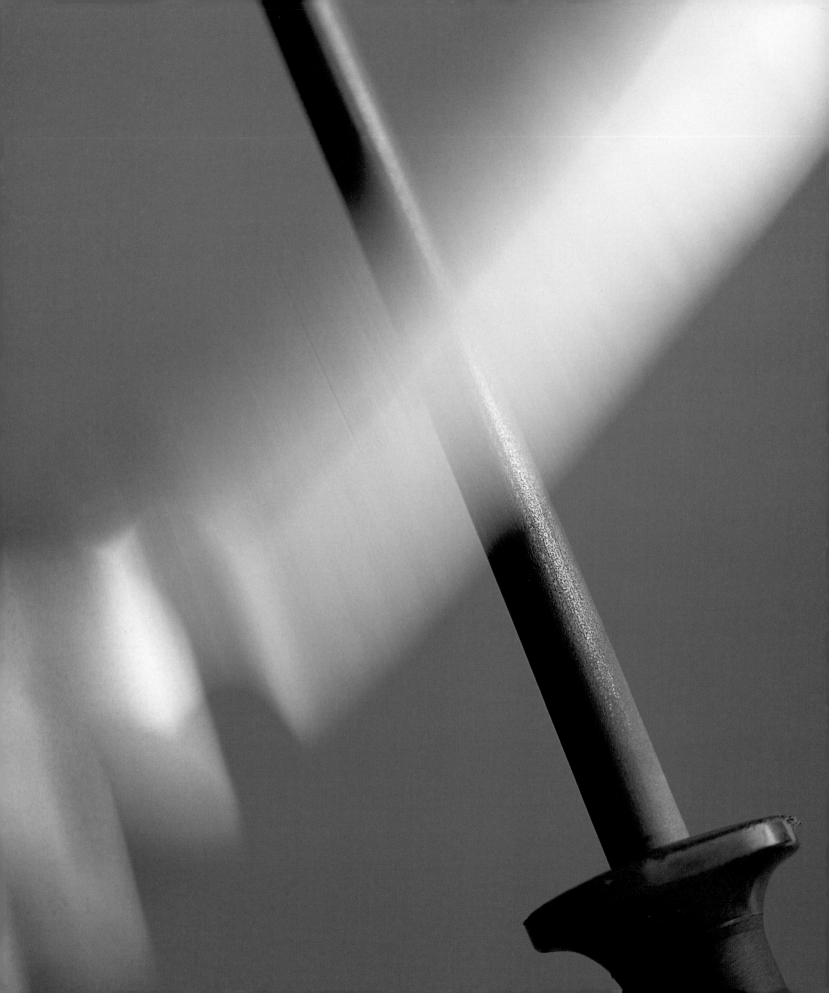

Mighty Meat

Meat is good for you in so many ways. It provides an excellent concentrated source of protein as well as offering many valuable nutrients. From the cook's point of view, meat is amazingly versatile – the wide variety of interesting cuts can be prepared and cooked in myriad ways to suit any occasion, budget or time available, and will provide a huge range of wonderful flavours and different textures. To add to the choice, there are lean venison and tasty wild boar, both becoming more widely available, plus more unusual meats such as ostrich, and savoury preserved and processed meats. All of these can be enjoyed as part of a healthy, well-balanced diet.

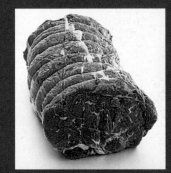

Meat in a healthy diet

Meat is a delicious, versatile way to get the vital protein, vitamins and minerals we need to be at our best. It can be healthily lean, too, if you choose wisely.

Protein – the body builder

Everyone needs protein, to grow and build up strength, to continually replenish body tissues, and to maintain good health. Every part of our bodies – muscles, bones, skin, hair and nails – depends on it. To fulfil this important role, an adult woman needs about 45 g protein daily, while an adult man needs 55 g. Eating meat is an excellent way to obtain the protein we require.

Although a regular protein intake is needed for optimum health, the daily requirement isn't really very much, and most of us eat far more than this. In fact, on a healthy well-balanced 'plate', protein foods should occupy only about one-sixth of the space – the largest part of the plate should be filled with starchy carbohydrates and fruit and vegetables. This turns traditional meal planning of 'meat with 2 veg' on its head – meat and other protein foods should be just one of the many component parts of a meal, not the major part of it.

Vital vitamins

A regular intake of vitamins is essential for good health. Meat provides many of them.
• Vitamin A is required for growth and normal development; it also protects against infection, and aids healthy skin, eyes and night vision. The active form of vitamin A, retinol, is found in meat, especially liver and other offal. Retinol is readily absorbed and used by the body.
• Vitamin D, combined with calcium, works to keep bones and teeth strong and healthy. Red meat is one of the richest natural sources of vitamin D in the diet.

• B vitamins are vital for all cell function in the body, but especially for healthy nerve and blood cells. Meat supplies most of the eight vitamins in the group. Of special importance is B_{12}, as foods of animal origin are the principal dietary source.

A comparison of the protein content of 100 g (3½ oz) boneless lean meat with other protein foods

beef		**veal**	
fillet steak, grilled	29 g	escalope, pan-fried	33 g
mince, cooked	25 g		
sirloin, roasted	32 g	**venison**	
		roasted	36 g
lamb			
cutlets, grilled	28 g	**other protein foods**	
leg, roasted	31 g	Cheddar cheese	25.5 g
loin chops, grilled	29 g	chicken breast, roasted	25 g
		cod fillet, baked	21 g
pork		eggs (2), poached	12.5 g
fillet, grilled	33 g	lentils, boiled	8.8 g
leg, roasted	35 g	red kidney beans, boiled	8.4 g
loin chop, grilled	32 g	tofu, uncooked	8.1 g

Essential minerals

Meat supplies many minerals, in particular iron and zinc.
• Iron is essential for the formation of the red blood cells that carry oxygen around the body – iron deficiency causes tiredness and anaemia. Women and teenage girls are prone to anaemia if their bodies do not absorb enough iron to cover losses of blood during menstruation and childbirth. Eating red meat makes a valuable contribution to the iron we need.
• Zinc is vital for normal growth and the healthy functioning of the immune and reproductive systems. It is also important

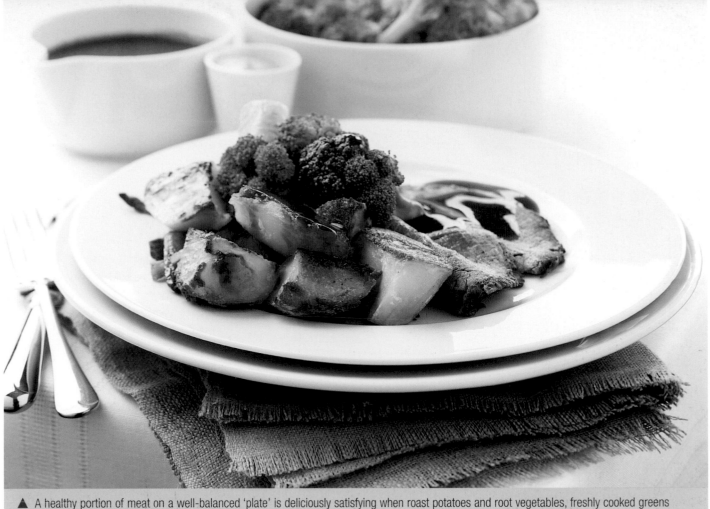

▲ A healthy portion of meat on a well-balanced 'plate' is deliciously satisfying when roast potatoes and root vegetables, freshly cooked greens and a tasty gravy are served alongside.

for healthy skin, especially where skin healing is necessary.

Among the best sources of zinc are red meat (beef and lamb in particular) and liver. Zinc is also found in wholegrain cereals, such as wholemeal bread, but the zinc in meat is more readily absorbed by the body. To make the maximum amount of zinc available, combine meat and cereals in the same meal. A good example of this is spaghetti bolognese – meat is in the sauce and cereal (wheat) is in the pasta.

Iron – a question of absorption

Much of the iron we eat is not properly or completely absorbed by our bodies. This is particularly true of the iron found in plant foods, which need to be eaten with vitamin-C rich fruits and vegetables in order for iron absorption to be maximised. The iron found in meat is a different kind. Called haem iron, it is easily absorbed by the body, and does not need to be combined with other foods.

• Meat also supplies three microminerals: copper and phosphorus, needed for a healthy respiratory tract and healthy bones, and selenium, which acts as an antioxidant. Only tiny amounts of these are required to help maintain good health.

What about vegetarians?

A properly balanced vegetarian diet is very healthy, but some people (young girls in particular) stop eating meat and eat only the salad or vegetables in a meal, so missing out on many vital nutrients. Others may eat too much cheese as a substitute for meat, not realising that the fat content can be very high. Sufficient protein and other essential nutrients can be obtained from combinations of pulses, cereals, vegetables, fruits and nuts, and you need to know about these if you have a vegetarian in the family. Vegans, who eat no animal products, need to eat some foods fortified with vitamin B_{12}, to be sure of not missing out on this vital nutrient.

Making the best choice

As a top source of protein, we don't need to eat much meat to benefit from it, so it makes sense to select the best we can afford.

A healthy variety

All the main kinds of meat – beef, veal, lamb and pork – are excellent sources of protein. They also provide the same vitamins and minerals, although in slightly differing amounts. For example, although all red meat is rich in B vitamins, pork, ham and bacon are especially rich in vitamin B_1, and beef is rich in B_{12}. So it's best to eat a variety of different meats to be sure you derive the maximum nutritional benefits on offer.

The fat issue

Despite its positive contribution to the diet, meat is often criticised for its fat content. Saturated fat in particular has given meat a bad name, and this has caused some people to consider omitting meat from their diets altogether. In fact, only about half of the fat in meat is saturated – much less than it used to be, thanks to modern breeding techniques.

Animal welfare and consumer choice

In the UK, comprehensive guidelines, backed by legislation, control animal welfare and all procedures throughout the food chain, including meat production. But in response to consumer demand, farm assurance schemes, such as the RSPCA's Freedom Food Standards, have been established, specifically to safeguard animal welfare, and food produced under these schemes is clearly labelled. Organic meat, from farms where the routine use of antibiotics is prohibited and the content of animal feed is rigorously controlled, is becoming more popular, and many other farms are changing to outdoor 'free-range' production instead of indoor intensive-rearing systems. When choosing meat, read the label or ask the butcher about the supplier, bearing in mind that all meat is equally nutritious.

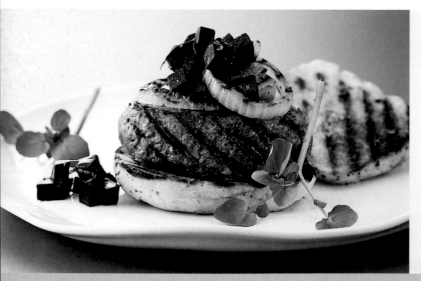

▲ Lean minced beef is low in fat and yet rich in zinc, iron and vitamins B and D.

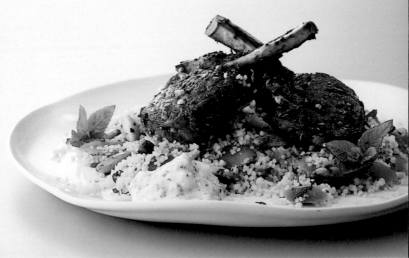

▲ Lamb provides lots of B vitamins, zinc and iron.

The remaining fat content is unsaturated – primarily the monounsaturated kind with a little polyunsaturated.

Fat is very high in calories – twice as many per gram as either carbohydrate or protein – and overconsumption of saturated fat is a major cause of health concerns, such as weight problems, coronary heart disease and some cancers. This is why nutrition experts recommend that we reduce the total amount of fatty foods we eat. According to current Department of Health guidelines, only 33% of our total daily calories should come from fat (of any kind), and of that a maximum of 10% should be from saturated fat. For an adult woman this means a daily maximum amount of 71g fat, of which 21.5 g can be saturated; for an adult man the daily amount is 93.5 g fat, of which 28.5 g can be saturated.

Eating moderate portions of lean meat can help to keep fat intake within healthy limits, while still providing all the benefits that meat has to offer.

Cutting along the seam

Seam butchery is a technique of butchering that reduces the amount of fat in meat. It involves the removal of individual muscles by following the seams in the carcass. As a result, any visible fat between the seams can be cut away and discarded before sale to produce very lean, boneless cuts. These are ready-trimmed and portioned for immediate use.

Fat content of 100 g (3½ oz) boneless lean meat*

	Total fat	Saturates	Mono-unsaturates	Poly-unsaturates
beef				
mince, lean	9.6 g	4.2 g	0.4 g	0.4 g
rump steak	4.1 g	1.7 g	1.7 g	0.3 g
sirloin	4.5 g	2.0 g	1.9 g	0.2 g
topside	2.7 g	1.1 g	1.2 g	0.2 g
lamb				
leg	8.3 g	3.8 g	3.2 g	0.4 g
pork				
leg	2.2 g	0.9 g	0.9 g	0.4 g
loin steaks	3.4 g	1.2 g	1.3 g	0.6 g
venison				
average	1.6 g	0.8 g	0.4 g	0.4 g

* The total fat figure includes fatty compounds and other fatty acids in addition to saturates and mono and polyunsaturates.

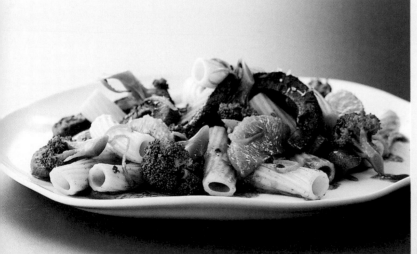

▲ Liver is rich in iron and vitamins A, B and D, and eating it just once a week can be beneficial.

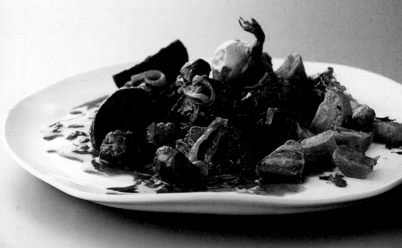

▲ Venison has twice as much iron as beef, and it is a good source of vitamins and minerals. It is also very low in fat.

The big four

Beef, veal, lamb and pork, and their offal, are excellent sources of protein and they provide many other essential nutrients too.

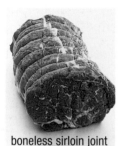
boneless sirloin joint

Beef

Beef comes from steers or bullocks reared to 18 months old or from heifers not required for breeding. The meat should be open-grained and moist with a good red colour. If it is a darker, reddish-brown, it will have been hung or aged for at least 2–3 weeks and will have a fuller, 'beefier' flavour.

Beef is both an excellent source of zinc and a useful source of iron. It also provides vitamins from the B group (particularly B_{12}) and is a useful source of vitamin D.

● Sirloin, foreribs, topside and thick flank (top rump) are the traditional beef joints for roasting. Lean and tender fillet can also be roasted, either whole or cut into smaller joints. When

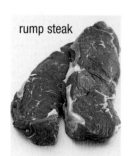
rump steak

buying a boneless joint allow 100–170 g (3½–6 oz) per person, or 225–340 g (8–12 oz) for meat on the bone. These raw weights allow for any waste in preparation and for loss of weight during cooking. An average cooked portion size is 85–100 g (3–3½ oz).

● Brisket and silverside are joints that become tender and succulent with long, slow cooking, so they are ideal for a pot roast – cooked in one large piece in a casserole with liquid, vegetables and flavourings.

● Sirloin, rump and fillet steaks are tender enough for quick cooking methods such as grilling, griddling, barbecuing and frying. Grilling is the healthiest way to cook steaks, as no extra fat is needed. Griddling on a ridged cast-iron grill pan or a

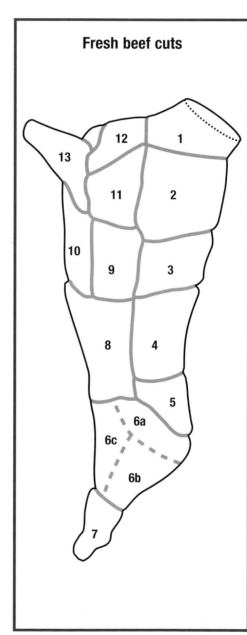

Fresh beef cuts

1. neck
2. chuck, including blade
3. forerib
4. sirloin, including fillet (joint and steak)
5. rump (rump steak and skirt)
6. round:
   (a) topside
   (b) silverside
   (c) thick flank or top rump
7. leg
8. flank
9. thin rib
10. brisket
11. top or thick rib
12. clod
13. shin

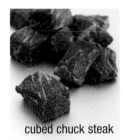
cubed chuck steak

heavy-based non-stick frying pan is almost as good, as long as you use the minimum amount of an oil such as olive or sunflower. A good tip is to get the pan hot before you put the meat on to cook. Steak can also be cut into cubes for kebabs, or into strips for stir-fries.

● Shin, leg, neck and clod (from the neck) are tougher cuts, being muscular or weight-bearing in the animal, so they need long, gentle stewing to make them tender. There is no limit to the different vegetables, herbs and spices that can be used in meaty stews to provide delicious flavour combinations, and the slow cooking allows plenty of time for the meat to become beautifully tender.

● Back or thick ribs, chuck and blade, sold as 'braising steak', are not as tough as stewing cuts such as shin, but too tough for grilling or griddling. They are ideal for stews and casseroles.

Veal

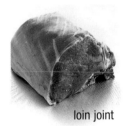

loin joint

Veal is the meat of a young calf 18–20 weeks old. It should be a very pale cream or delicate pink colour with virtually no fat. This leanness is good from the nutritional point of view, but it does mean that some veal dishes need a liquid or sauce to make them more moist and juicy. Veal has a very similar nutritional profile to beef, although it provides only about half the amount of iron.

● Leg is a prime lean cut for roasting – allow 225 g (8 oz) per person when buying meat on the bone. A boned and stuffed leg is even better, because the stuffing helps to make the meat moist and tasty.

● Fillet and topside, both cut from the leg, can be roasted successfully as joints, but are often cut into slices across the grain and beaten thin to make escalopes and schnitzels.

● Rump is usually cut into medallions or escalopes. Being thin cuts, these are perfect for very quick pan-frying.

escalopes

● Loin makes an excellent roasting joint on the bone, or boned, stuffed and rolled. Chops and cutlets are lean and tender, and can be roasted, grilled, pan-fried or braised.

● Shoulder, when boned and stuffed, makes a good roasting cut, but the meat is more usually removed from the bone, trimmed of fat and cut into cubes for use in pies and stews. With long, gentle cooking it becomes very tender.

● Shin, from the legs, is good in stews, the best known being the Italian osso buco.

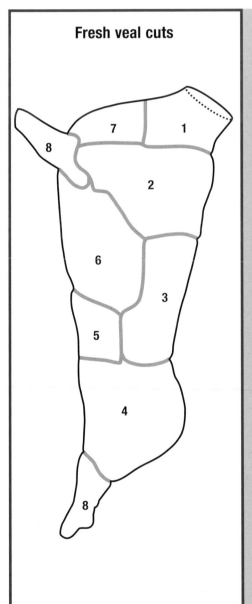

Fresh veal cuts

1. neck
2. shoulder or chuck
3. loin (joint, chops and cutlets)
4. leg, including rump, fillet and topside
5. thick flank
6. breast
7. clod
8. shin or knuckle

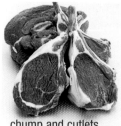
leg

Lamb

Of all the red meats, lamb is the one that has benefited the most from the new cutting and preparation techniques. More fat is now removed from the meat before being sold, and prepared new cuts are ideal for quick meals for one or two people. Early in the season, the meat from young lambs is a paler pink than that of older animals and it has a finer grain.

Lamb is an excellent source of vitamin B_{12} and zinc, a good source of vitamin B_1 (thiamin) and a useful source of iron.

• Leg, loin, best end of neck and shoulder are all excellent joints for traditional roasts on the bone. The leg can also be boned and 'butterflied', or opened out flat, and then grilled or barbecued. Loin is often boned, stuffed and rolled for roasting – many shops sell it ready-prepared. Best end of neck can be roasted as a whole rack of 6–7 cutlets or, for a special occasion, two racks can be joined, either as a guard of honour or a crown roast. Most butchers prepare these to order, and will stuff the centre of a crown roast if you like, although you may prefer your own stuffing. Allow 85–170 g (3–6 oz) per person when buying boneless meat and 225–340 g (8–12 oz) if the meat is on the bone.

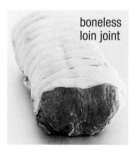
chump and cutlets

• Neck fillet, best end of neck cutlets, steaks cut from the top of the leg, and chump, loin and double loin chops are all excellent for grilling. The same cuts can also be cooked on a ridged cast-iron grill pan or in a non-stick frying pan using a little oil. Loin and chump chops are also good for roasting, as are lamb steaks, either on or off the bone. Lean and tender neck fillet and boneless leg steaks are perfect cut into cubes for kebabs or thin strips for stir-fries. If they are marinated before cooking, the meat will be extra succulent and tasty.

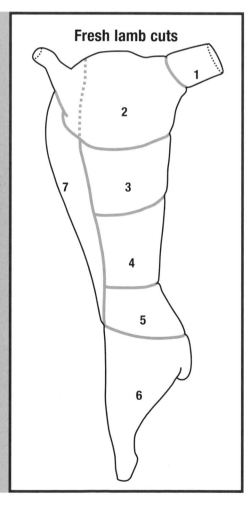

Fresh lamb cuts

1. neck and scrag
2. shoulder and middle neck (neck fillet)
3. rib or best end of neck (rack, crown roast and cutlets)
4. loin (joint and chops)
5. chump (chops)
6. leg (joint and steaks)
7. breast

Pork

boneless loin joint

The meat of the pig is sold fresh as pork, used in fresh meat products such as sausages, preserved as bacon and ham and in salami-type sausages, and used cooked in pies. Due to modern selective breeding techniques, pork is now leaner than it used to be – there is less fat within the tissues of the meat and the layer of back fat is very thin – which makes it a very healthy choice. Fresh pork should be smooth and pink, not at all grey or damp-looking.

Pork is an excellent source of vitamin B_{12} and a good source of zinc and vitamins B_1 (thiamin) and B_6.

• Leg, shoulder (hand and spring) and loin are the most popular lean cuts for roasting. Any fat on the joint can be removed before cooking or left on so it bastes the meat during roasting – stand the joint on a rack in the roasting tin so the fat drips through. The skin on a pork joint will also help to keep the meat moist during roasting, but it's best not to eat too

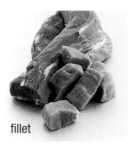
fillet

much of the crisp crackling that forms as it is very high in saturated fat – 45 g fat in every 100 g (3½ oz) of crackling. (The skin should not be left on when moist cooking methods such as casseroling and stewing are used, or the fat underneath it will melt into the cooking liquid.) Leg and loin can also be boned and stuffed before roasting. For a boneless roasting joint, allow 85–170 g (3–6 oz) per person; for a joint on the bone, allow 225–340 g (8–12 oz).

• Fillet, also called tenderloin, is very lean and tender, as its name suggests. It can be roasted whole, but it is most often cut into thin slices or strips for pan-fries and stir-fries, and into cubes for casseroles and kebabs.

Fresh pork cuts

1. spare rib (joint and chops)
2. loin, including fillet or tenderloin (joint and chops)
3. chump (joint and chops)
4. leg
5. belly
6. shoulder or hand and spring

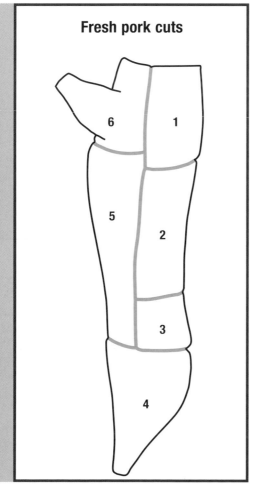

• Loin and chump chops can be roasted, or they can be grilled or pan-fried. The meat is lean and can dry out easily, so it is a good idea to coat it with a glaze or baste it during cooking, or use a moist cooking method such as braising. Loin chops may include the kidney, which adds extra flavour and more iron.
• Leg and shoulder (hand and spring) make good pot roasts, ending up deliciously moist and tender.

Nutrient-rich offal

Offal includes liver, kidneys, heart, tongue, sweetbreads, brains and trotters. Liver and kidneys are still popular, but other types of offal are not as widely eaten as they used to be, although they can be delicious. All offal is very nutritious, but liver, heart and kidneys are the stars, rich in iron and B vitamins, especially B_3 and B_{12}, and vitamins A and D. As vitamins A and D can be stored in the body, just one 85 g (3 oz) serving of offal once a week will build up and restore stocks. If you're not too keen on offal, you can combine it with other meats, say in a steak and kidney pie or in a pâté.

• Calf's liver is very tender and delicate in flavour. It is best pan-fried, stir-fried or grilled. Lamb's liver has a fairly strong flavour. It, too, can be grilled, but is better used in a casserole or stew. Pig's liver has the strongest flavour of all and a soft texture. Although it is suitable for casseroles, it is the favourite for pâtés and terrines.
• Lamb's kidneys are small and tender with a good flavour. They can be grilled or fried. Allow 2 kidneys per portion. Ox, calf's and pig's kidneys have a stronger flavour and are good in casseroles and stews. Allow 1 or 2 per person, depending on size.
• Whole ox heart is good stuffed and roasted, and it can also be sliced and cooked in stews and casseroles. Lamb's heart is more tender than calf's, but both can be stuffed and braised or roasted.
• Tongue may be pickled before cooking and pressing. Small lamb's tongues can be pressed together in a casserole, or they can be sliced and served cold.
• Fried calf's and lamb's sweetbreads are a traditional delicacy. Ox sweetbreads are tougher, and are best used in stews and stuffings.
• Calf's brains are considered to be the best and are traditionally served poached with a sauce. Lamb's brains are usually used in stews.
• Trotters are the feet of pigs or sheep. They can be boiled or grilled for eating hot, or simmered in a stock to help set it for an aspic.

Ring the changes

Preserved and processed meats are packed with flavour, so a little goes a long way. Exotic meats like venison and buffalo are low in fat, so are great additions to your diet.

Ever-popular bangers

Individual butchers make their own fresh sausages according to traditional recipes, and these vary from one part of the country to another, but the content is regulated and the type of meat and the percentage of it must be declared, with details of any preservatives, additives and flavourings used. To be sure of what you are buying, read the labels on the packets, or information displayed in the butcher's cabinet, paying particular attention to the fat content. Sausages with a high meat content are the best healthy choice.

Pork and beef are the most common meats used for sausages, but lamb, venison, wild boar, chicken and other speciality sausages are also available. The best low-fat cooking methods are grilling, barbecuing and baking on a rack in the oven, but sausages can also be cooked on a ridged cast-iron grill pan or in a non-stick frying pan. They are very good in casseroles and stews, and chopped up in sauces for pasta.

An ABC of special sausages

There is a wonderful variety of sausages from all parts of the world, many of them with unusual and exciting flavours. Each country has its own specialities, some of which need cooking and others not.

- Black pudding (boudin noir in French) is made from pig's blood (sheep's blood in Scotland), fat, cereals such as oatmeal, and flavourings. It is usually sliced and shallow-fried, grilled or baked.
- Bratwurst is a German smoked sausage made from pork or veal. It is usually grilled or fried.
- Chorizo is a Spanish pork sausage. There are both smoked and unsmoked varieties, and they may be spicy hot. Some can be sliced and eaten raw while others require cooking. A small quantity of chorizo will add lots of flavour to a stew or sauce.
- Frankfurters are long, slim smoked sausages made from a mixture of beef and pork. They can be heated in hot water, grilled or lightly fried, or added to casseroles.
- Salamis of innumerable kinds come from all over Europe. Most are made from pork, but some are a mixture of meats. All are 'matured' for at least a few weeks, which dries them out, and most are ready to eat.
- Toulouse sausages, made from coarsely chopped pork, are an essential ingredient of a traditional French cassoulet.

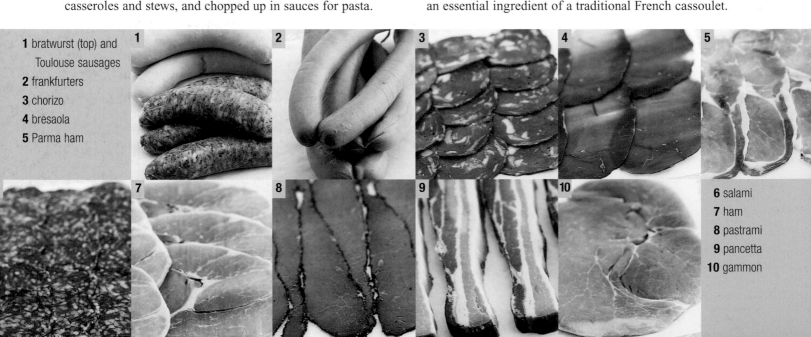

1 bratwurst (top) and Toulouse sausages
2 frankfurters
3 chorizo
4 bresaola
5 Parma ham
6 salami
7 ham
8 pastrami
9 pancetta
10 gammon

Cured for flavour

When meat is preserved by air-drying, salting, smoking or steeping in brine, it is described as 'cured'. Such meat is deliciously savoury, but it is often high in salt and saturated fat, so it is best not to eat too much of it too often. For some of the curing processes, preservatives such as sodium nitrate are used, which can be converted into undesirable nitrites in the body. To counteract the nitrites' effect, it is a good idea to eat cured meats with plenty of vitamin C-rich fruits and vegetables.

• Bacon is the cured meat from the back or side of the pig and may be unsmoked ('green') or smoked. Different smoking methods provide a variety of flavours. Rashers of back bacon are much leaner than streaky.

• Bresaola is cured raw beef from Italy. It is sold in wafer-thin slices to be used in antipasti, but it can be chopped and used in salads and other dishes. It has a strong, gamey flavour.

• Most of the corned beef eaten in Britain today is imported canned from Argentina and is compressed cured and cooked beef. It can be served chilled and thinly sliced with a salad or in sandwiches, or chopped and cooked with potato to make corned beef hash.

• Gammon is a type of bacon that is often sold in thick slices or steaks, or as joints. Collar, forehock, prime back, middle gammon and gammon hock are the best gammon joints for boiling or baking.

• Ham is the cured hind leg of the pig. There are many kinds, according to the breed of pig, its diet and type of cure – many flavours can be added during the curing process. Some hams are simply salted, while others are also smoked. York, Suffolk and Bradenham are famous British hams.

• Pancetta is a streaky bacon from Italy, often used chopped in dishes such as spaghetti carbonara, and in sauces, soups and casseroles. It comes smoked or unsmoked.

• Pastrami is brisket of beef cured with sugar, spices and garlic, then smoked. It is served very thinly sliced.

• Prosciutto crudo is salted, air-dried ham from Italy. Prosciutto di Parma (Parma ham) is the most famous – and the most expensive. After a long time maturing, it is usually sliced very thinly and served raw, although it can be chopped and used to flavour risottos and sauces for pasta. It can be used as a leaner alternative to bacon rashers.

Something different

Many large supermarkets stock rabbit and venison as do some butchers and game suppliers. You can also get them by mail order. Very unusual meats such as ostrich, kangaroo and buffalo are more often to be found only on restaurant menus, but may well become more widely available in the future. As with all other meats, strict welfare and production methods are enforced for all these speciality meats.

Rabbit Both wild and domesticated rabbits are sold, and the doe meat is said to be the best. The flesh is pale in colour, with a mild flavour. Nutritionally rabbit is similar to beef, except that it has far less zinc. Each rabbit provides 6–8 pieces, which can be roasted or used in casseroles and stews. Rabbit can be used in any chicken recipe.

Hare Hare is similar to rabbit, being jointed in the same way and offering the same nutritional benefits, but it has stronger-tasting, darker flesh. A whole hare can be stuffed and roasted to serve 6–8 people or joints can be used in casseroles or stews.

Venison Venison is very low in fat, and extremely nutritious. It provides more protein than any of the main types of meat, and has twice as much iron as beef. It is also tender and full of flavour. The leg and saddle are the choicest cuts for roasting, and an average joint will serve 8–10 people. Venison is also sold as lean steaks for pan-frying or grilling. Diced venison makes delicious stews, casseroles and game pies. Minced venison can be used in any recipe for minced beef.

Wild boar The lean meat of the wild boar is full of rich flavour. Marinating before cooking helps to make the meat deliciously moist, and also mellows its rather strong taste. It can be used in recipes for pork or venison.

Ostrich Ostrich is a good low-fat source of protein – it contains less saturated fat than other meats. It is now mostly imported and can be bought in a few specialist stores around the country.

Kangaroo A protected species in the wilds of Australia, kangaroo is bred in captivity under strict food standard regulations for home and export sales. Its meat is low in fat, and is an excellent source of iron and zinc. The flavour is similar to hare and the meat is very tender. It can be used in recipes for chicken.

Buffalo A few specialist butchers shops in Britain sell buffalo fillet. It is an excellent source of protein, and is very low in calories and fat compared with beef and chicken. The fillet is best marinated in wine and herbs and then roasted, or cut into steaks and pan-fried.

Bringing out the best in meat

Animals are bred and butchered to keep saturated fat to a minimum, making meat a healthy choice. Shop carefully and use healthy cooking methods for best results.

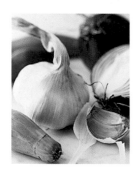

Buying for quality

When buying meat, it helps to be an informed shopper.

• Get to know your local independent butcher or the butcher in your supermarket who will prepare meat to suit your own requirements if you don't see exactly what you want on the shelves.

• Choose well-trimmed lean joints and cuts that look fresh and moist and have a good, healthy colour.

• Check the 'use-by' date on packaged meats.

• Many butchers and supermarkets sell ready-prepared meats such as kebabs, beef olives, stir-fry strips and marinated cuts. These are very convenient to use, but be sure to check what is in them before you buy. Read labels carefully, comparing amounts of saturated fat, sodium, preservatives and additives in different products and brands, and opting for the ones that contain the least of these.

• Some stores label meat as 'lean choice' or something similar. It is worth asking what this means exactly, as it may not be as lean as you think.

• Check the fat content of minced or ground beef, and choose the leanest available. Better still, buy lean meat and mince it yourself in a food processor or mincer, or ask the butcher to mince it for you. If a recipe doesn't require fine mince, you can chop good-quality meat with two sharp chef's knives to make a coarse, home-made version.

Keeping fat to a minimum

You can reduce the total fat content of a dish with a few simple preparation techniques.

• Before cooking, trim off any visible fat from steaks, chops and cutlets, and from cubes of meat that are to be used in a casserole or stew. For joints that are to be roasted, you may want to leave a thin layer of fat on so that it bastes the meat during cooking, to keep it moist, but be sure to set the joint on a rack in a roasting tin. This way the meat won't be sitting in its own fat during cooking.

• When making casseroles and stews, don't coat the pieces of meat with flour before browning them at the start of cooking because the flour will absorb any excess fat in the dish during cooking. It is better to brown the meat uncoated, then thicken the well-skimmed cooking liquid at the end if necessary.

• After cooking casseroles and stews, be sure to remove any fat from the surface. A bulb baster is the ideal gadget for this, although you can also use a spoon to skim off the fat, or blot it with kitchen paper. Another idea is to drop in a few ice cubes: fat will solidify round them and they can then be lifted out.

• After roasting, drain off and discard all the fat from the roasting tin before using the meat juices to make a gravy or sauce. A gravy strainer or separator, which is a jug with a spout rising from the bottom, is a great help.

• If possible, make casseroles and stews ahead of time and chill them in the fridge overnight. Any fat will rise to the surface and solidify in a layer that can be easily lifted off before the meat dish is reheated for serving.

• You can 'dry-fry' minced or ground meat in a non-stick frying pan without any fat. Turn and break up the meat as it browns, then tip it into a sieve to drain off all the fat that has come out of the meat. Chopped vegetables such as onion, celery and carrot can be dry-fried with the mince too.

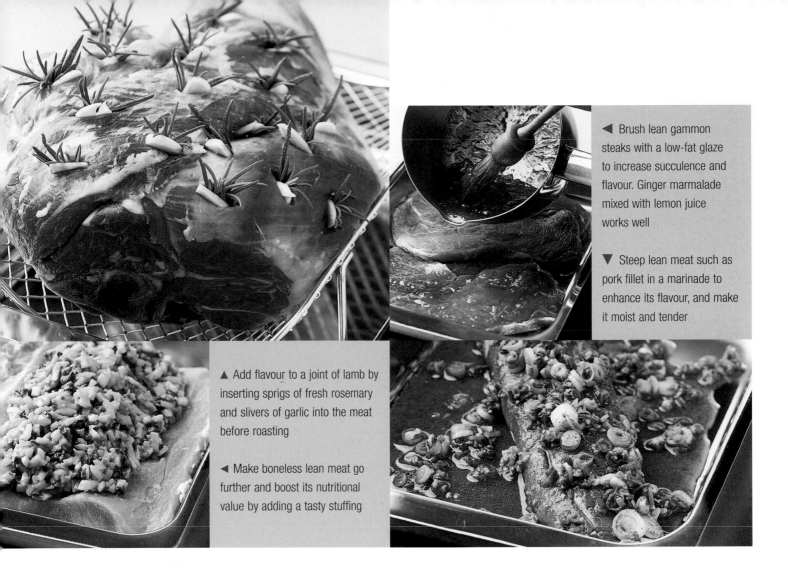

◀ Brush lean gammon steaks with a low-fat glaze to increase succulence and flavour. Ginger marmalade mixed with lemon juice works well

▼ Steep lean meat such as pork fillet in a marinade to enhance its flavour, and make it moist and tender

▲ Add flavour to a joint of lamb by inserting sprigs of fresh rosemary and slivers of garlic into the meat before roasting

◀ Make boneless lean meat go further and boost its nutritional value by adding a tasty stuffing

For tender results

Lean meat is not self-basting because it does not have fat 'marbled' throughout the flesh, so you need to take care that it doesn't dry out and become tough during cooking.

• If lean cuts such as steaks and escalopes are pounded before cooking, they will cook very quickly and have less time to dry out. Pounding also helps to break down tough fibres and make the meat more tender. To pound raw meat, use a meat mallet or a rolling pin, and cover the meat with cling film or greaseproof paper first to prevent the meat from tearing.

• You can add moisture and flavour to lean meat and help to tenderise it with a marinade. For tough cuts try including pineapple, figs or papaya in the marinade – these fruits contain enzymes that can have a beneficial tenderising effect on meat. Apricots and prunes have a similar effect, although they do not work quite so well. For best results, leave the meat in its marinade for at least 4 hours, at room temperature.

Punchy flavourings and stuffings

Rather than cooking or serving meat with a rich sauce or gravy, you can add wonderful flavours with herbs, garlic, spices and seasonings, and tasty glazes made from ingredients such as mustard, honey, fruit juice and soy sauce.

Stuffings are an absolute boon for a health-conscious cook. They enhance the flavour of meat and make a moderate amount seem very satisfying, and they can add valuable starchy carbohydrate in the form of bread or rice, plus vitamins, minerals and fibre when vegetables and fruits are included. A stuffing can be pushed inside a joint or a chop, usually in the space left after removing the bone, or you can spread it over boneless meat and then roll the meat up around it. Balls of stuffing can be cooked alongside the meat.

Cooked to perfection

Traditional cooking methods for meat are still justifiably popular, but stir-frying, barbecuing or cooking in a ridged grill pan use a minimum of fat and are fast.

Roasting

Roasting is a straightforward method for meat – the joint or other cut is simply cooked uncovered in the oven relatively slowly. The trick is to choose the right cuts, which should be reasonably tender, and to prevent them from drying out so they remain moist and succulent. Here are some useful tips.

- To help keep a boned joint in a good shape and make sure it cooks evenly, tie it with string.
- Place the meat on a rack in a roasting tin so that the largest cut surfaces of the meat are exposed and any fat is on the top. As the fat melts during roasting it will baste the meat.
- If the meat is very lean, baste it with the hot fat in the roasting tin from time to time during cooking. Alternatively, cover the joint with foil or cook it in a roasting bag. Better still, use a special roasting tin with a dimpled lid – a little water is poured into the base of the tin at the beginning of cooking, and then the lid is removed towards the end, to allow the meat to brown. Roasting like this gives very succulent and tender results – perfect every time.
- Once the roasting time is completed, it can be difficult to judge if the meat is actually cooked – the outside may look perfect and deliciously browned, but the inside might still be a bit undercooked. The most accurate test for doneness is by checking the internal temperature with a meat thermometer. Some thermometers are inserted into the meat at the beginning of cooking and left until the end, while others are pushed into the joint about 10 minutes before the end of the calculated cooking time, to take an 'instant reading'. Always make sure that the point of the thermometer goes into a thick part of the meat, not into fat or next to bone.

Grilling

When meat is cooked on the rack under a grill, any fat will drip away from the meat and into the pan below, which makes grilling one of the healthiest methods of cooking. The only drawback is that very lean meat can dry out during grilling.

- Brush a little oil over all surfaces of the meat before cooking, or baste it during cooking with a mixture containing oil. You can also add moisture by marinating the meat beforehand, depending on how much time you have.

Roasting times and temperatures

The cooking time for roasting meat is based on the weight of the joint, so weigh the meat – after stuffing if there is any – and then calculate the cooking time according to the chart below. The times given are suitable for meat on or off the bone. If you buy one of the special small 'mini-roasts', follow the cooking instructions on the packaging. Also check packet instructions if you are using a roasting bag. The ideal temperature for roasting is 180°C (350°F, gas mark 4). Meat thermometer temperatures are shown in square brackets.

---

beef and lamb

rare	20 minutes per 450 g (1 lb) plus 20 minutes [60°C/140°F]
medium	25 minutes per 450 g (1 lb) plus 25 minutes [70°C/160°F]
well-done	30 minutes per 450 g (1 lb) plus 30 minutes [80°C/175°F]

---

veal

well-done	30 minutes per 450 g (1 lb) plus 30 minutes [80°C/175°F]

---

pork

medium	30 minutes per 450 g (1 lb) plus 30 minutes [80°C/175°F]
well-done	35 minutes per 450 g (1 lb) plus 35 minutes [85°C/180°F]

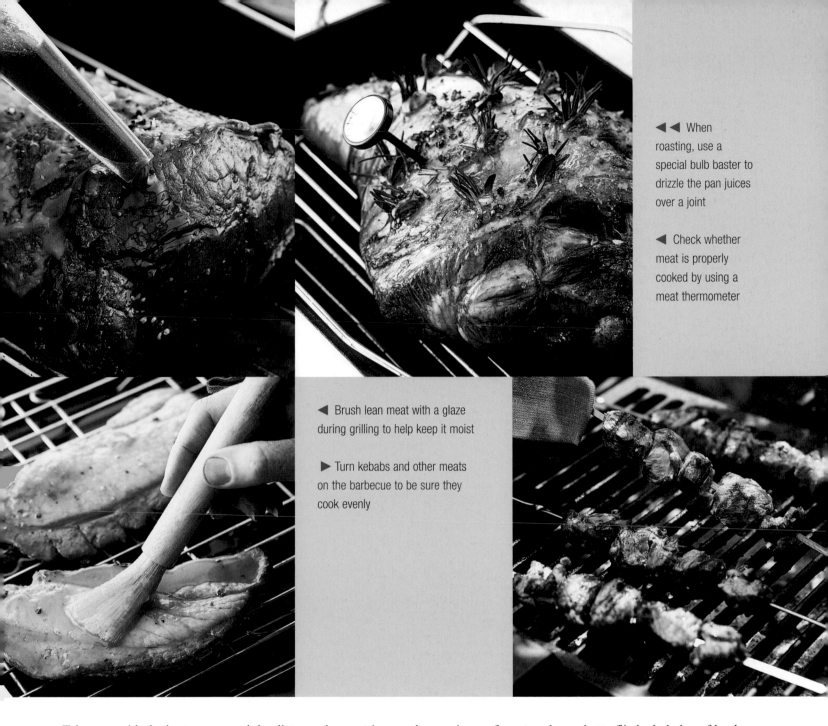

◄◄ When roasting, use a special bulb baster to drizzle the pan juices over a joint

◄ Check whether meat is properly cooked by using a meat thermometer

◄ Brush lean meat with a glaze during grilling to help keep it moist

► Turn kebabs and other meats on the barbecue to be sure they cook evenly

• Take care with the heat source and the distance the meat is from it. If the heat is too fierce and the meat too close to it, the outside of the meat will be browned before the inside is properly cooked. To gauge timing accurately, preheat the grill.

Barbecuing

Anything that can be grilled can also be barbecued, so when the weather is fine, use the barbecue to cook steaks, chops, cutlets, sausages, home-made burgers and kebabs, as well as larger pieces of meat such as a butterflied whole leg of lamb.

• To help keep lean meat moist and give it a good flavour, marinate it before cooking, and baste it with a little oil or a flavourful mixture while it is on the barbecue grid. Use a special long-handled brush for basting, as the fire is very hot and oil and fat dropping onto the hot coals will spit.

• The heat of the fire is important for successful cooking. If the coals are too hot the meat may char on the outside and yet still be raw in the centre. To safeguard against this, wait until all the flames have died down and the coals have turned from red to grey before putting the meat on to cook.

• Always make sure the meat is thoroughly cooked and piping hot before serving. If you are in any doubt with thick cuts of meat, you can always use a meat thermometer to check the internal temperature.

Griddling

This is a confusing term because it's actually a method of frying. A special ridged cast-iron grill pan is used over a high heat on top of the cooker – the pan's ridges give the meat charred stripes on the surface, which is why it is sometimes referred to as 'char-grilling', especially by chefs. Griddling is an excellent healthy way to cook steaks, chops, escalopes and other lean cuts because very little oil is needed and the meat is cooked very quickly. Also, the stripes on the meat make it look attractive and taste delicious.

• Use a pan with a thick base – the heavier the better.

• Heat the pan thoroughly before you put in the meat, usually for 10 minutes.

• Griddling causes a lot of smoke, so be sure to turn the extractor fan on high.

Frying

There are other healthy methods of frying besides griddling.

• Dry-frying, which uses no fat at all, is the healthiest option for more fatty meat such as mince, sausages and bacon – their natural fat melts out and prevents the meat from sticking to the pan. All you need is a good non-stick frying pan. After cooking, drain mince in a sieve; take sausages and bacon from the pan with a draining spoon and drain well on kitchen paper.

• Shallow-frying, or pan-frying, is excellent for thin cuts of meat. Use a heavy non-stick pan and heat it before adding just a little oil to prevent sticking. The oil can be applied in a drizzle or rubbed on with a wad of kitchen paper. Even better, spray on the oil from a special mister, which gives a very light and even coating to the pan. Be sure the oil is hot before you put in the meat so that it browns quickly and doesn't absorb the oil. Then you can reduce the heat to finish the cooking, if necessary.

• Stir-frying in a wok uses the minimum amount of oil, and the meat is cut into thin strips so that it cooks very quickly. It's an excellent way to combine a small amount of meat with rice or noodles and lots of vegetables, to make a quick meal in one pan. Groundnut oil is good for stir-frying because it can be heated to a high temperature without burning, but you can also use sunflower, corn or olive oil. For extra flavour, add a little walnut or sesame oil too. If you haven't got a wok, you can use a deep frying pan or sauté pan instead.

Stewing, braising, casseroling and pot roasting

These are slow, moist methods of cooking at low temperatures, either in the oven or on top of the cooker. They help to tenderise the less expensive, more coarse-grained cuts of meat like beef brisket, pork shoulder and lamb chump chops. Braising traditionally uses slices of meat, while stews and casseroles use cubes. Whole large pieces or joints and pieces of meat on the bone make succulent pot roasts.

• Use a well-flavoured stock and/or wine, cider or beer, plus lots of herbs and spices, to get the best flavour. Add lots of vegetables to provide extra interest and nutritional value.

• Starchy carbohydrates such as rice, pasta and dumplings can be added near the end of cooking, to add nutritious bulk and help 'stretch' meat. Or you can turn a casserole or stew into a satisfying meal-in-a-pot by topping it with a thick layer of sliced potatoes about an hour before cooking time finishes. Cook uncovered so the potatoes turn crisp and golden brown.

Microwaving

Using a microwave speeds up meat cookery and can be very successful, especially if your oven has a browning element or browning dish to give the meat an attractive appearance. Follow the manufacturer's instructions for cooking times as these vary according to the model and power of each machine.

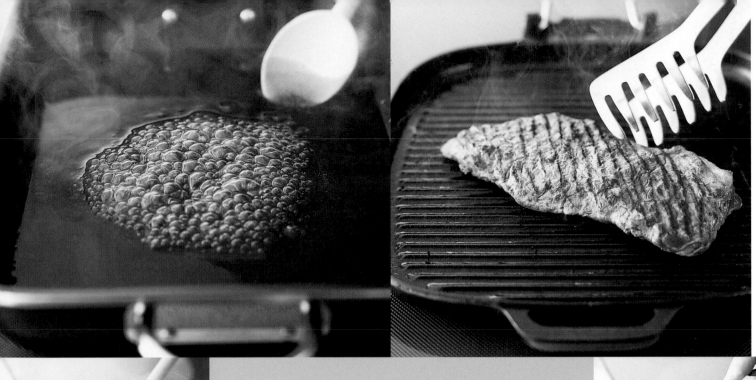

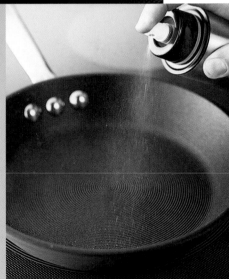

▲ Make a nutritious gravy from the cooking juices of roast meat

◀ Dry-fry minced meat at the beginning of cooking so the fat will melt out. It can then be strained off and discarded

▼ Stir-frying in a wok is quick and very healthy as it uses a very small amount of oil

▲ A cast-iron grill pan gives meat an attractive 'griddled' look, and it needs hardly any fat

▶ To use the minimum amount of oil, spray it from a special mister

▼ Long, slow casserole cooking with vegetables and flavourings makes cheaper cuts of meat very tender

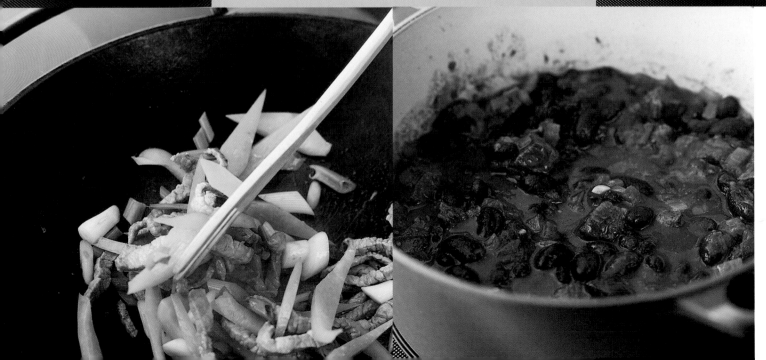

Safe handling

Raw meat can contain bacteria that cause food poisoning, so it must be handled and prepared with care. Follow these simple precautions to keep meat safe.

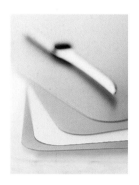

Effective hygiene

To safeguard against bacteria transferring from raw meat to other foods:
- Wash hands, equipment and surfaces before and after handling raw meat.
- Use separate chopping boards and knives for cutting and preparing raw meat.

Storing meat in the fridge

For storage, keep raw meat in its original wrapping, transfer it to a covered dish or wrap it in fresh cling film or foil. Be sure to store raw and cooked meats separately, and place raw meat on the lowest shelf. This will avoid contamination from blood that might drip from the raw meat. Check regularly that your fridge is running no higher than 5°C (41°F).

Storing meat in the freezer

Before shopping, it's a good idea to turn the switch to 'super-freeze' or 'fast-freeze' if you know that you will be freezing a lot of items on your return. If the freezer is very cold – lower than the standard temperature of −18°C – meat will freeze more quickly. This helps to prevent ice crystals from forming, which would otherwise spoil the texture of the meat. Wrap steaks, chops and similar items individually in cling film or foil for easy separation later. Be sure to label each packet clearly with contents and date.

If you are buying meat that is already frozen, make it your last purchase and hurry home to place it in the freezer quickly before it starts to thaw. Taking a cool box with you is a great help, especially in hot weather.

Thawing meat

Meat is best thawed in its wrappings in the fridge, but for speed you can use a microwave oven – check manufacturer's instructions. Meat must be completely thawed before cooking, and once thawed, it should be cooked as soon as possible. Never re-freeze raw meat. However, after cooking, it can be re-frozen. For example, you can thaw frozen braising steak, cook it in a casserole and then freeze the casserole.

Enjoying the leftovers

Any leftovers of cooked meat or a cooked meat dish should be cooled quickly (no longer than 2 hours at room temperature), then covered and placed in the fridge. Once cold they can be frozen. A cooked meat dish should only be reheated once. Make sure it is piping hot in the centre. Frozen cooked meat dishes must be completely thawed before thorough reheating.

Storage times for raw meat

	Fridge	Freezer
beef	3 days	9–12 months
lamb	3 days	6–9 months
pork	2 days	4–6 months
bacon rashers	3 days	1 month
vacuum-packed bacon rashers (unopened)	1–2 weeks	3 months
bacon joints	3 days	3 months
minced meat and offal	1 day	3 months
sausages	3 days	3 months

Note: The freezer storage times are a guide to the times beyond which the flavour and texture of meat may deteriorate, even though it is still safe to eat. It is preferable to have a quick turnover.

Meat stock

A home-made stock beats cubes, powders and pastes from the flavour point of view and it is also salt-free, which many of the chilled stocks sold in supermarkets are not. When you use the stock in a recipe you can add salt to taste, depending on the other ingredients.

Beef, veal or lamb stock

Makes about 1.2 litres (2 pints)

900 g (2 lb) meat bones (beef, veal or lamb), chopped
2 sprigs of fresh thyme
2 sprigs of parsley
1 large bay leaf
7.5 cm (3 in) piece celery
2 onions, roughly chopped
2 celery sticks, roughly chopped
2 carrots, roughly chopped
4 peppercorns

Preparation time: 20 minutes, plus chilling
Cooking time: 5–6 hours

1 Place the bones in a large saucepan and add about 2 litres (3½ pints) water, enough to cover the bones. Bring to the boil, skimming off the scum as it rises to the surface.

2 Tie the thyme, parsley, bay leaf and celery into a bouquet garni and add to the pan with the onions, celery, carrots and peppercorns. Cover and simmer gently for 5–6 hours.

3 Strain the stock through a sieve into a bowl, discarding the bones and vegetables. Leave to cool, then chill until the fat has risen to the surface of the stock and solidified. Lift the fat off the surface and discard before using the stock.

Some more ideas

● If you prefer a richer, brown stock, first roast the bones in a 230ºC (450ºF, gas mark 8) oven for 40 minutes.

● For a non-bone stock, brown a 125 g (4½ oz) piece of stewing beef or lean boneless lamb or pork in 1 tbsp sunflower oil in a large saucepan. Remove the meat, and add 1 onion, 1 carrot and 1 celery stick, all roughly chopped, to the pan. Brown the vegetables, then pour in 2 litres (3½ pints) water and bring to the boil. Replace the meat and heat until simmering again, skimming as necessary, then add 2 bay leaves, 1 sprig each of parsley and fresh thyme, 10 black peppercorns and ½ tsp salt. Reduce the heat, cover and simmer for 2 hours. Strain, cool and remove the fat as above. This will make about 1.2 litres (2 pints).

● After chilling the stock and removing the fat, you can boil it until reduced and concentrated in flavour, then cool and freeze it in ice-cube trays to make frozen 'stock cubes'. These can then be packed together in a freezer bag and used individually – simply add them frozen to hot liquids in soups, casseroles and stews. They will melt almost instantly.

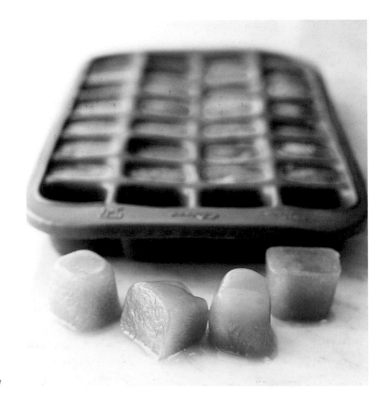

Thai-style stir-fried beef with mango

This colourful dish is bursting with fresh flavours and deliciously contrasting textures. The dressing is completely oil-free, so although both the beef and nuts contain fat and the beef is stir-fried in a little oil, the dish is still light on the fat front. Also, no extra salt is needed because of the spicy dressing and saltiness of soy sauce.

Serves 4

400 g (14 oz) lean steak, such as sirloin

3 garlic cloves, finely chopped

1 tsp caster sugar

2 tsp soy sauce

1½ tbsp sunflower oil

Ginger and honey dressing

2 tsp paprika

2 tsp mild Mexican-style chilli powder

1½ tbsp clear honey

2.5 cm (1 in) piece fresh root ginger, grated

4 tbsp rice vinegar or cider vinegar

juice of 1 lime or lemon

Salad

1 ripe but firm mango, peeled and cut
   into strips

2 ripe but firm plums, sliced

¼ medium-sized red cabbage, shredded

55 g (2 oz) watercress leaves

½ cucumber, cut into matchsticks

½ red pepper, cut into thin strips

3–4 spring onions, cut into diagonal pieces

45 g (1½ oz) mixed fresh mint and coriander

2 tbsp coarsely chopped roasted unsalted
   peanuts

Preparation time: 30 minutes

Cooking time: about 10 minutes

1 To make the dressing, put the paprika, chilli powder, honey, ginger and vinegar in a saucepan and slowly add 250 ml (8½ fl oz) of water, stirring. Bring to the boil, then reduce the heat and simmer for 5 minutes. Remove from the heat and stir in the lime or lemon juice. Set aside.

2 Combine all the salad ingredients, except the peanuts, in a large shallow serving dish and toss gently together until evenly mixed. Set aside.

3 Cut the steak into thin strips for stir-frying. Put the steak in a bowl with the garlic, sugar and soy sauce and mix together so the strips of steak are seasoned. Heat a wok or non-stick pan on a high heat, then add the oil. Add the beef and stir-fry until the strips are evenly browned and cooked to taste.

4 Spoon the stir-fried beef over the top of the salad. Drizzle the dressing over the top and sprinkle with the peanuts. Serve immediately.

Some more ideas

● Add cubes of fresh or canned pineapple (canned in juice rather than syrup) or kiwi fruit to the salad, to increase the fruit content.

● Spice up the salad with very thin strips of fresh red chilli – particularly if you have a cold, as scientists have suggested that eating chillies can help to alleviate nasal congestion.

● For a vegetarian version, omit the beef and increase the quantity of peanuts to 150 g (5½ oz). Peanuts are an excellent source of protein and contain less saturated fat than meat.

Plus points

● All orange and red fruit and vegetables, such as mango, red cabbage and red peppers, are excellent sources of beta-carotene and vitamin C – both antioxidants that help to protect against heart disease and cancer. The vitamin C aids the absorption of valuable iron from the steak.

● Apart from adding its delicious spiciness to the dressing, ginger also aids digestion.

Each serving provides

kcal 265, protein 27 g, fat 8 g (of which saturated fat 3 g), carbohydrate 20 g (of which sugars 18 g), fibre 3 g

✓✓✓	B_{12}, C
✓✓	A, B_6, iron, zinc
✓	B_1, B_2, E, folate, niacin, copper

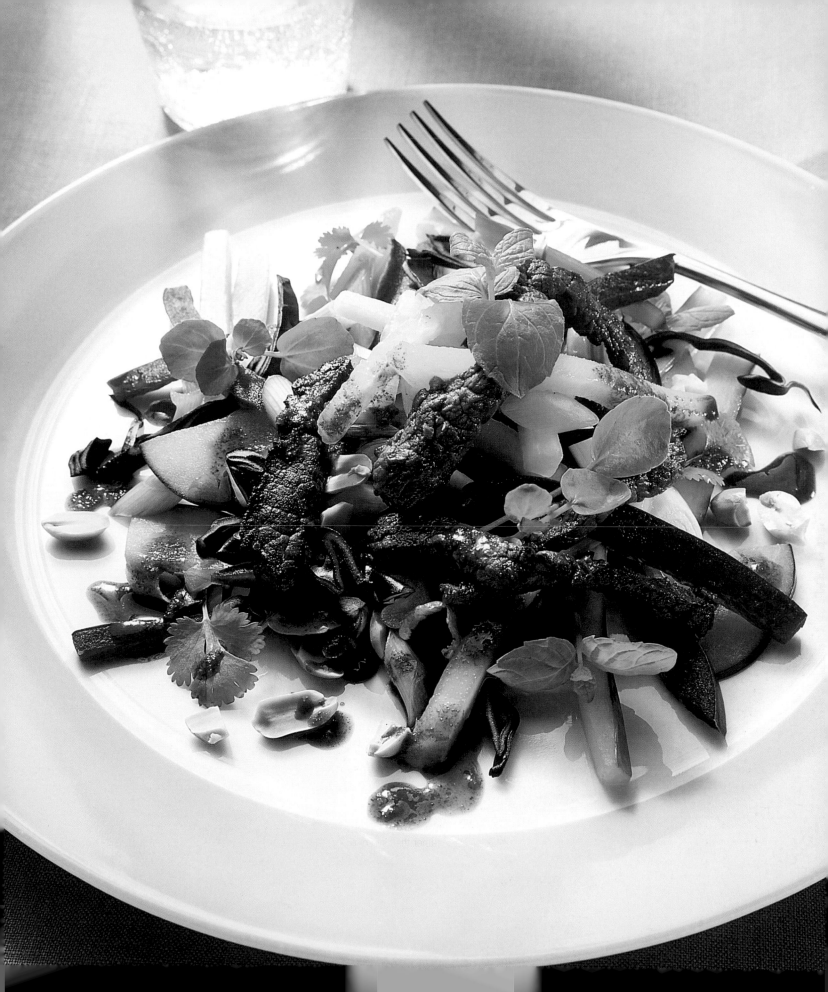

Aromatic beef curry

This will satisfy even the most demanding curry addict. Lean and tender sirloin steak is quickly cooked with lots of spices, tomatoes, mushrooms and spinach, with yogurt added to give a luxurious feel. Served with cardamom-spiced rice, it makes a really healthy and nutritious meal.

Serves 4

1 tbsp sunflower oil

1 large onion, thinly sliced

150 g (5½ oz) button mushrooms, sliced

400 g (14 oz) sirloin steak, trimmed of fat and cut into thin strips

1½ tsp bottled chopped root ginger in oil, drained

2 garlic cloves, crushed

½ tsp crushed dried chillies

2 tsp ground coriander

¼ tsp ground cardamom

½ tsp turmeric

¼ tsp grated nutmeg

1 can chopped tomatoes, about 400g

1 tsp cornflour mixed with 1 tbsp water

300 g (10½ oz) plain whole-milk yogurt

1 tbsp clear honey

125 g (4½ oz) young spinach leaves

juice of ½ lime

2 tbsp chopped fresh coriander, plus extra leaves to garnish

Cardamom rice

340 g (12 oz) basmati rice, well rinsed

1 cinnamon stick

8 whole green cardamom pods, cracked

juice of ½ lemon

salt

Preparation time: 10 minutes
Cooking time: 20 minutes

1 Heat the oil in a large saucepan and add the onion and mushrooms. Cook over a high heat for 2 minutes or until the onion slices begin to colour.

2 Add the beef together with the ginger, garlic, chillies, ground coriander, cardamom, turmeric and nutmeg. Cook for 2 minutes, stirring well, then add the tomatoes with their juice and the cornflour mixture. Bring to the boil, stirring. Stir in the yogurt and honey. Bring back to the boil, then reduce the heat, cover and simmer gently for 20 minutes.

3 Meanwhile, prepare the cardamom rice. Put 450 ml (15 fl oz) cold water in a saucepan and bring to the boil. Add the rice, cinnamon stick and cardamom pods. Bring back to the boil, then cover tightly and cook for 10 minutes or until the rice is tender. Drain off any excess water and return the rice to the saucepan. Stir in the lemon juice and keep covered until the curry is ready to serve.

4 Stir the spinach, lime juice and chopped coriander into the curry and allow the leaves to wilt down into the sauce. To serve, spoon the curry over the rice and garnish with fresh coriander leaves.

Plus points

- Cardamom is believed to be helpful for digestive problems, such as indigestion, flatulence and stomach cramps.
- Mushrooms are low in fat and calories and provide useful amounts of the B vitamins niacin, B_6 and folate. They are also a good source of copper.
- Along with its many other nutritional benefits, beef provides vitamins from the B group and is a useful source of vitamin D, which is found in relatively few foods.

Each serving provides

kcal 590, protein 36 g, fat 11 g (of which saturated fat 4 g), carbohydrate 86 g (of which sugars 16 g), fibre 2 g

✓✓✓	iron, zinc
✓✓	A, B_6, B_{12}, C, calcium, copper, potassium
✓	B_1, B_2, E, folate, selenium

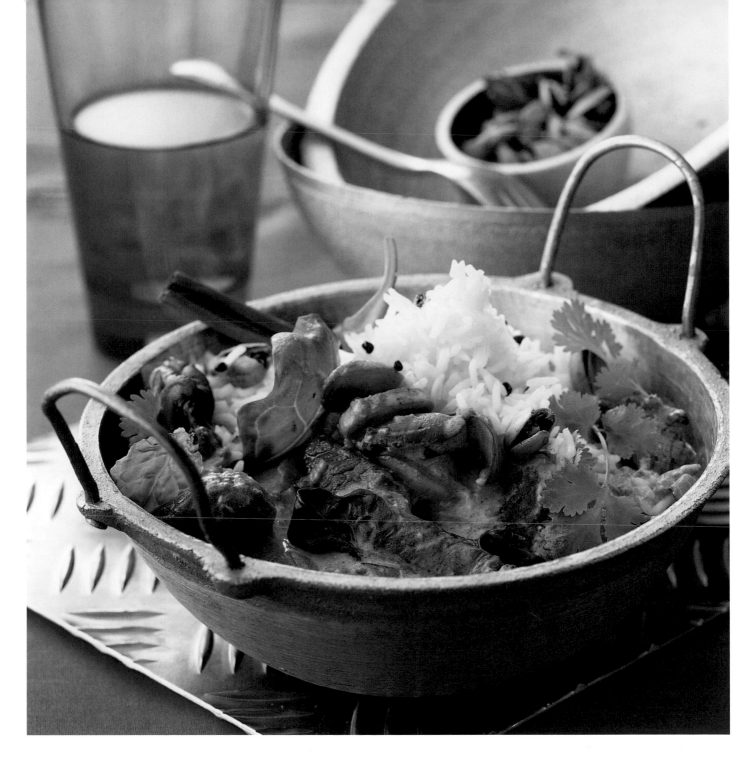

Some more ideas

• If you like a hot curry, add a halved fresh red chilli to the sauce towards the end of the cooking time. The chilli can be left in the sauce or discarded before serving.

• Make a Thai-style pork and potato curry. Soften the onion and garlic in the oil with 200 g (7 oz) new potatoes, scrubbed and cut into small cubes, for 5 minutes. Stir in 300 g (10½ oz) pork fillet (tenderloin), thinly sliced, and 2 tbsp Thai red curry paste. Cook for 2 minutes or until browned. Add the canned chopped tomatoes, 150 ml (5 fl oz) vegetable stock and 100 g (3½ oz) ready-to-eat dried apricots, chopped. Bring to the boil, then cover and simmer for 20 minutes or until the pork is tender. Mix ½ tsp cornflour with 1 tbsp cold water and stir into the curry with 150 g (5½ oz) plain whole-milk yogurt, 1 tsp caster sugar and the spinach. Cook until the leaves wilt down into the sauce, then serve on plain rice.

Perfect pot roast

This long-simmered, one-pot meal is wonderfully satisfying. It can be prepared ahead, so it's perfect for family dinners as well as informal entertaining. Serve with a crunchy mixed salad and bread.

Serves 6

1 tsp extra virgin olive oil

1 kg (2¼ lb) piece boneless beef chuck, about 7.5 cm (3 in) thick, trimmed of fat and tied

2 large onions, finely chopped

1 celery stick, finely chopped

3 garlic cloves, crushed

250 ml (8½ fl oz) dry red or white wine

1 can chopped tomatoes, about 225 g

1 large carrot, grated

1 tsp chopped fresh thyme

450 ml (15 fl oz) beef stock, preferably home-made (see page 153)

600 g (1 lb 5 oz) new potatoes, scrubbed and quartered

340 g (12 oz) celeriac, cut into 2.5 cm (1 in) cubes

340 g (12 oz) swede, cut into 2.5 cm (1 in) cubes

4 carrots, about 280 g (10 oz) in total, sliced

salt and pepper

3 tbsp chopped parsley to garnish

Preparation and cooking time: 4 hours

Each serving provides

kcal 399, protein 43 g, fat 12 g (of which saturated fat 4 g), carbohydrate 33 g (of which sugars 15 g), fibre 8 g

✓✓✓	A, B$_1$, B$_6$, B$_{12}$, C, folate, niacin, zinc
✓✓	B$_2$, iron
✓	selenium

1 Preheat the oven to 160°C (325°F, gas mark 3). Heat the oil in a large flameproof casserole. Add the beef and brown it over a moderately high heat for 6–8 minutes or until it is well coloured on all sides. Remove the meat to a plate.

2 Reduce the heat to moderate. Add the onions, celery and garlic and cook, stirring frequently, for about 3 minutes or until the onions begin to soften. Add the wine and let it bubble for about 1 minute, then add the tomatoes with their juice and the grated carrot. Cook for a further 2 minutes.

3 Return the beef to the casserole together with any juices that have collected on the plate and the chopped thyme. Tuck a piece of greaseproof paper or foil around the top of the meat, turning back the corners so that it doesn't touch the liquid, then cover with a tight-fitting lid. Transfer the casserole to the oven and cook for 2½ hours.

4 About 20 minutes before the end of the cooking time, bring the stock to the boil in a deep saucepan with a lid. Add the potatoes, celeriac, swede and sliced carrots. Cover and simmer gently for 12–15 minutes or until they are starting to become tender.

5 Meanwhile, remove the beef from the casserole and set aside. Remove any fat from the cooking liquid, either by spooning it off or by using a bulb baster, then purée the casseroled vegetables and liquid in a blender or food processor until smooth. Season to taste.

6 Drain the potatoes and other root vegetables, reserving the liquid. Make a layer of the vegetables in the casserole, put the beef on top and add the remaining root vegetables and their cooking liquid. Pour over the puréed sauce. Cover the casserole and return to the oven to cook for 20 minutes or until the root vegetables are tender.

7 Remove the beef to a carving board, cover and leave to rest for 10 minutes. Keep the vegetables and sauce in the oven turned down to low.

8 Carve the beef and arrange on warmed plates with the vegetables and sauce. Sprinkle with the parsley and serve immediately.

Plus points

● Swede is a member of the cruciferous family of vegetables. It is a useful source of vitamin C and beta-carotene and rich in phytochemicals that are believed to help protect against cancer.

● A freshly dug potato may contain as much as ten times more vitamin C than one that has been stored.

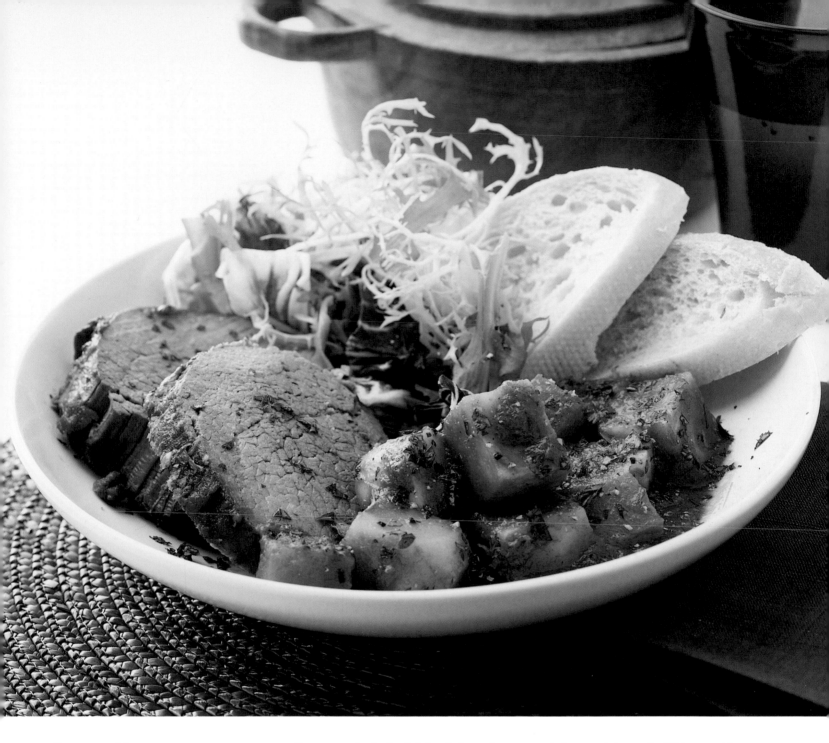

Some more ideas

• Brisket can be used instead of chuck, as can topside of beef.

• Any leftover beef can be chopped or shredded and mixed with the sauce and/or a freshly made tomato sauce, then served over spaghetti or other pasta.

• Substitute a boneless gammon joint, soaked if necessary, for the beef. Soften 1 chopped onion in 1 tsp extra virgin olive oil with 2 chopped garlic cloves (omit the celery). Add the wine (use white) and gammon (there is no need to brown it first). Omit the tomatoes, grated carrot and thyme and add 750 ml (1¼ pints) unsalted vegetable stock, 3 cloves, 1½ tsp mustard powder and 1 strip of orange zest. Cover and simmer for 1¼ hours, adding the root vegetables after 25 minutes. When the meat is cooked, transfer it to a carving board as in step 7. Strain the cooking liquid and remove the fat, then boil rapidly until reduced to 600 ml (1 pint). Stir in 2 tbsp cornflour mixed with 1½ tbsp cold water and boil until the liquid has thickened. Finish as in the main recipe.

Sesame pork and noodle salad

With its typical Chinese flavours – ginger, sesame, soy sauce and rice vinegar – this salad makes a delectable lunch or supper dish. It is very nutritious as most of the vegetables are raw. For the best effect, cut the pepper, carrot and spring onions about the same thickness as the noodles.

Serves 4

400 g (14 oz) pork fillet (tenderloin)

2 tsp grated fresh root ginger

1 large garlic clove, finely chopped

1½ tsp toasted sesame oil

3 tbsp light soy sauce

2 tbsp dry sherry

2 tsp rice vinegar

225 g (8 oz) fine Chinese egg noodles

1 red pepper, seeded and cut into matchstick strips

1 large carrot, cut into matchstick strips

6 spring onions, cut into matchstick strips

250 g (8½ oz) bean sprouts

150 g (5½ oz) mange-tout

2 tbsp sesame seeds

1 tbsp sunflower oil

Preparation and cooking time: 45 minutes

Each serving provides

kcal 454, protein 33 g, fat 13 g (of which saturated fat 3 g), carbohydrate 51 g (of which sugars 9 g), fibre 5 g

✓✓✓	A, B₁, B₆, B₁₂, C, E, niacin
✓✓	B₆, folate, copper, iron, zinc
✓	potassium, selenium

1 Trim all visible fat from the pork fillet. Cut the pork across into slices about 5 cm (2 in) thick, then cut each slice into thin strips.

2 Combine the ginger, garlic, sesame oil, soy sauce, sherry and vinegar in a bowl. Add the pork strips and toss to coat, then leave to marinate while you prepare the other ingredients.

3 Put the noodles in a large mixing bowl and pour over enough boiling water to cover generously. Leave to soak for about 4 minutes, or according to the packet instructions, until tender. Drain well and tip back into the bowl. Add the red pepper, carrot, spring onions and bean sprouts.

4 Drop the mange-tout into a pan of boiling water and cook for about 1 minute or until just tender but still crisp. Drain and refresh under cold running water. Add the mange-tout to the noodle and vegetable mixture and toss to mix. Set aside.

5 Toast the sesame seeds in a large frying pan over a moderate heat for 1–2 minutes or until golden, stirring constantly. Tip the seeds onto a piece of kitchen paper. Heat the sunflower oil in the frying pan, increase the heat slightly and add the pork with its marinade. Stir-fry for 4–5 minutes or until the pork is no longer pink.

6 Add the strips of pork and any cooking juices to the noodle and vegetable mixture, and stir gently to combine. Divide among 4 shallow bowls, sprinkle with the toasted sesame seeds and serve.

Plus points

● In the past, pork has had a reputation for being rather fatty, but this is certainly no longer the case. Over the last 20 years, in response to consumer demands, farmers have been breeding leaner pigs. Pork now contains considerably less fat, and it also contains higher levels of the 'good' polyunsaturated fats. The average fat content of lean pork is less than 3%, much the same as that contained in skinless chicken breast.

● The vegetables in this dish provide a good variety of different nutrients, in particular vitamin C and beta-carotene.

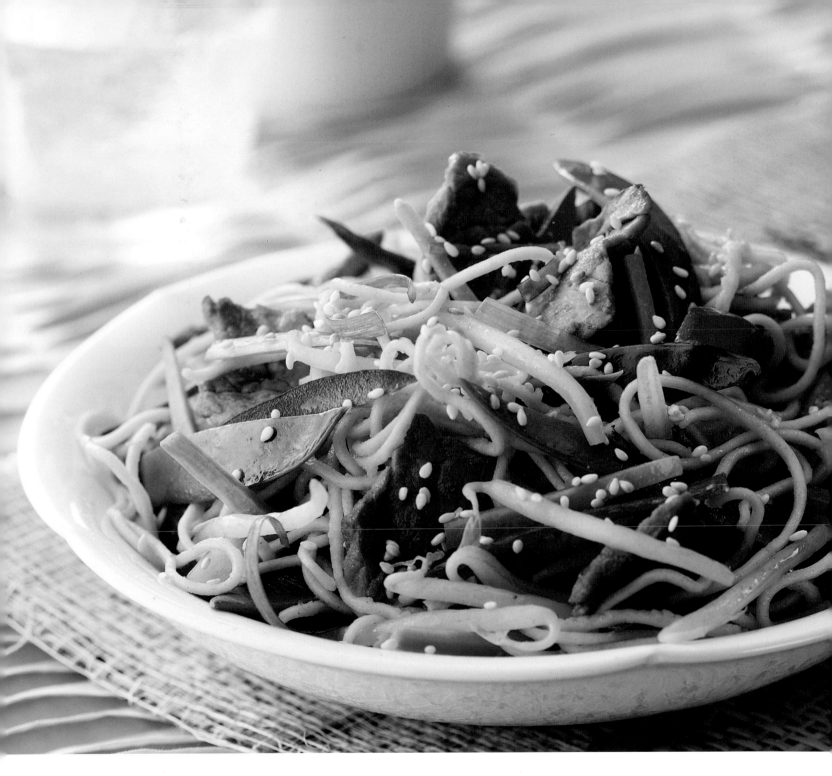

Another idea

● For a sesame pork and rice noodle salad, use 250 g (8½ oz) rice noodles instead of egg noodles. Soak them as in the main recipe, then mix with the red pepper, carrot and spring onions (omit the bean sprouts and mange-tout).

Cut off the leaves from 200 g (7 oz) small pak choy and reserve; cut the stalks across into 1 cm (½ in) thick slices. Drain the marinade from the pork and reserve. Heat 1 tbsp extra virgin olive oil in a frying pan and stir-fry the pork with 125 g (4½ oz) baby corn, cut in half

lengthways, for 1½ minutes. Add the pak choy leaves and stalks, and stir-fry for 1 minute or until the leaves just begin to wilt and the pork is cooked. Tip into the bowl with the noodles and vegetables. Heat the reserved marinade in the frying pan, pour it over the salad and toss well.

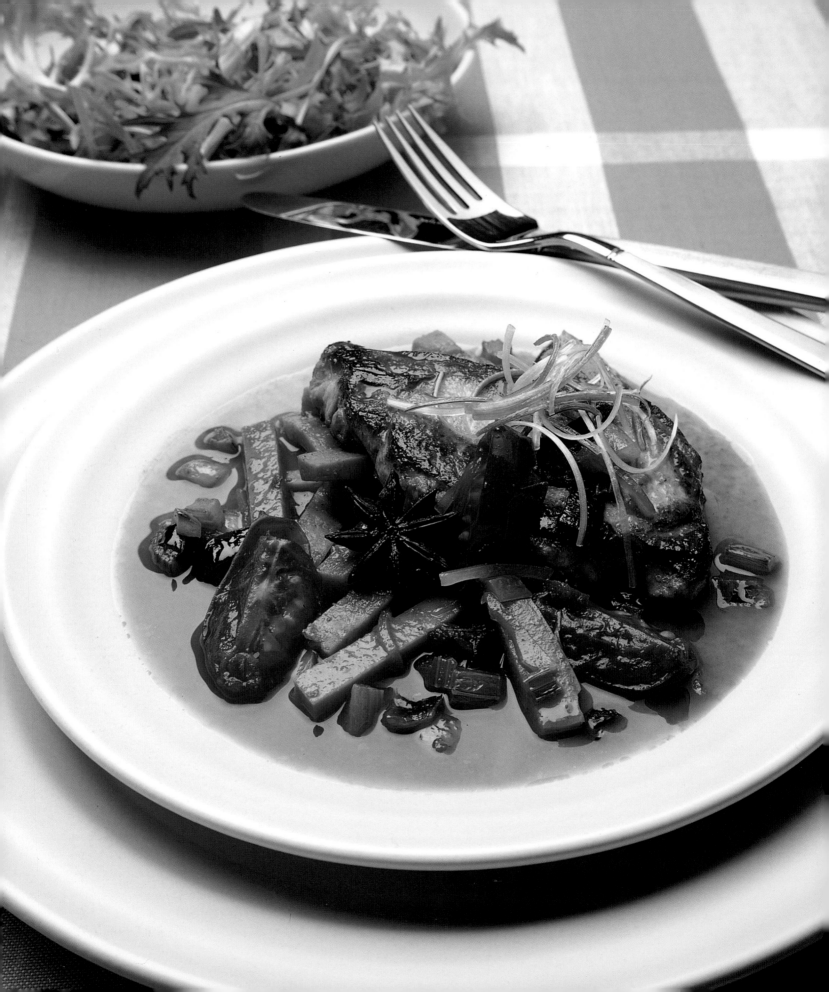

Spiced pork with sweet potatoes

This thoroughly modern casserole is a delicious example of fusion cooking, marrying ingredients and flavours from diverse cuisines. Oriental spices, sweet potatoes and fruit flavours go very well with the lean pork. Add bean sprouts and spring onions to a simple green salad to make a crisp, refreshing accompaniment.

Serves 4

1 tbsp sunflower oil

4 pork loin steaks or boneless pork chops, about 140 g (5 oz) each, trimmed of fat

1 red onion, coarsely chopped

2 celery sticks, chopped

1 large orange-fleshed sweet potato, about 400 g (14 oz), peeled and cut into sticks

150 ml (5 fl oz) sweetened cranberry juice

150 ml (5 fl oz) chicken stock, preferably home-made (see page 113)

1 piece of preserved stem ginger, drained and cut into fine sticks

1 tbsp thick-cut orange marmalade

1 tbsp dry sherry

1 tsp Chinese five-spice powder

2 star anise

4 plum tomatoes, quartered lengthways

salt and pepper

3 spring onions, shredded, to garnish

Preparation time: 30 minutes

Cooking time: about 30 minutes

Each serving provides

kcal 340, protein 34 g, fat 9 g (of which saturated fat 2 g), carbohydrate 32 g (of which sugars 16 g), fibre 4 g

✓✓✓	B₁, C
✓✓	A, B₆, B₁₂, E, iron, phosphorus, zinc
✓	B₂, folate, niacin, selenium

1 Heat the oil in a large flameproof casserole or deep sauté pan. Add the pork steaks and brown them for 3–4 minutes on each side. Transfer the pork to a plate and set aside.

2 Add the onion and celery to the oil remaining in the casserole and cook, stirring, over a moderate heat for 2–3 minutes. Add the sweet potato, cover the pan and sweat the vegetables for 3–4 minutes or until softened.

3 Stir in the cranberry juice drink, stock, ginger, marmalade, sherry, five-spice powder, star anise and a little salt and pepper. Bring to the boil, then reduce the heat and return the pork to the casserole. Cover and cook gently for 15 minutes.

4 Add the tomatoes to the casserole, cover and cook gently for a further 5 minutes or until the tomatoes are lightly cooked, but still hold their shape. Taste for seasoning, adding more salt and pepper if necessary, and serve, garnished with spring onions.

Some more ideas

• Add 400 g (14 oz) cubed pumpkin or butternut squash instead of the sweet potato, and 1 small bulb of fennel, chopped, instead of the celery sticks.

• Tomato rice goes well with this casserole. Bring 200 ml (7 fl oz) water to the boil and add 225 g (8 oz) rinsed basmati rice, 1 can chopped tomatoes, about 400g, with the juice and 4 chopped sun-dried tomatoes. Cover and cook gently for 10 minutes or until the rice is tender and has absorbed all the water.

• For a rich fruit casserole, add 200 g (7 oz) pitted, ready-to-eat prunes and 2 cored and thickly sliced dessert apples instead of the tomatoes. Omit the sherry.

Plus points

• Sweet potatoes have a delicious natural sweetness that intensifies during storage and cooking. Although they contain slightly more calories than ordinary white potatoes – sweet potatoes have 87 kcal per 100 g (3½ oz), white potatoes 75 kcal – they are low in fat.

• Sweet potatoes are also an excellent source of beta-carotene and they provide good amounts of vitamins C and E.

• Lean pork has a lower fat content than beef or lamb. It is a good source of zinc and it provides useful amounts of iron.

Mexican pork

Lean pork marinated in a zesty Mexican spice and citrus mixture is griddled until succulent, then sliced thinly and served in soft flour tortillas. The finishing touch is a fresh avocado salsa.

Serves 4

400 g (14 oz) pork fillet (tenderloin), trimmed of fat

2 tsp extra virgin olive oil

2 onions, thickly sliced

2 peppers (1 red and 1 yellow), seeded and cut into chunks

4 large tomato-flavoured flour tortillas

Citrus marinade

3 garlic cloves, chopped

juice of 1 lime

juice of ½ grapefruit or 1 small blood orange

2 tsp mild chilli powder

1 tsp paprika

½ tsp ground cumin

¼ tsp dried oregano or mixed herbs such as herbes de Provence

pinch of ground cinnamon

3 spring onions, chopped

1 tbsp extra virgin olive oil

Avocado and radish salsa

1 avocado

3 radishes, diced

1 garlic clove, chopped

1 ripe tomato, diced

juice of ½ lime, or to taste

1 spring onion, chopped

1 tbsp chopped fresh coriander

salt and pepper

Preparation and cooking time: about 50 minutes, plus at least 30 minutes marinating

1 Mix together all the ingredients for the marinade in a shallow dish. Add the pork fillet and turn to coat. Cover and marinate for at least 30 minutes, or overnight.

2 To prepare the salsa, halve, stone and peel the avocado, then mash the flesh in a bowl. Add the remaining salsa ingredients and mix well, then season to taste. Cover and chill until serving time.

3 Preheat the oven to 180°C (350°F, gas mark 4). Heat a ridged cast-iron grill pan or non-stick frying pan over a moderate heat until hot. Remove the meat from its marinade and pat it dry with kitchen paper. Brush the pan with the olive oil, then add the pork and sear on all sides.

4 Push the pork to one side and add the onions and peppers to the pan. Cook for 12–15 minutes or until the vegetables are tender and lightly charred and the pork is cooked through.

5 Meanwhile, wrap the tortillas, stacked up, in foil and put into the oven to warm for 5–10 minutes.

6 Remove the grill pan from the heat. Lift out the pork and cut it into thin strips, then return it to the pan and mix with the onions and peppers.

7 To serve, pile the pork, onions and peppers into the tortillas, roll into cone shapes and top with salsa.

Plus points

• Avocados are high in calories, mainly from the monounsaturated fat they contain. This is the same type of fat that makes olive oil so highly recommended for the prevention of coronary heart disease. Avocados are also a useful source of vitamin E, an important antioxidant, and of vitamin B_6.

• Cooking garlic destroys some of the allicin, one of the beneficial phytochemicals it contains, so for maximum health benefits it is best eaten raw.

• There is plenty of vitamin C in this dish, from the peppers and tomatoes in particular. Vitamin C plays a major role in maintaining a healthy immune system.

Each serving provides

kcal 437, protein 30 g, fat 17 g (of which saturated fat 4 g), carbohydrate 46 g (of which sugars 11 g), fibre 6 g

✓✓✓	A, B_1, B_6, B_{12}, C, E, niacin
✓✓	folate, iron
✓	calcium, potassium, zinc

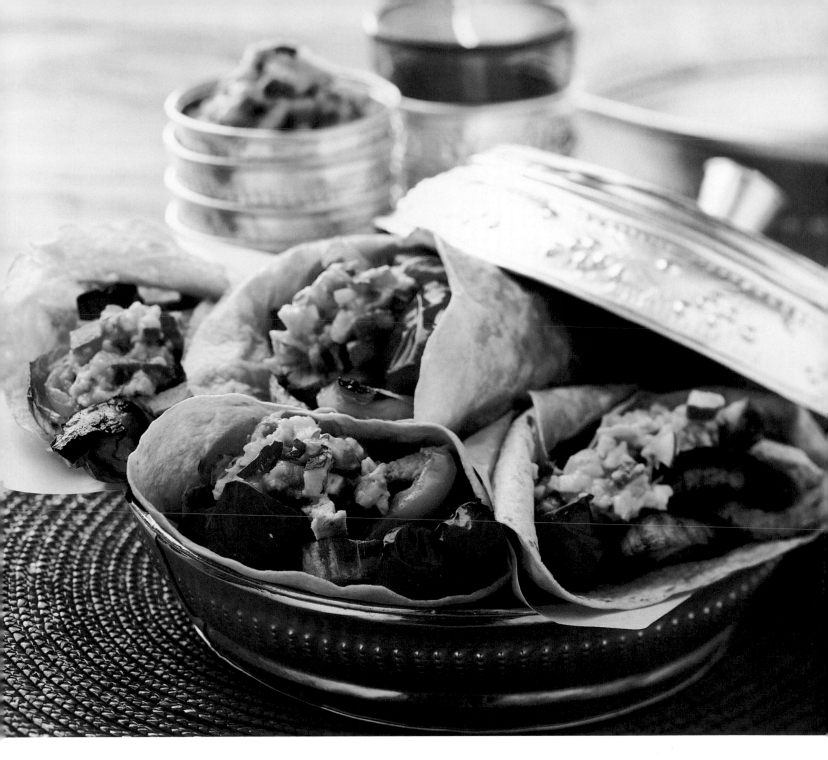

Some more ideas

• Fillet, rump or sirloin of beef can be used instead of pork.

• If you can't get tomato-flavoured flour tortillas, any kind of soft flour tortilla can be used. If you prefer, you can warm them through on top of the cooker. Spray or sprinkle each one with a few drops of water, then heat in a non-stick frying pan for 15–30 seconds on each side. As each tortilla is done, wrap loosely in a clean tea towel to keep warm.

• For a change from the avocado salsa, serve with a fruity salsa. Mix together 300 g (10½ oz) sliced seedless green grapes, 1 seeded and diced satsuma or other small citrus fruit, 1 diced (unpeeled) small crisp pear, ¼ seeded and chopped fresh red chilli, 3 chopped radishes, 1 chopped garlic clove, 1 thinly sliced spring onion, 1 tbsp each chopped fresh coriander and mint, 1 tsp sugar or honey and the juice of ½ lime or lemon. Serve chilled.

Oriental lamb and plum wraps

Packed with crisp raw vegetables and juicy fruit slices, these wraps make a refreshing alternative to rich Peking duck in a Chinese meal. They are ideal for entertaining because the lamb is equally good hot or at room temperature. Serve as a main dish, or as a starter for 8, with a bowl of thinly sliced cucumber.

Serves 4 (makes 16 wraps)

500 g (1 lb 2 oz) lean lamb neck fillets, trimmed of fat

1½ tbsp soy sauce

6 spring onions

¼ cucumber, about 150 g (5½ oz)

6 sweet red plums, about 340 g (12 oz) in total

16 large, crisp romaine or cos lettuce leaves

16 rice paper wrappers

Sesame dipping sauce

5 tsp toasted sesame oil

1 tbsp finely grated fresh root ginger

½ tbsp sesame seeds

2 tsp soy sauce

1 tsp caster sugar

Preparation and cooking time: 35 minutes

Each serving provides

kcal 360, protein 26 g, fat 22 g (of which saturated fat 9 g), carbohydrate 15 g (of which sugars 9 g), fibre 3 g

✓✓✓	B₁, B₆, B₁₂, E, niacin, zinc
✓✓	copper, magnesium
✓	A, B₂, C, folate, iron, potassium, selenium

1 First make the dipping sauce. Put all the ingredients in a screw-top jar and shake well. Set aside.

2 Cut each lamb fillet lengthways into three, then cut each piece into long, thin slices. Mix the slices in a bowl with the soy sauce and set aside.

3 Cut the spring onions lengthways in half, then shred them finely. Set a few aside for garnish and put the rest on a large platter. Cut the cucumber lengthways in half and scoop out the seeds with a teaspoon, then thinly slice the cucumber halves into half moons. Add to the platter.

4 Halve the plums and remove the stones. Cut the plums into long, thin slices. Add to the platter with the spring onions and cucumber.

5 Rinse and dry the lettuce leaves and remove the central stalks. Tear off 16 pieces large enough to fit in the centre of the rice paper wrappers. Finely shred the remaining lettuce and add to the platter of vegetables and plums.

6 Heat a large non-stick frying pan over a moderately high heat until hot. Add half of the lamb slices and stir-fry for 3–5 minutes or until the meat is cooked to your liking. Using a draining spoon, transfer the meat to a plate. Stir-fry the remaining lamb and spoon onto the plate. Keep warm.

7 Pour 1 cm (½ in) hot water into a dish large enough to hold the wrappers. Place a clean tea towel on the work surface. Working with 1 wrapper at a time, dip it in the water to soften for 20–25 seconds, then transfer to the tea towel and pat dry. Immediately put a lettuce leaf in the centre of the wrapper. Top with a spoonful of lamb, then some spring onions, cucumber, plums and shredded lettuce. Fold in both sides of the wrapper, then roll up. Repeat, to make 16 rolls altogether.

8 Shake the dipping sauce, then pour it into a small bowl. Arrange the wraps on plates and scatter over the remaining spring onions. Serve with the dipping sauce handed separately.

Plus points

● Although lamb still tends to contain more fat than other meats, changes in breeding, feeding and butchery techniques mean that lean cuts only contain about one-third of the fat that they would have 20 years ago. More of the fat is monounsaturated, which is good news for healthy hearts.

● Plums offer useful amounts of fibre and beta-carotene.

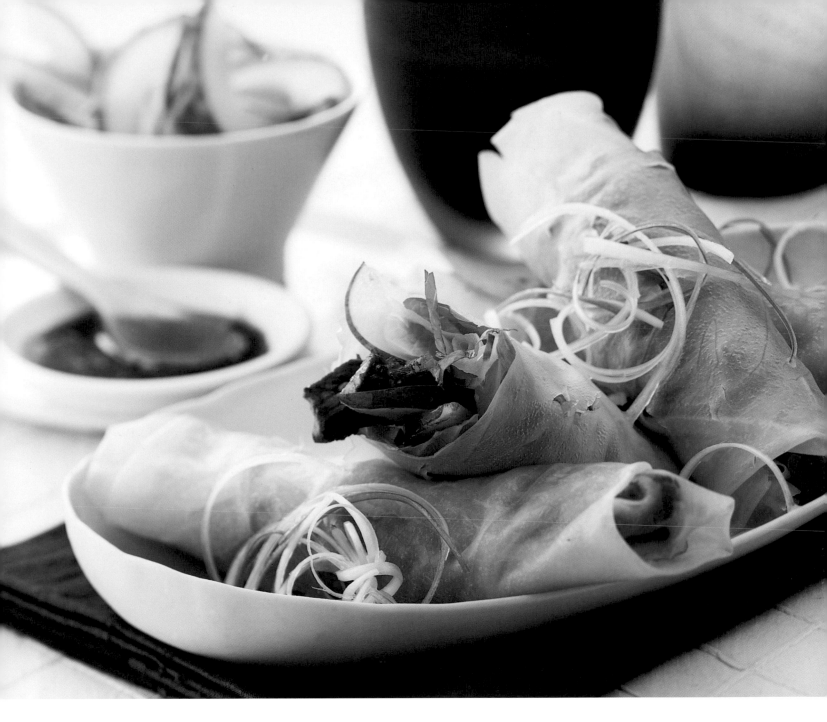

Some more ideas

- This is a good way to use up leftover roast lamb, beef or pork. Cut it into thin strips.
- Instead of the cucumber and plums, use 300 g (10½ oz) each grated carrots and courgettes.
- Other vitamin-packed raw vegetables to use with either the lamb, beef or pork versions include finely shredded peppers, bean sprouts, alfalfa, shredded mange-tout, and thinly sliced button mushrooms or enoki mushrooms.
- Sprinkle the filling with finely chopped fresh coriander, chives or parsley before rolling up the wrappers.
- Chopped, drained canned water chestnuts will add extra texture to the filling.
- Chilled mango or papaya slices can be used instead of the plums.
- Pickled ginger slices, available from Japanese food stores and some supermarkets, can replace the plums for a hot, zingy flavour.
- For an extra kick, spread a tiny dab of wasabi (Japanese horseradish) on each lettuce leaf.
- For an instant dipping sauce, you can use bottled plum sauce.
- For a spicy dipping sauce, add a good pinch of crushed dried chillies.

Greek lamb kebabs

Cubes of lamb flavoured with a mixture of garlic, lemon and fresh oregano are cooked on skewers and served with a Greek-style tomato and cabbage salad and pitta bread for a deliciously aromatic main dish.

Serves 4

1 tbsp extra virgin olive oil
2 large garlic cloves, crushed
juice of ½ lemon
1 tbsp chopped fresh oregano
450 g (1 lb) boneless leg of lamb, trimmed of
     all fat and cut into 2.5 cm (1 in) cubes
salt and pepper

Greek-style salad

6 tomatoes, thickly sliced
1 red onion, finely chopped
1 baby white cabbage, about 225 g (8 oz),
     core removed and thinly shredded
4 tbsp chopped fresh mint
¼ cucumber, halved and thinly sliced
juice of ½ lemon
1 tbsp extra virgin olive oil

To serve

4 pitta breads, cut into triangles
Greek-style yogurt (optional)

Preparation and cooking time: 30 minutes

Each serving provides

kcal 470, protein 32 g, fat 16 g (of which saturated fat 5 g), carbohydrate 52 g (of which sugars 10 g), fibre 5 g

✓✓✓	B₁₂, C
✓✓	A, B₆, E, iron, zinc
✓	B₁, folate, niacin, potassium

1 Preheat the grill or heat a ridged cast-iron grill pan. Put the olive oil, garlic, lemon juice and chopped oregano in a bowl and stir to mix together. Add the cubes of lamb and turn until very well coated. Thread the cubes onto 4 skewers.

2 Cook the lamb under the grill or on the grill pan for 7–8 minutes or until tender, turning frequently. Towards the end of cooking, warm the pitta bread under the grill or on the grill pan.

3 Meanwhile, make the salad. Put all the ingredients in a salad bowl and season with salt and pepper to taste. Toss together gently.

4 Serve the kebabs with the salad, pitta bread and yogurt.

Another idea

• To make chilli beef kebabs, use 4 beef fillet or sirloin steaks, about 400 g (14 oz) in total, cut into 2.5 cm (1 in) cubes. Mix together 1 tsp chilli powder, ¼ tsp ground cumin, 1 tbsp extra virgin olive oil, 2 large garlic cloves, crushed, the juice of ½ lime and seasoning to taste. Coat the steak cubes on all sides with the spice mixture, then thread onto 4 skewers. Cook with 1 large sliced onion under the grill or on the ridged grill pan for 4–6 minutes or until tender, turning frequently. Take the skewers from the pan and continue cooking the onion until tender. Meanwhile, to make the salad, mix 1 can red kidney beans, about 410g, drained and rinsed, with 1 large diced avocado, the juice of 1 lime, 1½ tbsp extra virgin olive oil, ½ red onion, very finely chopped, 1 fresh green chilli, seeded and finely chopped, 300 g (10½ oz) cherry tomatoes, halved, and 15 g (½ oz) chopped fresh coriander. Season to taste and add a pinch of caster sugar. Remove the steak from the skewers and divide with the onion among 8 warmed flour tortillas. Add 1 tbsp bottled Caesar salad dressing and some of the salad to each tortilla, and roll up into wraps. Serve with the rest of the salad.

Plus points

• Lamb is a rich source of B vitamins, needed for a healthy nervous system. It is also a good source of zinc and iron.
• Cabbage belongs to a family of vegetables that contain a number of different phytochemicals that may help to protect against breast cancer. They are also a good source of vitamin C and among the richest vegetable sources of folate.
• Onions, along with chicory, leeks, garlic, Jerusalem artichokes, asparagus, barley and bananas, contain a type of dietary fibre called fructoligosaccarides (FOS). This is believed to stimulate the growth of friendly bacteria in the gut while inhibiting the growth of bad bacteria.

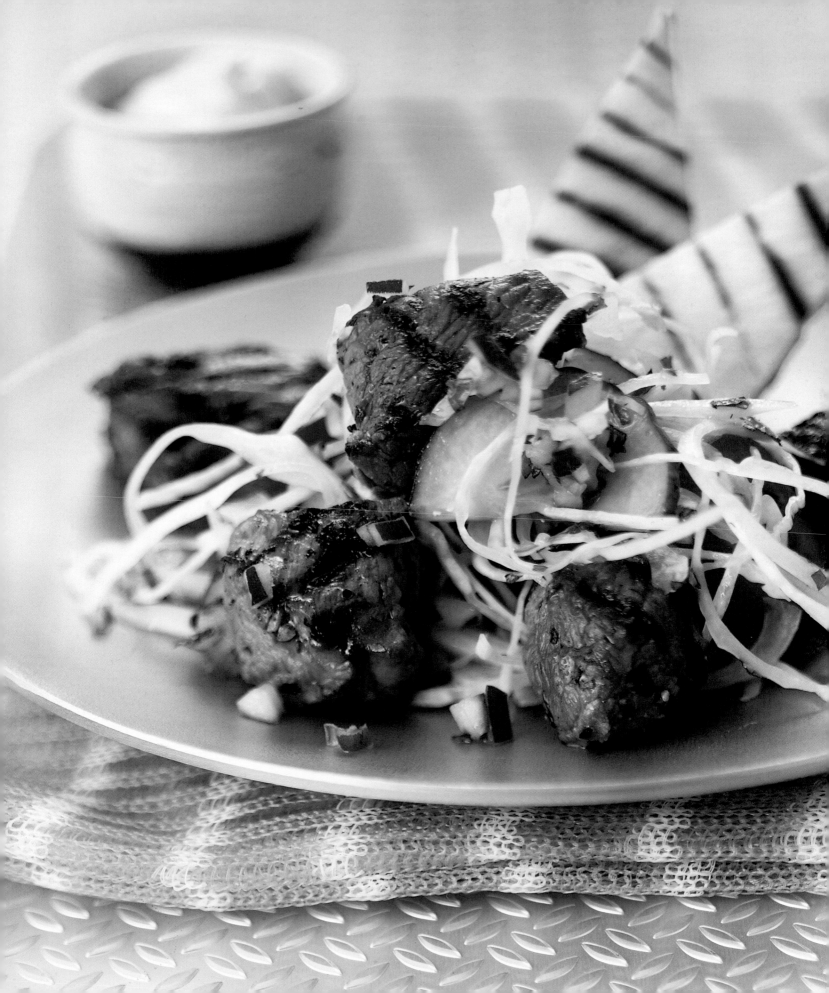

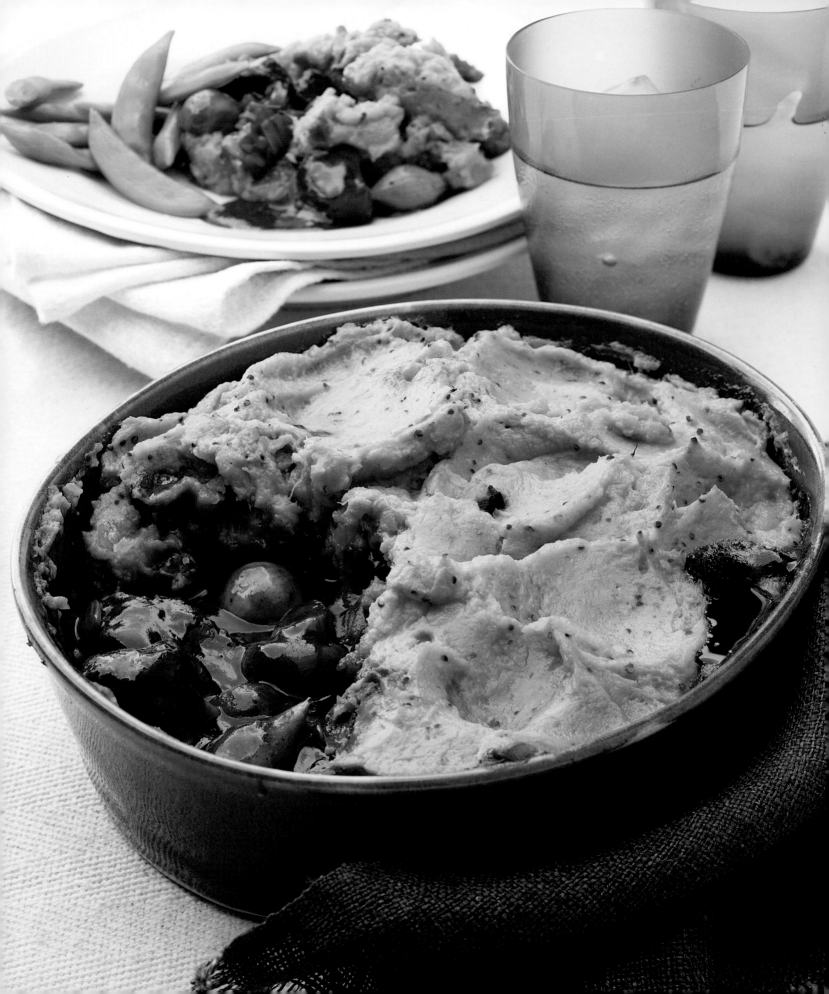

Venison and mushroom pie

A sweet potato mash flavoured with mustard and orange is the colourful top for this winter pie. Underneath is a hearty and rich-tasting filling of lean venison simmered in red wine with baby onions and button mushrooms. Some simple green vegetables are all that's needed to balance this delicious dish.

Serves 4

2 tbsp extra virgin olive oil

200 g (7 oz) small button onions, peeled and left whole

500 g (1 lb 2 oz) boneless haunch of venison or venison shoulder, diced

150 g (5½ oz) baby button mushrooms

3 celery sticks, thickly sliced

1 tbsp fresh thyme leaves

300 ml (10 fl oz) full-bodied red wine

150 ml (5 fl oz) strong beef stock

1½ tbsp cornflour

salt and pepper

Sweet potato mash

1 kg (2¼ lb) sweet potatoes, cubed

1 tbsp wholegrain mustard

grated zest and juice of 1 orange

Preparation time: 1¼ hours

Cooking time: 20 minutes

Each serving provides

kcal 500, protein 33 g, fat 9 g (of which saturated fat 2 g), carbohydrate 64 g (of which sugars 19 g), fibre 8 g

✓✓✓	A, C, E, copper, zinc
✓✓	B₁, iron, potassium, selenium
✓	B₂, B₆, folate, niacin, calcium

1 Heat the oil in a large saucepan and add the onions. Cover and cook over a low heat for 8–10 minutes, shaking the pan occasionally, until the onions are lightly browned all over.

2 Remove the onions to a plate using a draining spoon. Add the venison to the pan and cook, uncovered, over a moderately high heat for 2–3 minutes or until the cubes are well browned.

3 Add the onions, mushrooms, celery and thyme. Pour in the wine and stock. Bring to the boil, then reduce the heat. Cover and simmer for 45 minutes or until the venison is tender.

4 Meanwhile, steam the sweet potatoes for 25 minutes or until tender. Alternatively, cook them in boiling water for 15 minutes, then drain.

5 Preheat the oven to 190°C (375°F, gas mark 5). Tip the sweet potatoes into a bowl and mash with the mustard, orange zest and juice, and salt and pepper to taste. Set aside.

6 Blend the cornflour with 2 tbsp cold water. Stir into the venison mixture and cook, stirring, until lightly thickened. Season to taste. Spoon the filling into a 1.2 litre (2 pint) pie dish.

7 Spread the sweet potato mash over the venison filling to cover it completely. Bake for 20 minutes. Serve the pie hot.

Some more ideas

- The pie can be made ahead and chilled, then reheated in a preheated 190°C (375°F, gas mark 5) oven for 45 minutes or until piping hot.
- Cover the venison filling with a potato and butternut mash. Steam 500 g (1 lb 2 oz) each peeled potatoes and butternut squash for 25 minutes, or cook in boiling water for about 15 minutes, until tender. Mash with 15 g (½ oz) butter and 2 tbsp snipped fresh chives.
- For a rabbit pie, lightly brown 400 g (14 oz) boneless diced rabbit in 1 tbsp extra virgin olive oil with 100 g (3½ oz) diced smoked bacon. Add 2 large sliced leeks, 3 sliced carrots and 2 parsnips, cut into chunks. Stir in 300 ml (10 fl oz) white wine, 150 ml (5 fl oz) chicken stock and 1 tbsp Dijon mustard. Simmer, covered, for 45 minutes. Cover with the sweet potato mash, or the potato and butternut mash, and bake as in the main recipe.

Plus points

- Venison is a particularly low-fat meat, containing even less fat than chicken. It is a rich source of B vitamins and contains twice as much iron as beef.
- Sweet potatoes are an excellent source of beta-carotene. They contain more vitamin E than any other vegetable and are a good source of vitamin C.

Fresh Eggs and Dairy Foods

Milk has been enjoyed as a nutritious food for thousands of years, not only as a high-vitality drink but also in the multitude of cheese, yogurt, cream and butter products made from it. Supplying protein and many vitamins and minerals, in particular calcium, milk and other dairy products can play a vital part in maintaining good health for everyone in the family. Eggs, too, are an important food to include in a healthy, well-balanced diet, providing high-quality protein and plenty of other beneficial nutrients – and all in a very convenient little package.

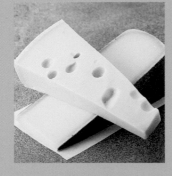

Healthy eggs, milk and cheese

Eggs and dairy products are rich in high-quality protein, vitamins and essential minerals such as calcium.

Why eat eggs, milk and cheese?

Since animals were first domesticated thousands of years ago, we have used their eggs and milk as food. Today, hen's eggs and cow's milk are the most common, but we can also enjoy duck, quail and goose eggs, as well as dairy products – such as cream, yogurt, butter and cheese – made from the milk of sheep, goats and water buffalo.

Most of us use eggs and some form of dairy products in the kitchen every day, and these staple foods have a lot to offer nutritionally.

● Eggs and dairy products, apart from cream, provide high-quality protein – protein that contains all 8 of the essential amino acids. A regular intake of protein is needed for optimum health.

● Eggs are a useful source of vitamins A, B_{12}, E and niacin, as well as providing zinc, potassium, magnesium, calcium, selenium and iodine. They also contain iron, although it is not in a form that is easily absorbed by the body.

● Dairy products provide conjugated linoleic acid, which may help to protect against heart attacks.

● Milk, yogurt and cheese are rich in calcium, phosphorus and B vitamins, especially B_2 and B_{12}. They also contain some zinc and magnesium.

● Full-fat milk, cream and many cheeses are a valuable source of vitamin A.

● Yogurt offers excellent amounts of potassium and iodine.

Calcium throughout life

One of the key reasons for including dairy products in the diet is that they are rich in calcium. Although this vital mineral is available in some other foods, such as dark leafy greens, nuts and seeds, it appears in the greatest quantities and in the most readily assimilated form in dairy products. As long as there is an adequate intake of vitamin D (from eggs and oily fish as well as the action of sunlight on skin), the body can take full advantage of the calcium on offer.

● Children and teenagers need plenty of calcium to maintain optimum bone and tooth development, while pregnant and breastfeeding women need calcium to perform the same task for their baby.

● Young adults should ensure a good supply of calcium to help build 'peak bone mass', which is reached at around the age of 30. The larger and stronger the bones, the more able they will be to cope with bone demineralisation in later life.

● Adults, particularly women, need a good intake of calcium to help maintain optimum bone density throughout life, which in turn will help to minimise the effects of osteoporosis after the menopause.

● High-calcium dairy products are good for oral health. In a recent study, people who regularly ate at least 3 portions of dairy products a day had a 50% reduction in the risk of gum

---

When you need a little extra …

There are certain times in our lives when we have special dietary needs, and eating eggs and a good variety of dairy products is an excellent way to meet these extra requirements.

● Small children need extra calcium to help the growth of healthy bones and teeth.

● From the ages of 15–18, teenagers need around 10% more calories than adults.

● Pregnant and breastfeeding women need extra calcium and vitamins A, B and D. Women need to increase their daily calorie intake by about 200 kcal during the last 3 months of pregnancy and by about 500 kcal while breastfeeding.

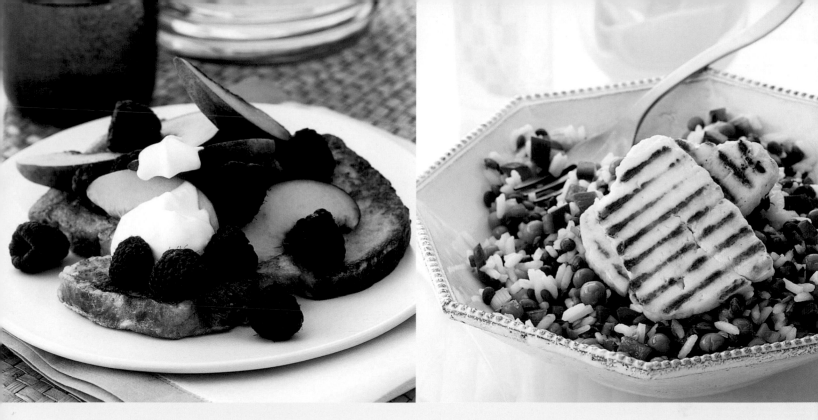

▲ For a special breakfast or brunch, dip brioche into egg and a little milk, fry until golden brown and serve with raspberries, sliced peaches and Greek-style yogurt

▲ Toss some Puy lentils with rice in a chilli dressing and top with griddled slices of halloumi cheese

▼ Layer a fresh plum purée with a creamy mixture of fromage frais and bio yogurt for a delectable dessert

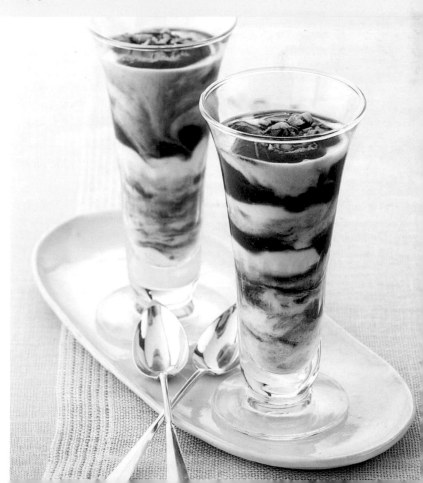

disease and tooth decay. And it has been shown that eating cheese after a meal helps to protect against dental erosion.

Minerals are principally found in the non-fat part of milk, so semi-skimmed and skimmed milk contain more calcium than full-fat varieties.

Disproving the bad press

In recent years our consumption of eggs and dairy products has declined, mainly because they are perceived to be high in cholesterol and saturated fat. In fact, this reputation is largely undeserved. For example, for most people, eating foods that contain cholesterol, as eggs do, will not have an adverse effect on blood cholesterol levels and so does not increase the risk of heart disease. With regard to fat in dairy products, many have a medium or low fat content. And with all the positive benefits of dairy products, even higher-fat items such as hard cheeses are well worth including in a healthy diet.

Nutritious and versatile eggs

Eggs offer many health benefits as well as being one of the cheapest forms of protein. Not only are they indispensable in many recipes, but they are great on their own, too.

The goodness of eggs

Eggs are designed by nature to be a complete food package for the growing chick. This means they contain a wide range of essential nutrients, including protein (12.5 g per 100 g/ 3½ oz), plenty of minerals, such as calcium, iodine, iron, magnesium, potassium, zinc and selenium, and vitamins A, D, E and many from the B group. Eggs are not high in fat, and almost two-thirds of the fat present is unsaturated – 47% of it monounsaturated and 12% polyunsaturated.

A small hen's egg, weighing about 50 g (scant 2 oz), contains 75 kcal, a medium egg 85–90 kcal and a large egg about 100 kcal. Most of the calories, fat and nutrients – and all of the cholesterol – are in the yolk. The white (albumen) is 88% water, with the rest mostly protein, plus a good amount of potassium and vitamin B_2.

The cholesterol question

Too much cholesterol in the blood can increase the risk of coronary heart disease, and because of this some people have had reservations about eating eggs – eggs are fairly high in dietary cholesterol, with about 217 mg in a medium egg. However, it is now recognised that the amount of fat you eat, particularly saturated or trans fats, will have more effect on blood cholesterol levels than cholesterol intake through food. The current advice is that people in normal health can eat up to 7 eggs a week. (People being treated for high blood lipids and cholesterol may receive different advice and should consult their doctor, dietician or nutritionist.)

Brown, white, pale blue, green, pink ...

Most hen's eggs are brown or white, although there are other colours appearing in supermarkets now. The colour of the shell makes no difference to the nutritional or cooking quality of the egg – it is purely a reflection of the breed of hen. The colour of the yolk, too, may vary from egg to egg, and largely depends on the hen's diet. For example, a deep yellow yolk can be an indication of an egg from an organic or free-range hen that has been fed on maize. However, the feed for battery hens is sometimes adulterated with artificial colourings to give the yolks a similar deep yellow colour.

Types of egg

Although the majority of eggs consumed are hen's, we can also eat eggs from other birds such as ducks, geese and quails. **Bantam's eggs** are small and tasty, and usually have a white shell. Bantams are a smaller variety of hen.

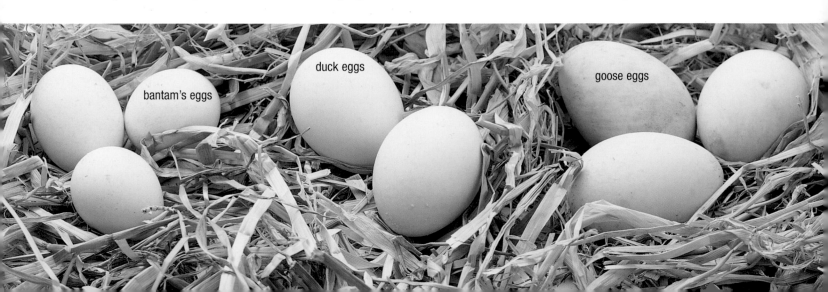

bantam's eggs

duck eggs

goose eggs

Duck eggs are much larger than hen's eggs and have a stronger flavour. They are slightly higher in fat, protein and cholesterol, and are also higher in iron and vitamins A, B group and D. Duck eggs can generally be used in cooking in the same ways as hen's eggs, although the strong flavour should be borne in mind. For safety, however, it is best not to use them in recipes that require lightly cooked eggs – they should be boiled for at least 10 minutes. Unless otherwise stated on the box, they are likely to come from intensively reared ducks.

Goose eggs are the largest of all the eggs you are likely to find on sale. They have a similar flavour and nutritional profile to hen's eggs, and can be used in all hen's egg recipes and basic dishes. They are likely to be free range.

Hen's eggs are graded according to size – small, medium, large and extra large or very large. About 90% of commercial eggs come from battery-reared hens. Barn eggs come from hens that are still very intensively farmed but are not confined to cages. Free-range hens are allowed more space and some outdoor living, although conditions can vary widely.

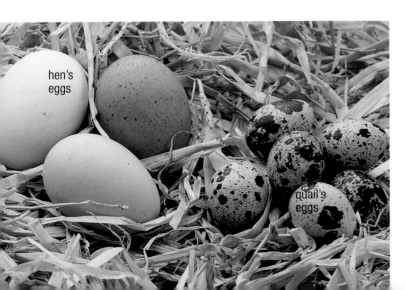

hen's eggs

quail's eggs

Organic eggs come from hens that are reared according to strict dietary stipulations. Labels such as 'farm fresh' and 'country' hint at a natural upbringing for the hen but are meaningless – usually these eggs come from battery hens.

Quail's eggs are tiny, with pretty speckled shells and a delicate flavour. Almost all quail's eggs sold are from battery-farmed birds. They have a similar nutritional composition to hen's eggs, with 6 quail's eggs being roughly equivalent to 1 hen's egg. Use them in the same way as you would hen's eggs, bearing in mind that because of their size cooking times will be shorter.

Egg storage

Eggs should be stored in the fridge, and it is best to leave them in their box so you can keep an eye on the date stamp, using older eggs first. They can usually be kept for up to 3 weeks. Don't store them next to strong-smelling foods – as their shells are porous they easily pick up odours and even flavours. They should also be kept away from possible contaminants such as raw meat and poultry.

Checking eggs for freshness

Most egg boxes are marked with a packing date rather than a laying date, so it is important to bear in mind that the eggs may have been several days old when they were packed. For an indication of the egg's age, look at the 'best before' date: on those with the Lion stamp, this will be 3 weeks after the egg was laid. This 21-day standard is not a legal requisite, so on other non-Lion-stamped eggs the best before date could be up to 28 days from laying.

When a fresh egg is cracked open, it will have a round, plump yolk and a thick white that clings closely to the yolk, with a thinner outer layer that spreads out around the inner white only a short way. The older the egg, the flatter the yolk and the flatter, thinner and runnier the white will be. Eggs that have gone bad have an unmistakable sulphurous smell.

To check if a raw egg in its shell is fresh, immerse it in a glass of cold water: if it lies horizontally at the bottom it is very fresh; if it begins to point upwards it is about a week old; if it stands vertically it is stale. A fresh egg tends to feel heavy in the hand, because the older the egg, the more water inside it will have evaporated.

Cooking eggs

It's hard to imagine a more versatile ingredient than the egg. It forms the basis for pancakes and other batters, helps to set savoury and sweet tarts, and enriches and flavours most cakes and many desserts. Egg yolks are indispensable for thickening sauces, and whisked egg whites add volume and lightness to soufflés and many other dishes.

In some cases, the age of an egg may affect the success of a dish. Very fresh eggs give the best results when poaching and frying, and are also a better choice for soft-boiling, omelettes, scrambling and general cooking. However, very fresh eggs (only a few days old) are not ideal for hard-boiling, as the shell and the membrane just underneath it will be hard to peel off. Eggs 1–2 weeks old are the best for hard-boiling.

Once you have mastered these basic cooking methods, you will have the foundation for a wide range of meals at your fingertips. Timings given are for hen's eggs.

Boiling

Put a medium egg (at room temperature) into a saucepan with tepid water to cover. Bring to the boil, then reduce the heat and simmer for 3–4 minutes for soft-boiled and 7 minutes for hard-boiled. Large eggs will take 4–5 minutes for soft-boiled and 8 minutes for hard-boiled.

Remove the egg with a slotted spoon. If soft-boiled, remove the 'cap' or top of the shell straightaway, to arrest the cooking process. Place hard-boiled eggs in a bowl of cold water to cool (this helps to prevent a black ring forming around the yolk), then peel them when cool enough to handle.

Poaching

Bring a frying pan of water at least 4 cm (1½ in) deep to a simmer. If you like, add 1 tsp vinegar to the water to help speed the coagulation of the albumen and thus preserve the shape of the egg (you will not need the vinegar if your eggs are very fresh). Carefully break the eggs into the water one at a time (or break each one into a cup and slide it into the water). Poach for about 3 minutes, by which time the whites should be set and the yolks still a bit runny (poach for another minute if you prefer the yolk to be set). Towards the end of the cooking, baste the yolks with the simmering water. Lift out each egg with a draining spoon and, with the egg still on the

spoon, rest it on some kitchen paper for a few seconds to absorb any water. If you like, trim the edges of the egg with kitchen scissors to neaten any straggly bits of white, then serve. Poached eggs can be kept in the fridge for a day and reheated for 1 minute in hot water.

Scrambling

Break the eggs into a bowl and add 1 tbsp semi-skimmed milk per egg, plus salt and pepper to taste. Whisk thoroughly to combine. Heat a small knob of butter in a non-stick saucepan over a moderate heat. When it has melted, pour in the egg mixture and cook, stirring frequently, until the eggs are almost set but still soft and glossy looking. Remove from the heat, as the eggs will continue to cook in the heat of the pan – take care not to overcook or the eggs will become dry and grainy.

Scrambled eggs can also be cooked in a double saucepan or heatproof bowl set over a pan of hot water.

Baking (en cocotte)

Lightly oil or butter 7.5 cm (3 in) ramekin dishes and break an egg into each one. (For a more substantial dish, put a little smoked fish or lightly cooked spinach or mushrooms in the ramekins first.) Season and top with a small knob of butter. Set the dishes in a baking tin and pour enough boiling water into the tin to come halfway up the sides of the ramekins. Bake in a preheated 180°C (350°F, gas mark 4) oven for 10–15 minutes or until set. Serve hot.

Frying

Melt a small knob of butter in a non-stick frying pan over a moderate heat. Break the eggs into the pan, then reduce the heat a little and cover the pan. Fry for 4–6 minutes or until the eggs are cooked to your taste. Alternatively, do not cover the pan and instead, when the whites are set, carefully flip the eggs over using a fish slice. Fry for about 30 seconds longer.

Making a folded French omelette

Whisk 2 eggs in a bowl with 1 tbsp cold water and seasoning to taste. Melt a small knob of butter in a 15–18 cm (6–7 in) non-stick omelette or frying pan over a high heat, swirling it around as it melts. When the butter is foaming, add the egg mixture. After a few seconds, tilt the pan and use a spatula to

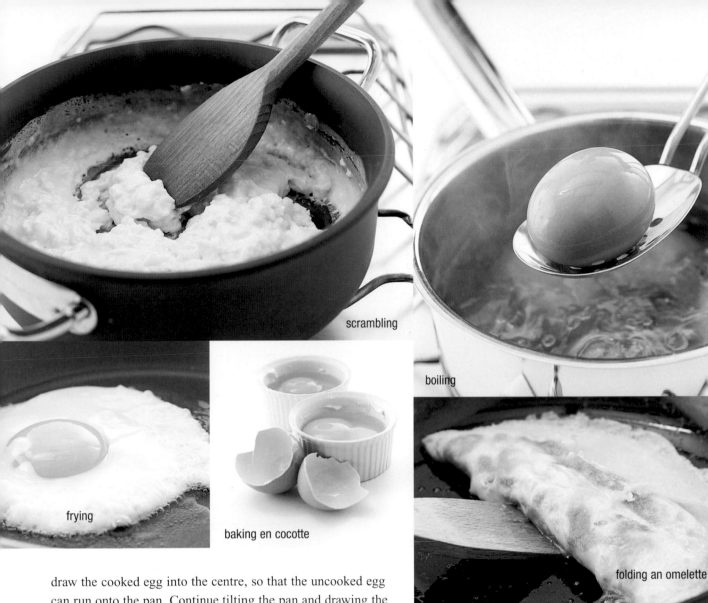

scrambling

boiling

frying

baking en cocotte

folding an omelette

poaching

draw the cooked egg into the centre, so that the uncooked egg can run onto the pan. Continue tilting the pan and drawing the cooked egg in, to build up a plump omelette. When there is very little runny egg left, add any filling, such as grated cheese, diced tomatoes, cooked vegetables and so on, then leave the omelette undisturbed for about 10 seconds so that it can set and become golden on the base. Remove from the heat and use the spatula to fold one-third of the omelette over towards the centre. Slide the omelette across the pan and roll it onto a serving plate (the folds should be underneath as the omelette lands on the plate).

To make a soufflé omelette, separate the eggs and beat the yolks with seasoning to taste. In a separate bowl, whisk the whites until stiff, then fold them into the yolks. Cook in the butter until set and golden on the base, without moving the egg mixture in the pan, then transfer to a preheated grill to finish cooking and set the top.

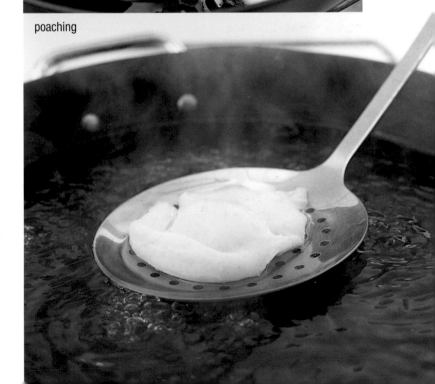

Fresh foods from the dairy

Milk offers valuable nutrients in an easy-to-enjoy form. It is also the basis of butter and cream – two of life's luxuries that should be used with some discretion.

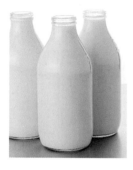

Milk

The many different types of milk available to us today are in sharp contrast to what the milkman brought 50 or so years ago. We can now choose to drink cow's milk, or that of other animals, such as goats, sheep or even water buffalo, and we can opt for lower-fat versions.

All fresh milk should be kept, covered, in the fridge and used by the date on the lid or carton. Exposure to sunlight destroys vitamin B$_2$, so bottles of milk should not be left on the doorstep all day. Cow's milk and goat's milk freeze well in their cartons or in freezer containers; they can be kept for up to 1 month.

Breakfast milk, sometimes labelled Channel Island milk, comes from Jersey and Guernsey cows and is richer in fat than ordinary full-fat milk.

Condensed milk, available in both full-fat and skimmed versions, is made by heating milk to remove some of the water content and then adding sugar to act as a preservative. The thick, heavily sweetened milk, which will keep for several months, has a toffee-like taste.

Dried milk is made by evaporating skimmed milk. The resulting powder can be stored for several months, and is simply mixed with water to reconstitute it. Since the advent of UHT milk, this method of keeping milk long term is not used so much.

Evaporated milk is a concentrated version of full-fat or skimmed milk that has been heated to remove much of its water content, and then sterilised so that it will keep well.

It is slightly darker than fresh milk and has a 'cooked' flavour. **Full-fat milk**, or whole milk, is milk from the cow with nothing added and nothing taken away. It retains all of the fat-soluble vitamins that are lost from semi-skimmed and skimmed milk, although it is slightly lower in calcium than they are. Children should be given full-fat milk after the age of 1 year, although semi-skimmed milk can be introduced gradually after the age of 2, and skimmed milk usually after the age of 5, if the child's nutrient intake is otherwise adequate and growth is satisfactory. **Goat's milk**, available in full-fat, skimmed and long-life versions, is slightly creamier than cow's milk but has a similar taste. Some people find it easier to digest than cow's milk.

Nutritional content of milk and cream per 100 ml (3½ fl oz)

	kcal	fat (g)	protein (g)	calcium (mg)
Milk				
breakfast	78	4.8	3.6	130
condensed (full-fat)	333	10.1	8.5	330
evaporated (full-fat)	151	9.4	8.4	290
full-fat	66	3.9	3.2	115
goat's (full-fat)	60	3.5	3.1	100
semi-skimmed	46	1.8	3.3	120
sheep'	95	6.0	5.4	170
skimmed	33	0.1–0.3	3.3	120
Cream				
clotted	586	63	1.6	37
crème fraîche	380	40	2.4	50
double	449	48	1.7	50
single	198	19	2.6	91
soured	205	20	2.9	93
whipping	373	39	2.0	62

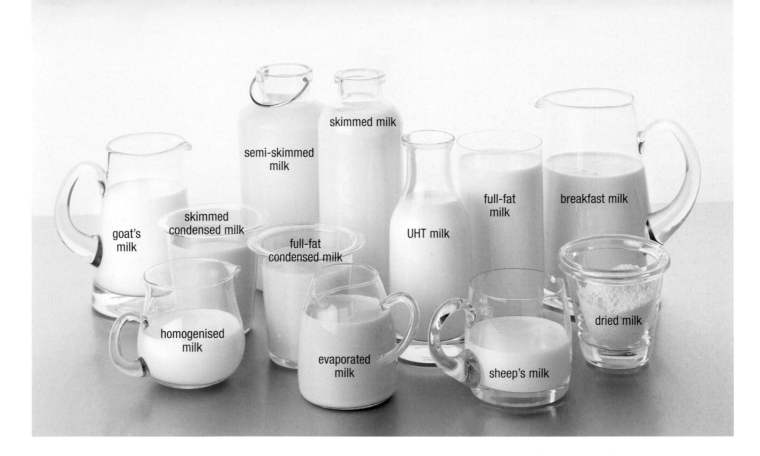

semi-skimmed milk

skimmed milk

full-fat milk

breakfast milk

goat's milk

skimmed condensed milk

UHT milk

full-fat condensed milk

dried milk

homogenised milk

evaporated milk

sheep's milk

Homogenised milk has been treated to distribute the fat evenly. If full-fat milk is not homogenised, it will separate into layers, with the cream on top and semi-skimmed milk underneath.

Pasteurised milk has been flash-heated for 5 seconds to destroy most of the bacteria naturally present and to improve its keeping qualities. Almost all of the milk sold in the UK is pasteurised. Most of the vitamin content is retained, although some beneficial bacteria are lost.

Semi-skimmed milk has had about half of its fat removed, taking more than half the fat-soluble vitamins with it but leaving the calcium and protein. It is a good compromise for people who prefer a slightly richer taste than skimmed milk but who find full-fat milk too creamy.

Sheep's milk, which is usually higher in fat than goat's milk, may also be suitable for people who find cow's milk difficult to digest. However, it is not widely available.

Skimmed milk has had almost all of the fat removed, giving it a rather thin, watery consistency. It has lost the fat-soluble vitamins A, D and E, but retains most of its other nutrients, such as calcium and protein.

UHT (ultra-heat-treated) milk has been pasteurised and then subjected to heat to kill off any bacteria present – a process that may also reduce the vitamin B content, although it does

not affect the flavour. A carton of UHT milk can be kept at room temperature for up to 6 months, but once opened it should be stored in the fridge like fresh milk.

Lactose intolerance

A high proportion of the world's population is not able to digest the lactose (milk sugars) in milk because of a deficiency in the enzyme lactase – this enzyme breaks down the lactose in the digestive system. The undigested lactose remains in the gut, where it can cause long-term health problems. Avoiding lactose is the usual answer for such people. Lactose is found in the milk and milk byproducts of cows, goats and sheep. Some people with lactose intolerance find they can tolerate goat's and sheep's milk better than cow's milk. Acidophilus milk, which is pasteurised cow's milk to which *Lactobacillus* bacteria have been reintroduced, is easier to digest than ordinary cow's milk, and may provide another alternative. Some cheeses, including Brie, Edam and pecorino, contain only very small amounts of lactose and may therefore be tolerated. If you think you may be lactose-intolerant, seek advice from your doctor before making any changes to your diet.

Cream

Cream is the fat that rises to the surface of fresh milk and is skimmed off. Generally, the thicker the cream, the higher the fat content. All the different types contain useful amounts of vitamin A, calcium and phosphorus.

Fresh cream should be kept, covered, in the fridge and used by the date on the carton.

Clotted cream, traditionally made in the West Country, is the thickest and richest of the dairy creams. Its pale yellow colour and thick texture are obtained by heating full-fat milk to evaporate some of the liquid and then skimming off the creamy crust. Clotted cream is usually served as an accompaniment to desserts and to top scones rather than used in cooking.

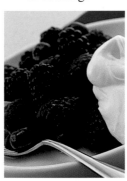

Crème fraîche, originally from Normandy in France, has a similar taste to soured cream but is less acidic. Because it is treated with a lactic culture it is very thick, although surprisingly its fat content is lower than that of double cream. Crème fraîche keeps well and is a good all-round cooking cream, as it never separates when boiled. A half-fat version is available, which often includes thickeners and other additives.

Double cream is high in fat, so is best used sparingly. As it can be boiled, it is added to sweet and savoury sauces to enrich them. It can also be whipped to a soft or firm consistency.

Single cream cannot be whipped, but is good for pouring and for using in cooking when you want a richer texture or flavour than milk can provide. Extra-thick single cream has a similar texture to very lightly whipped double cream.

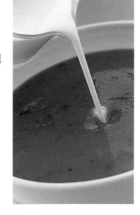

Smetana is similar to soured cream but is made from single cream and skimmed milk, and is therefore lower in fat than soured cream.

Soured cream is fresh single cream that has been soured and slightly thickened by the addition of lactic acid-producing bacteria, giving it a tangy flavour. The souring also makes it easier to digest than single cream.

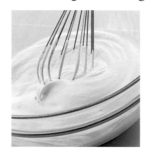

Whipping cream is slightly less rich than double cream and is quicker and easier to whip, with a consistent, light result. It can be mixed with lower-fat dairy products such as plain yogurt to make a rich-tasting but lower-calorie alternative to whipped cream.

Butter

Butter is made by churning cream. It is a good source of the fat-soluble vitamins A and D, and it contains 15 mg calcium per 100 g (3½ oz). It is also high in saturated fat, at 67% of its total fat content, and in calories (727 kcal per 100 g/3½ oz). Half-fat butter, which contains half the fat and calories of standard butter, is available; it is not suitable for baking.

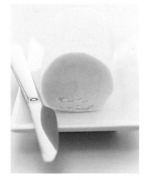

Several studies show that the natural fats in butter do not have an adverse effect on blood cholesterol levels in the same way as the artificial trans fats in many commercial hydrogenated margarines and low-fat spreads. So a little butter eaten within an overall healthy diet is not such a bad thing, and there is nothing to compare with the flavour it brings.

● Buy good-quality butter – its taste, colour and texture will be superior. The cream used to make French butter has often been treated with a lactic culture, which gives it more flavour.

● Salt improves the keeping qualities of butter in the fridge.

● Butter should be stored in a lidded butter dish or in its own wrapping in the fridge. If kept out at room temperature it will soon go 'off' and taste rancid, and must be discarded.

● Butter freezes well. Salted butter can be kept for 3 months, and unsalted butter for 6 months.

● For spreading, let butter come to room temperature, or try special 'spreadable' butter that can be used straight from the fridge. If the butter is soft, you'll spread less of it on bread.

● Butter burns at high temperatures so it is generally not used on its own for frying. Instead, it is best mixed with oil.

Milk and egg sauces

These simple sauces form the basis for many other dishes or are served alongside. If you dress them up with flavourings – cheese and herbs in the basic white sauce, orange zest or liqueur in the custard, for example – they can really make an impact and turn a meal into something special.

Basic white sauce

Makes about 600 ml (1 pint), to serve 4

55 g (2 oz) butter
55 g (2 oz) plain flour
600 ml (1 pint) semi-skimmed milk
salt and pepper

Preparation time: 5 minutes
Cooking time: 5 minutes

1 Melt the butter in a heavy-based saucepan over a low heat. Remove from the heat and stir in the flour. Gradually pour in the milk, stirring or whisking constantly.

2 Return the pan to the heat and bring to the boil, still stirring or whisking. Reduce the heat and simmer the sauce gently for 5 minutes, stirring occasionally. Taste and season with salt and pepper. Serve or use immediately.

Another idea

• For a low-fat cornflour-thickened white sauce, omit the butter and flour, and instead mix 4 tbsp cornflour to a smooth paste with a little of the milk. Heat the remaining milk to boiling point, then pour a little of it onto the cornflour mixture, stirring. Return this to the milk in the saucepan. Bring to the boil, stirring, until the sauce thickens, then simmer for 3 minutes. This makes a thick sauce; for a thinner one, use 3 tbsp cornflour.

Custard

Makes about 600 ml (1 pint), to serve 4

4 egg yolks
4 tsp cornflour
4 tbsp caster sugar
600 ml (1 pint) semi-skimmed milk

Preparation time: 5 minutes
Cooking time: 5 minutes

1 Put the egg yolks, cornflour and sugar in a bowl and beat until smooth.

2 Pour the milk into a saucepan and bring to the boil, then slowly pour it onto the egg yolk mixture, stirring thoroughly.

3 Return the mixture to the saucepan and cook over a low heat, stirring constantly, until it thickens to a custard consistency. It should reach 82°C (180°F) on a cooking thermometer. Remove from the heat and strain into a bowl. Serve hot or leave to cool before using or serving.

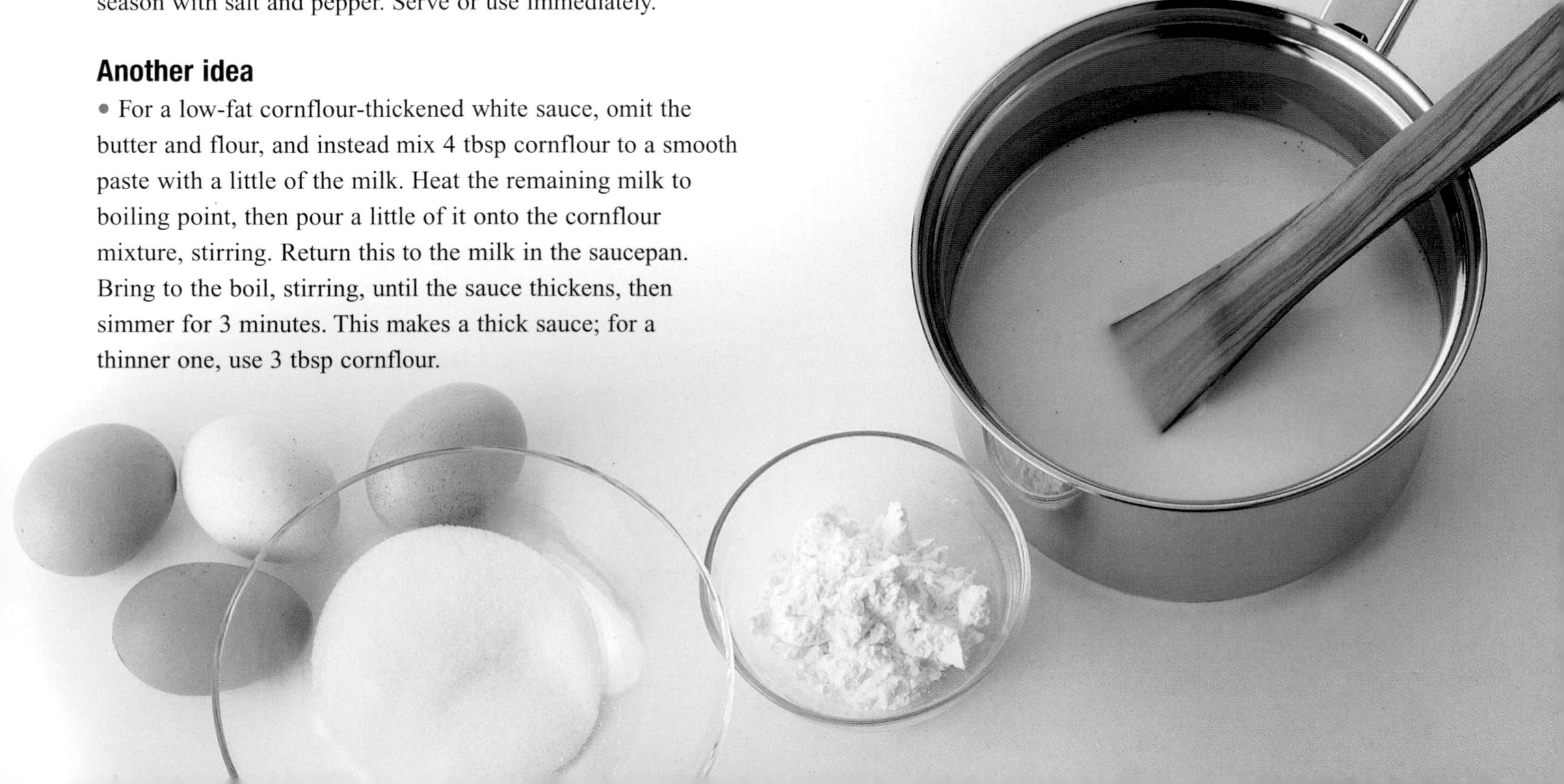

Culturing milk into yogurt

Yogurt offers many dietary benefits – it is rich in nutrients and contains bacteria that are helpful to both the digestive and immune systems.

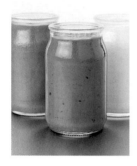

The benefits of yogurt

Yogurt is a thick, creamy, slightly acidic-tasting dairy product, made by curdling (or fermenting) warmed pasteurised milk with lactic acid cultures (bacteria). It is easily digested and some people can tolerate it better than milk. The nutritional profile of yogurt varies according to what type of milk it is made from, how it is produced and what is added to it, but generally it is a good source of protein, B vitamins and calcium, and is low or fairly low in fat.

Most yogurts on sale are 'live' (although this is not always stated on the label), which means they contain living bacteria that are beneficial to the digestive system – usually Lactobacillus bulgaricus and Streptococcus thermophilus. Bio yogurt contains a slightly different bacterial culture, aimed specifically at redressing the natural balance of the gut flora.

There is evidence that if the gut is colonised sufficiently with friendly bacteria, there may be an improvement in conditions such as candida and in stomach upsets such as diarrhoea and flatulence. They may also help to prevent problems such as cow's milk allergy and eczema in infants, and help to strengthen the immune system. Eating plenty of yogurt is sometimes recommended after a course of antibiotics, which can reduce the amount of beneficial bacteria in the gut.

Yogurt should be stored, covered, in the fridge. Unopened, it will keep until its 'use-by' date; once opened it should be used within 1–2 days. It is not suitable for freezing.

If yogurt is to be added to a dish that is cooked over a high heat, it needs to be stabilised first with a little cornflour, to prevent it from separating.

Types of yogurt

Most of the different kinds of yogurt are available both plain (or natural) and flavoured. Many flavoured yogurts contain artificial sweeteners or sugar, flavourings and colourings, plus gelatine and other thickeners. The best contain only plain yogurt plus natural flavourings such as fruit purées.

Full-fat or whole-milk yogurt is rich and creamy. It can be used as a lower-fat alternative to cream in many dishes, adding a delightful piquant taste.

Goat's milk yogurt, which is becoming more widely available, has a pleasant, mild taste. It may be suitable for people who cannot eat cow's milk products. Low-fat, full-fat and bio versions are produced.

Greek-style yogurt is traditionally made from full-fat sheep's milk, though cow's milk versions are also available. It is strained to remove some of the liquid, making it very thick and rich, with a delicious creamy flavour – and a higher fat content than other yogurts. A 0% fat version is also available. Greek-style yogurt makes an excellent alternative to whipped cream as a topping for desserts. It can also be used in cooking.

Nutritional content of different yogurts per 100g (3½oz)

	kcal	fat (g)	protein(g)	calcium(mg)
full-fat	79	3	5	200
goat's milk, bio	105	7.3	5.5	159
Greek-style	115	9	6	150
low-fat plain	56	less than 1	5	190
sheep's milk	106	7.5	4.4	150

Low-fat yogurt, made from skimmed milk, is available in 'set' (firm) or 'stirred' (runny) versions. Bio low-fat yogurt tends to taste milder and creamier than non-bio varieties. Plain low-fat yogurt is a delicious ingredient for hot and cold dishes.
Sheep's milk yogurt, other than traditional Greek varieties, is not widely available.

Other cultured milk products

Cultured milk products are becoming increasingly popular as their nutritional benefits are recognised.

'Bio' milks are flavoured, sweetened milks to which the Lactobacillus bacteria have been added. They have similar health benefits to live yogurt.
Buttermilk is traditionally a byproduct of making butter – the whey left after churning. Nowadays, most buttermilk available in the shops is made by adding cultures to skimmed milk. It is low in calories and fat (37 kcal and less than 1 g fat per 100 ml/3½ fl oz) and, with its slightly acidic quality, is ideal for making scones and soda bread. It also makes a refreshing, easily digested drink.

Making yogurt

You can buy electric yogurt makers, either with 6 or 8 small pots or 1 large pot. These are simple and convenient to use, but it is also very easy to make yogurt without any special equipment. All you need is a little plain live yogurt and some milk – skimmed, semi-skimmed or full-fat, depending on how rich you want your yogurt to be. Use at least 600 ml (1 pint) milk – it is not really worth going to the trouble of making less yogurt than this.

• Bring the milk to the boil, then leave it to cool to blood heat, which is around 37°C (98°F) – a thermometer will help here.

• Stir 1 tbsp plain live yogurt into the milk, then pour it into a bowl or wide-necked flask. Cover and leave in a warm place such as an airing cupboard for 8–12 hours, by which time it will have set. Transfer to the fridge.

• Home-made yogurt can be used plain or you can flavour it as desired, with fresh fruit, fruit purée, honey, chopped nuts or a few drops of pure vanilla extract.

• To make Greek-style yogurt, once your yogurt has set put it into a large muslin bag, or a sieve lined with muslin, and suspend it over a bowl. Put it into the fridge. The liquid will drip through into the bowl, leaving you with firmer, thicker yogurt. The longer you let it drain, the more like a soft, fresh cheese it will become. Discard the liquid in the bowl, or use it in cooking as a tangy substitute for milk.

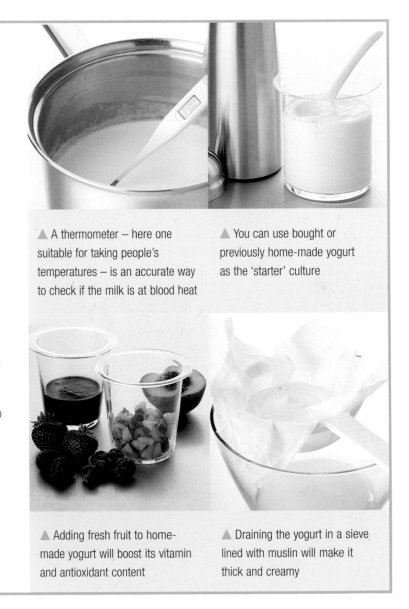

▲ A thermometer – here one suitable for taking people's temperatures – is an accurate way to check if the milk is at blood heat

▲ You can use bought or previously home-made yogurt as the 'starter' culture

▲ Adding fresh fruit to home-made yogurt will boost its vitamin and antioxidant content

▲ Draining the yogurt in a sieve lined with muslin will make it thick and creamy

Cheese variety

Cheese comes in an infinite variety of forms, flavours and textures, yet all cheese starts as milk. It is deliciously satisfying and nutritious, however you eat it.

How cheese is made

Cheese is most commonly made from cow's milk, but goat's, sheep's and water buffalo milk are also used – and even the milk of reindeer, asses, mares and camels in some parts of the world. The simplest forms of cheese are made by coagulating, or curdling, the milk. This can happen naturally – warm milk left out long enough becomes sour and then curdles into whitish lumps (curds) in a thin liquid called whey, which is drained off. However, for commercial production a bacterial culture or starter is usually added to sour the milk, and rennet is used to aid the curdling.

Traditionally, rennet is a substance obtained from the stomach lining of young calves. However, nowadays many cheeses are produced with a vegetarian microbial starter or a genetically engineered rennet, both of which are suitable for a vegetarian diet.

The curds are sometimes heated or scalded and, in the case of hard cheeses, pressed to remove more whey.

Then they are moulded or shaped, salted and left to ripen or mature under controlled conditions. The ripening or maturing process may take anywhere from several weeks to years, depending upon the cheese-maker and the type of cheese.

Cheese in a healthy diet

Since most cheeses are a concentrated food, they are a particularly rich source of the nutrients they offer. So just a little can have a big impact on the vitamins, minerals and protein in a meal.

In general, the harder the cheese, the more dense it is and therefore the more protein, B-group vitamins, calcium and phosphorus it will contain – and the more calories. The exception to this rule are soft cheeses, such as cream cheese and mascarpone, which are higher in calories than hard cheeses as they contain a lot of cream. These cream cheeses tend to be quite low in protein and other nutrients, because the cream itself is low in most nutrients except vitamin A.

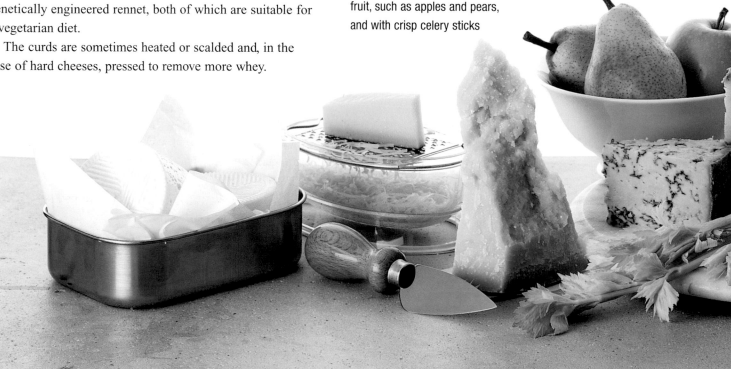

Cheese goes well with fresh fruit, such as apples and pears, and with crisp celery sticks

Nutritional value of typical cheeses per 100 g (3½ oz)

	kcal	fat (g)	protein (g)	calcium (mg)
Soft fresh cheeses				
cottage cheese	98	4	13.8	73
fromage frais (8%)	113	7.1	6.8	89
mozzarella	290	22	26	590
reduced-fat soft cheese	196	15	12	360
Semi-soft rinded cheeses				
Brie	320	26	19.2	540
Goat's and sheep's milk cheeses				
feta	250	20	15.6	360
goat's cheese (medium-fat)	339	28.5	11.7	185
Semi-hard and hard cheeses				
Cheddar (traditional)	412	34	26	720
Edam	334	26	26	770
Parmesan	452	32.7	39.4	1,200
Blue cheeses				
Danish blue	348	30	20	500
Stilton	412	36	22	320

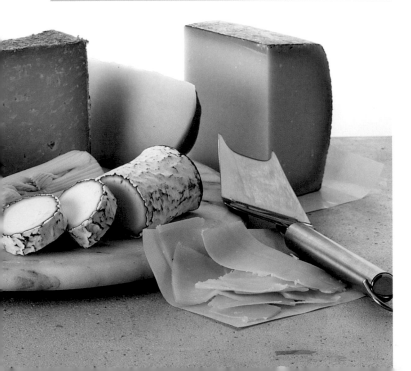

Cheese in the kitchen

Here are a few guidelines on choosing, storing and cooking.

• Buy only enough cheese to last you for about a week at a time; once cut, cheese tends to deteriorate.

• Avoid cheese that has been wrapped in cling film or similar, as it encourages a damp surface. Also, chemicals such as plasticisers in the film may transfer to the cheese.

• Keep soft fresh cheeses in the coldest part of the fridge and use within a few days of unwrapping or opening.

• Keep semi-soft, semi-hard and hard cheeses in a cool, but not too cool, place – for example, the least cold part of the fridge or a cool larder. Store either in a special cheese box with air vents, or wrapped in greaseproof paper or foil (don't wrap in cling film). Be sure not to leave any edges of cheese exposed or they will dry out and become inedible.

• If semi-soft rinded cheeses such as Brie and Camembert need to ripen a bit before being eaten, leave them (still wrapped in their original packaging) at room temperature for a few days. Once ripe, keep them in the fridge.

• Cream cheese and hard cheeses for cooking can be frozen for up to a month. Pack grated hard cheese in strong freezer bags. It is quite easy to remove just the amount you want, as the flakes stay fairly separate.

• The stronger the cheese, the less you need.

• If you want to use only a small amount of a high-fat cheese in sandwiches, make it go farther either by grating it or by cutting it thinly with a special cheese slice (available from kitchen shops). Chilling cheese before grating or slicing it will make the process easier.

• Before serving cheese as part of a cheeseboard or in a salad, bring it to room temperature, to maximise the flavour.

• Heat and prolonged cooking can spoil the texture of cheese and make it rubbery or stringy. If exposing cheese to a fierce heat, such as the grill, cook it as briefly as possible. When making a cheese sauce, add the cheese at the end of cooking and heat gently just to melt the cheese, stirring constantly.

• Add cheese to a sauce or other preparation before seasoning – most cheese is quite salty and you may find you don't need to add extra salt (taste to find out).

• If a cheese smells rancid or of ammonia, it is past its best. Cheese that tastes mouldy or rank, or that is slightly fizzy (soft cheeses), should be thrown out.

Soft fresh cheeses

These are unripened cheeses and generally need to be eaten as
soon as possible after purchase. Most of them are made from
cow's milk.

Cottage cheese consists of loose, soft curds mixed with a small
amount of cultured cream. It has a mild, slightly sweet and
tangy flavour, and is low in fat. There is also an even lower-fat
version (sometimes called 'diet' cottage cheese), which has no
cream added. Several flavoured varieties are also available.

Curd cheese is a low or medium-fat soft white cheese with a
slightly granular texture. It is made with a lactic acid starter,
which gives it a fresh, slightly sharp flavour.

Fromage frais originates from France, where it is sometimes
called fromage blanc. It has a fairly dense but soft texture,
making it ideal as a cream substitute. The normal (8%) version
has a little cream added, whereas the 0% fat version is, as the
name implies, virtually fat-free.

Mascarpone, an ultra-smooth cheese produced in Italy, has an
extremely high fat content (46 g fat and 450 kcal per 100 g/
3½ oz) because it is made from cream rather than milk.

Mozzarella, the cheese for pizza, is made differently from most
soft fresh cheeses – the curds are kneaded and stretched (or
spun in hot water) before being shaped into balls. This is why
mozzarella has an elastic texture when melted. It is mild and
delicate in flavour. Buffalo milk mozzarella and a smoked
mozzarella are also available.

Paneer, a low-fat fresh cheese made in India, is usually added
to curry. It is not easy to buy in the UK, but is simple to make
at home.

Quark, which originates from Germany, is a very low-fat
variety of curd cheese. Its nutrient profile is similar to 0% fat
fromage frais, but its flavour is slightly less creamy, and has a
hint of acidity.

Ricotta, a low to medium-fat cheese, is unusual in that it is
made from whey rather than curds – traditionally the whey
left over after making pecorino, a hard sheep's milk cheese
from Italy. Ricotta is mild and slightly sweet with a grainy,
soft texture.

Soft cheese, also called cream cheese, is smooth and mild.
It is available in full-fat and reduced-fat versions.

Soft and semi-soft rinded cheeses

This group includes surface-ripened cheeses, such as Brie and
Camembert, which produce a downy white mould on the skin,
and surface-washed cheeses, which are washed during the
ripening process with various types of liquid, from salt water
to brandy. They are soft or semi-soft and creamy underneath
the rind, and because of their higher water content tend to be
lower in fat than most hard cheeses.

Brie, from the French area of the same name, is made from
full-fat or semi-skimmed cow's milk and comes in flat, round
discs, which can be as large as 60 cm (2 ft) in diameter. The
creamy yellow interior may be full and mild in flavour or more
piquant, depending on how ripe the cheese is.

Camembert is another classic French cheese, similar to Brie
but smaller and with a stronger, more tangy flavour. It is
slightly lower in fat than Brie.

Neufchâtel, a full-fat cow's milk cheese from France, may be
ripened only briefly to give a delicate, bloomy rind, or left to
ripen until it is firm and pungent. It is available in different
shapes, most famously a heart.

Port-Salut was originally made by monks in France. It is an
orange rind-washed and pressed cheese with a creamy yellow
interior and mild but distinctive flavour.

Taleggio could be called the Italian equivalent of Brie, with a
similar nutritional profile. It has a deliciously creamy, fruity
flavour with a faintly nutty aroma. Sold in oblong blocks with
a pink rind, it melts well and is therefore useful in cooking.

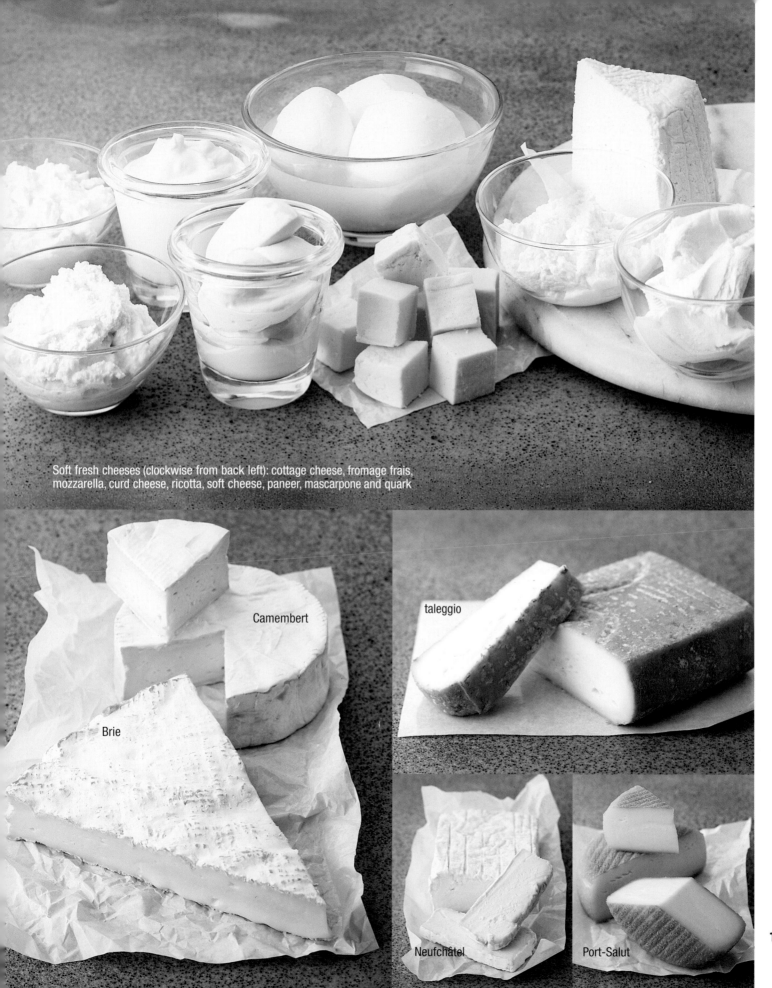

Soft fresh cheeses (clockwise from back left): cottage cheese, fromage frais, mozzarella, curd cheese, ricotta, soft cheese, paneer, mascarpone and quark

Camembert

Brie

taleggio

Neufchâtel

Port-Salut

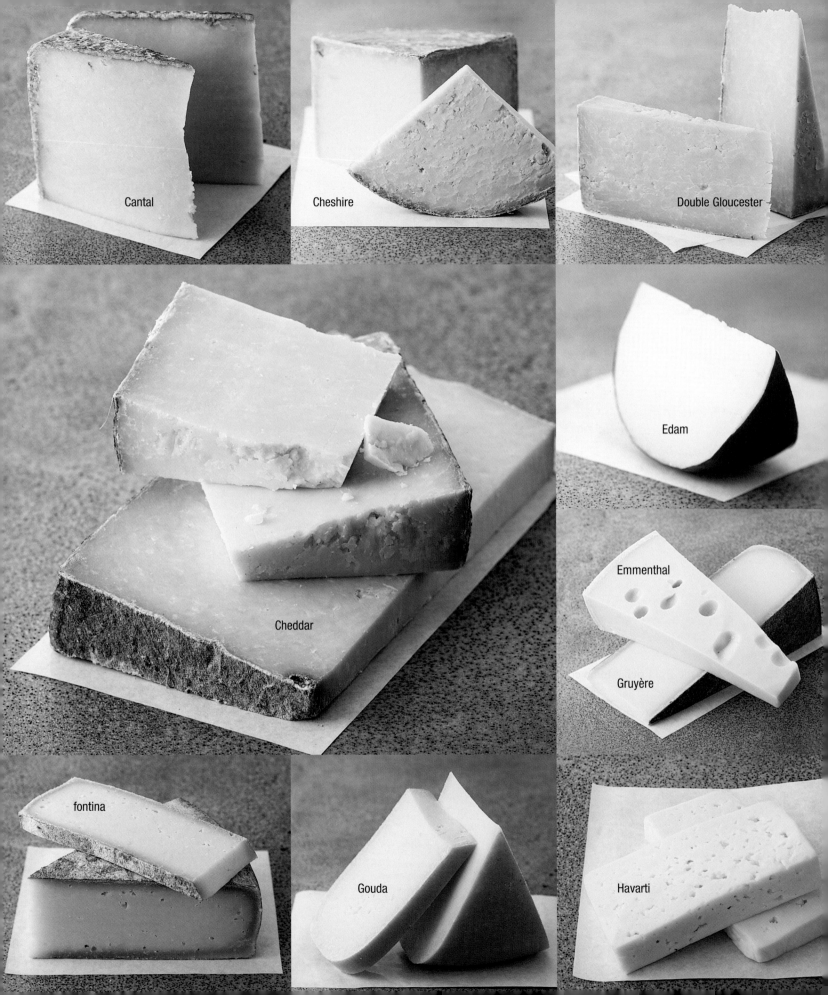

Cantal

Cheshire

Double Gloucester

Cheddar

Edam

Emmenthal

Gruyère

fontina

Gouda

Havarti

Semi-hard and hard cheeses

This large group contains all the cheeses that traditionally take a long time to mature. In general, the longer the maturing period, the harder and stronger the cheese will be. Some, such as Gruyère and Emmenthal, are made from scalded ('cooked') curds to produce a different texture. Most hard cheeses are pressed to help the draining process.

Cantal is a hard cheese made in the Auvergne region of France. Similar in appearance to a pale Cheddar, it may be mild, medium or strong, according to how ripe it is.

Cheddar, one of the world's greatest cheeses, originated in the Cheddar district of Somerset, but is now made all over the world. Factory-produced Cheddar tends to have an almost waxy consistency, while well-matured traditional farmhouse Cheddar has a very hard, slightly crumbly texture. The taste ranges from sweet and very mild in young cheeses to strong, sharp and savoury in those that are mature.

Cheshire is a hard English cheese that can be orange-red or white, depending on whether it has been coloured with the tasteless dye annatto. It is mild but slightly salty in flavour, with a crumbly, open texture.

Double Gloucester is a large, round English cheese made from full-fat cow's milk (Single Gloucester is made from partly skimmed milk). Like Cheshire, it is often dyed with annatto. The flavour is mild and rich, the texture smooth and creamy.

Edam, the well-known Dutch cheese, is yellowy-orange within its red or yellow wax coating. It is usually factory made, from semi-skimmed milk, and has a waxy, semi-hard texture. When young it can be quite bland, but matures to a mellow flavour.

Emmenthal, a hard, ivory-yellow Swiss or French cheese, is traditionally made from rich Alpine cow's milk. It comes in massive, brown-rinded wheels and has a waxy texture pitted with large holes. The flavour is mild, nutty and sweet.

Fontina, made from full-fat cow's milk, is a semi-hard cheese from Italy. It has a slightly nutty flavour and a creamy texture.

Gouda, produced in the Dutch town of the same name, is made from full-fat cow's milk, so it is slightly higher in fat and calories than Edam, to which it is very similar. Normally in a yellow wax coating, Gouda that has been matured for at least 7 years is coated with black wax.

Gruyère looks similar to Emmenthal but has fewer and smaller holes. Also from Switzerland, it has a stronger, nuttier flavour. Its good melting qualities make it very popular in cooking.

Havarti, from Denmark, is a semi-hard washed-rind cheese full of tiny holes. Made from full-fat cow's milk, it may be mild in flavour or strong and pungent when mature.

Lancashire is a semi-hard white cheese with a crumbly texture. Farmhouse Lancashire is made by a more laborious process than the factory version, which gives it a creamy, tangy flavour. Mass-produced Lancashire can be very bland.

Leicester is a hard cow's milk English cheese with a flaky texture. Its smooth, mellow flavour develops with age.

Parmesan, the world-famous Italian cooked, pressed cheese, is made with semi-skimmed cow's milk and is aged for at least a year (often much longer). Look for cheese marked parmigiano reggiano – this is the genuine article, made by traditional methods in the Emilia-Romagna region of Italy, with milk from cows fed only on grass or hay. Parmesan has a soft yellow colour, crumbly texture and slightly salty, rich taste. It is well worth buying a piece for shaving or grating, as the flavour is vastly superior to ready-grated Parmesan. It will keep for weeks in the fridge if well wrapped in foil.

Provolone is made like mozzarella. Young provolone, called dolce, has a very mild flavour, whereas piccante provolone, a hard cheese matured for up to 2 years, is much stronger and sharper. Smoked provolone is also available.

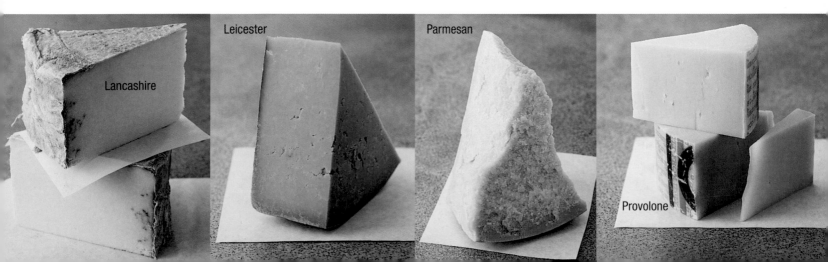

Lancashire

Leicester

Parmesan

Provolone

Goat's and sheep's milk cheeses

Traditionally, goat's and sheep's milk cheeses were made in areas where the land was unsuitable for cattle, and today some of the best still come from such places – mountainous regions or countries with a dry, harsh climate. Goat's cheeses are often labelled as 'chèvre', the French word for goat. They are generally lower in fat than cow's milk cheeses and have an unmistakably 'goaty' taste. Sheep's milk cheeses are more varied, ranging in style from Roquefort to pecorino.

Fresh goat's cheese (chèvre frais) is unripened, has no rind and is mildly tangy in flavour.

Soft or medium-fat goat's cheese, sometimes labelled medium mature, is white-rinded with a creamy interior

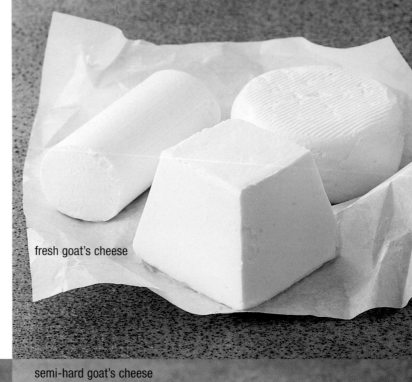

fresh goat's cheese

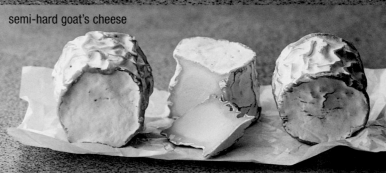

soft goat's cheese

semi-hard goat's cheese

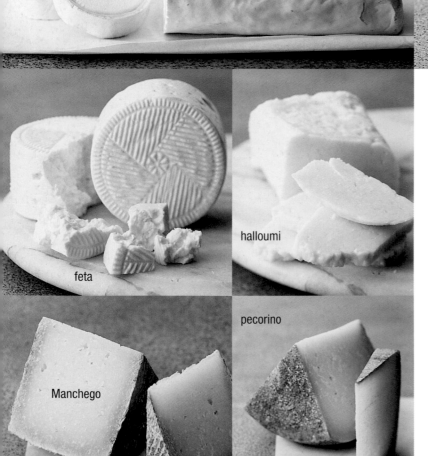

feta

halloumi

Manchego

pecorino

and a stronger flavour than fresh goat's cheese. It is usually log-shaped, which makes it easy to slice.

Semi-hard and hard goat's cheeses can be very pungent, with a soft and creamy or dry, crumbly interior and a firm rind. They are usually quite small – the French crottin-style cheeses can weigh as little as 25 g (scant 1 oz).

Feta, traditionally an unripened sheep's milk cheese from Greece, is now mass-produced in other countries. Much commercial feta contains a proportion of goat's and/or cow's milk and is slightly matured. White, moist and crumbly, with a piquant, salty flavour, it is sold in blocks packed in brine.

Halloumi, a medium-hard non-rinded cheese from Cyprus, has a slightly rubbery texture and a distinctive flavour that owes much to the addition of chopped mint. Like feta, halloumi is traditionally made from sheep's milk, but may now be made from a combination of milks. Unusually, it retains its shape when cooked, making it suitable for grilling or frying in slices.

Manchego, from Spain, is a hard waxed cheese sometimes pitted with tiny holes. Made from full-fat sheep's milk, it has a rich, mellow flavour with a sharp edge.

Pecorino is a hard, grainy-textured sheep's milk cheese made in Italy. The original variety is pecorino romano, which has a strong, salty flavour. Similar in character and nutritional value to Parmesan, it can be used in much the same way.

Blue cheeses

Blue cheeses are usually made by injecting the cheese with a penicillin mould in the early stages of the cheese-making process. Later, steel wires are inserted, creating tiny veins of air, which are then turned blue by the action of the mould.

Bleu d'Auvergne is a semi-hard French cheese that may be made with a mixture of cow's and goat's or sheep's milk. It has a piquant but not overly strong flavour and is usually sold wrapped in foil, since it has a very thin rind.

Cambozola, a German invention, is a creamy hybrid between Camembert and Gorgonzola. Although it is often described as blue Brie, it has a much higher fat content than Brie, since it contains added cream.

Dolcelatte, meaning 'sweet milk' in Italian, is the brand name of a creamy, mild commercial version of Gorgonzola.

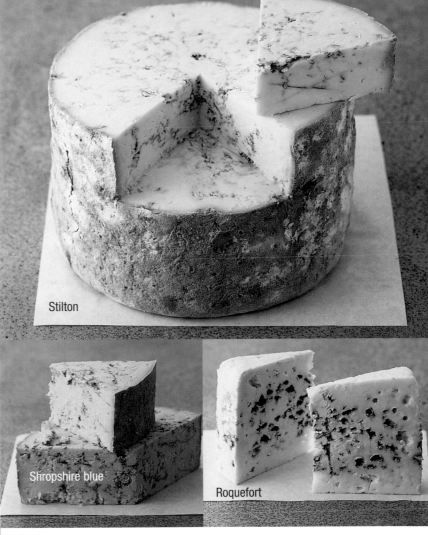

Stilton

Shropshire blue

Roquefort

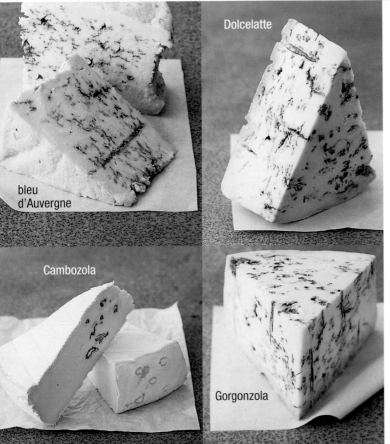

Dolcelatte

bleu d'Auvergne

Cambozola

Gorgonzola

Gorgonzola is a semi-hard cow's milk cheese from central Italy, with a slightly crumbly texture. Mass-produced versions can be quite mild, while farmhouse ones are more pungent.

Shropshire blue is deep orange-yellow with blue veining. Its strong, salty taste has an underlying hint of sweetness.

Roquefort comes from the region of the same name in France, where it is matured in limestone caves. A full-flavoured yet subtle, semi-soft blue cheese, with a smooth, creamy texture, it is made from full-fat sheep's milk. It is almost rindless.

Stilton, often described as the king of English cheeses, is a semi-hard, unpressed cheese made from full-fat cow's milk, traditionally with cream added. It varies in strength depending on how long it has been matured, but the flavour should be rich and piquant rather than sharp. Traditional farmhouse Stilton, moulded into tall cylinders, is strongest of all, with more grey-green veining than younger cheeses. Stilton can only be made in certain areas of central England.

Garlicky fresh cheese

This tangy, soft-textured yogurt cheese, flavoured with herbs and garlic, makes a healthy starter or snack, and is a great addition to a picnic basket, too. The garlic is blanched for a sweeter flavour. Serve with fresh vegetables for dipping, plus wholemeal bread, such as soda bread, to be spread with the cheese.

Serves 4

150 g (5½ oz) plain low-fat bio yogurt

150 g (5½ oz) fromage frais

2 large garlic cloves

1 tbsp snipped fresh chives

1 tbsp chopped parsley

2 tsp chopped fresh dill

1 tsp finely grated lemon zest

salt and pepper

To serve

1 head chicory, leaves separated

4 carrots, cut into 5 cm (2 in) sticks

1 bunch spring onions

4 celery sticks, cut into 5 cm (2 in) sticks

4 slices wholemeal soda bread, about 170 g
(6 oz) in total, cut into large chunks

Preparation and cooking time: 30–35 minutes,
plus overnight draining

Each serving provides Ⓥ

kcal 229, protein 10 g, fat 5 g (of which saturated fat 2 g), carbohydrate 40 g (of which sugars 15 g), fibre 5 g

✓✓✓	A
✓✓	C, calcium
✓	B₁, B₂, B₆, B₁₂, folate, niacin, copper, iron, potassium, zinc

1 Line a deep sieve with a double thickness of muslin and set over a bowl. Mix together the yogurt and fromage frais until smooth, then spoon into the muslin-lined sieve. Wrap the muslin over the top and put into the refrigerator. Leave to drain overnight.

2 The next day, drop the unpeeled garlic cloves into a small pan of boiling water and simmer for 3 minutes or until soft. Drain. Squeeze the garlic flesh out of the skins and mash or chop.

3 Unwrap the drained yogurt mixture and put it into a clean bowl (discard the liquid that has drained from the mixture). Add the blanched garlic, herbs and lemon zest to the yogurt cheese, and season with salt and pepper to taste. (The yogurt cheese can be kept, covered, in the fridge for 3–4 days.)

4 Spoon the yogurt cheese into a small bowl and set on a platter. Arrange the prepared vegetables and bread chunks around, and serve.

Some more ideas

• Thoroughly chill the yogurt cheese, then form it into a small 'barrel' shape. Roll in 75 g (2½ oz) finely chopped walnuts or hazelnuts to coat on all sides.

• For an olive and caper cheese, mash 45 g (1½ oz) feta cheese and stir into the freshly drained yogurt cheese together with ½ tsp crushed dried chillies, 1 crushed garlic clove, 1 tbsp chopped capers, 1 tbsp chopped black olives, 1 tbsp chopped fresh oregano and seasoning to taste. Serve as a starter or snack for 6, with the crudités and toasted pitta bread.

Plus points

• This home-made soft cheese is much lower in fat than similar commercial cheeses, yet it is just as tasty. There is no need to add salt to the mixture as the herbs, garlic and lemon provide plenty of flavour.

• Recently published research suggests that garlic has a role to play in reducing blood cholesterol levels and inhibiting blood clotting. Including garlic in the diet on a regular basis may therefore help to reduce the risk of heart disease and stroke.

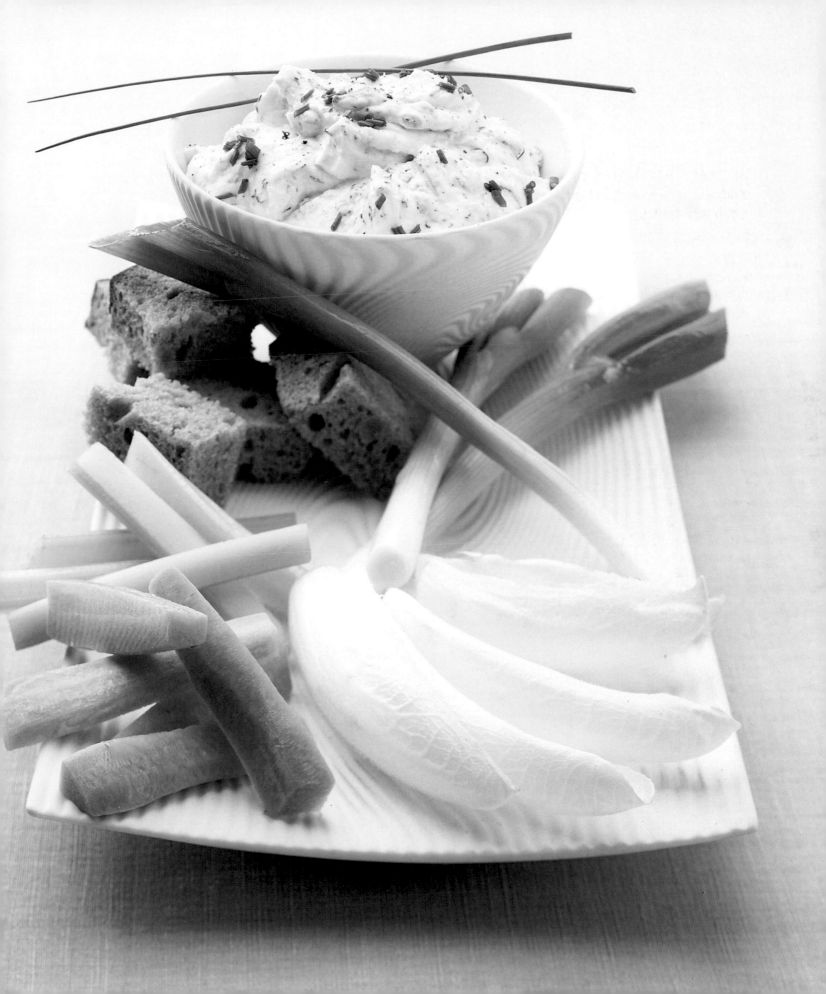

Eggs florentine

The term 'florentine' in a recipe title indicates that the dish uses spinach – in this case, poached eggs on a bed of spinach and leeks, coated with a cheese sauce. This updated version of the classic eggs florentine uses a lighter sauce thickened with cornflour rather than a butter and flour roux. Serve for supper with wholemeal toast.

Serves 4

20 g (¾ oz) cornflour

300 ml (10 fl oz) semi-skimmed milk

45 g (1½ oz) Gruyère cheese, finely grated

pinch of grated nutmeg

15 g (½ oz) butter

1 tbsp extra virgin olive oil

200 g (7 oz) baby leeks, thinly sliced

800 g (1¾ lb) baby spinach leaves

1 tsp vinegar

8 eggs

salt and pepper

paprika to garnish

Preparation and cooking time: 30 minutes

Each serving provides Ⓥ

kcal 386, protein 27 g, fat 26 g (of which saturated fat 9 g), carbohydrate 13 g (of which sugars 8 g), fibre 5 g

✓✓✓	A, B₁₂, C, E, folate, calcium
✓✓	B₆, B₂, B₆, niacin, iron, potassium, selenium, zinc
✓	copper

1 First make the sauce. Mix the cornflour to a smooth paste with a little of the milk. Pour the remaining milk into a non-stick saucepan and bring to the boil. Stir the boiling milk into the cornflour mixture, then pour back into the saucepan. Bring to the boil, stirring. Once the sauce has thickened, simmer for 2 minutes. Remove from the heat, stir in the Gruyère, and season with nutmeg, salt and pepper to taste. Cover the surface of the sauce with a piece of greaseproof paper to prevent a skin from forming and set aside in a warm place.

2 Heat the butter with the olive oil in a large saucepan. Add the leeks and cook gently for about 3 minutes, stirring, until beginning to soften. Add the spinach and stir. Cover the pan and continue cooking over a moderate heat for 2–3 minutes or until the spinach has wilted and the leeks are tender. Drain the vegetables in a sieve, pressing down with the back of a spoon to remove excess moisture. Return to the pan and season with salt and pepper to taste. Cover to keep warm.

3 While the vegetables are cooking, poach the eggs. Half fill a large frying pan with water and bring to simmering point. Add the vinegar. Break in 4 of the eggs, one at a time, and cook gently for 3–4 minutes, spooning the hot water over the yolks towards the end of the cooking time. Lift out the eggs with a draining spoon and drain on kitchen paper. Poach the remaining eggs in the same way.

4 Preheat the grill to high. Spread the leek and spinach mixture in an even layer in a large flameproof dish. Make 8 hollows in the vegetables using the back of a spoon and place a poached egg in each hollow.

5 Spoon the cheese sauce over the eggs. Lightly dust with paprika, then place the dish under the grill. Cook for 3–4 minutes or until the top is lightly browned. Serve at once.

Plus points

• Like other animal foods, eggs provide useful amounts of vitamin B₁₂. Free-range eggs tend to contain more than eggs from battery hens.

• Spinach is a good source of nutrients with antioxidant properties, including vitamins C and E and carotenoid compounds.

• Leeks belong to the onion family. They provide vitamin E, and the green part of the leek is a good source of beta-carotene.

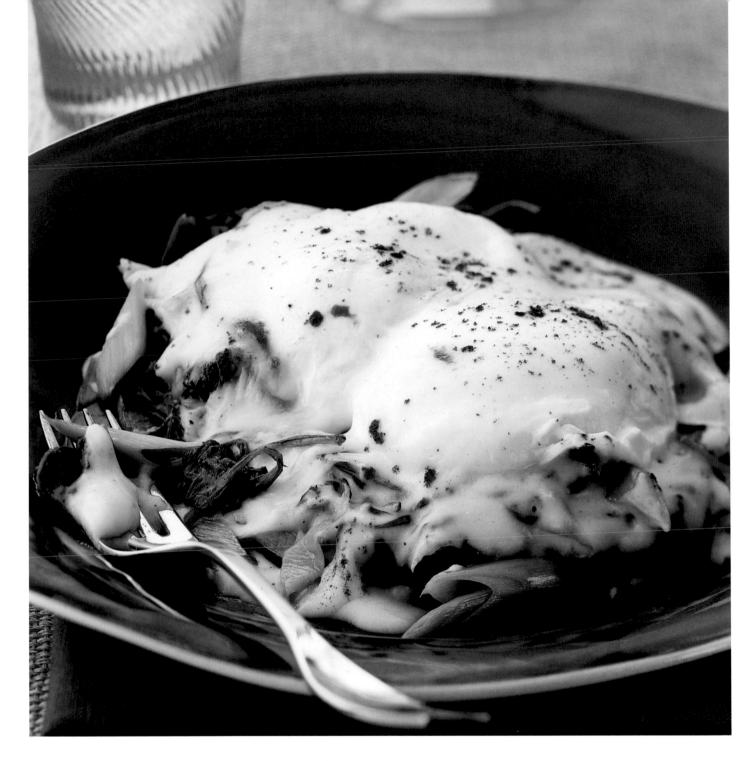

Another idea

• For bubble and squeak eggs, cook 400 g (14 oz) scrubbed and diced new potatoes in a large pan of boiling water for 7 minutes. Add 500 g (1 lb 2 oz) shredded spring greens to the pan and continue cooking for 4–5 minutes or until the vegetables are tender. Drain well, then return to the pan and crush together using a potato masher. Add 115 g (4 oz) diced cooked beetroot and carefully fold in. Season with salt and pepper to taste. Heat 1 tbsp extra virgin olive oil in a large non-stick frying pan with a flameproof handle. Transfer the vegetable mixture to the pan and spread it out evenly, pressing down with the back of a large spoon. Make 8 hollows in the vegetable mixture, then break an egg into each. Grate 55 g (2 oz) Lancashire cheese over the top, being sure to cover the whole surface. Cook under a preheated hot grill for 7–8 minutes or until the eggs are set. Serve hot, with French bread.

Smoked haddock soufflé

Light, fluffy soufflés rarely fail to impress, yet they are surprisingly easy to make. This recipe uses the fish-poaching milk to make the soufflé base, and fresh herbs and chopped tomatoes are added for a lovely flavour. Serve straight from the oven, with crusty wholemeal bread as an accompaniment.

Serves 4

300 g (10½ oz) smoked haddock fillet
300 ml (10 fl oz) semi-skimmed milk
1 tsp butter
1 tbsp Parmesan cheese
1 tbsp fine dry breadcrumbs
3 tbsp cornflour
3 eggs, separated
250 g (8½ oz) tomatoes, skinned, seeded and diced
1 tsp wholegrain mustard
2 tbsp finely chopped parsley
2 tbsp finely snipped fresh chives
1 egg white
salt and pepper

Preparation time: about 35 minutes
Cooking time: 35 minutes

Each serving provides

kcal 250, protein 25 g, fat 9 g (of which saturated fat 3 g), carbohydrate 19 g (of which sugars 6 g), fibre 1 g

✓✓✓	B_{12}
✓✓	A, niacin, selenium
✓	B_1, B_2, B_6, C, E, folate, calcium, copper, iron, potassium, zinc

1 Put the haddock and milk in a saucepan and heat until simmering. Simmer gently for about 8 minutes or until the fish will just flake when tested with a fork. Remove the pan from the heat and leave the fish to cool in the milk. When the fish is cool enough to handle, remove it and flake the flesh, discarding the skin and any bones. Set the poaching milk aside to cool.

2 Preheat the oven, with a metal baking sheet inside, to 190°C (375°F, gas mark 5). Lightly grease a 1.7 litre (3 pint) soufflé dish with the butter. Mix together the Parmesan and breadcrumbs, and sprinkle over the bottom and side of the dish, turning the dish to coat evenly. Shake out any excess crumb mixture and reserve.

3 Mix the cornflour with a little of the reserved, cold poaching milk to make a smooth paste. Heat the remaining milk in a small saucepan until almost boiling, then pour into the cornflour mixture, stirring constantly. Return to the pan and bring to the boil, stirring to make a thick sauce.

4 Pour the sauce into a large mixing bowl. Add the egg yolks, one by one, beating them thoroughly into the sauce. Stir in the flaked haddock, tomatoes, mustard, parsley, chives, and salt and pepper to taste.

5 In a clean, dry mixing bowl, whisk the 4 egg whites until stiff enough to hold soft peaks. Fold one-quarter of the whites into the sauce mixture to lighten it, then gently fold in the remaining whites.

6 Spoon the mixture into the prepared soufflé dish and sprinkle the top with the reserved Parmesan and breadcrumb mixture. Set the dish on the hot baking sheet and bake for about 35 minutes or until well risen and golden brown. Serve at once.

Plus points

• Haddock is a useful source of vitamin B_6. This vitamin helps the body to make use of protein from food and to form haemoglobin, which is the pigment in red blood cells.

• Milk is an excellent source of many essential nutrients, the majority of which are concentrated in the non-fat part of milk. Semi-skimmed and skimmed milk therefore contain more of these nutrients than full-fat milks.

• Thickening the soufflé base with cornflour, instead of the more traditional method using butter, helps to reduce the total fat content of this recipe.

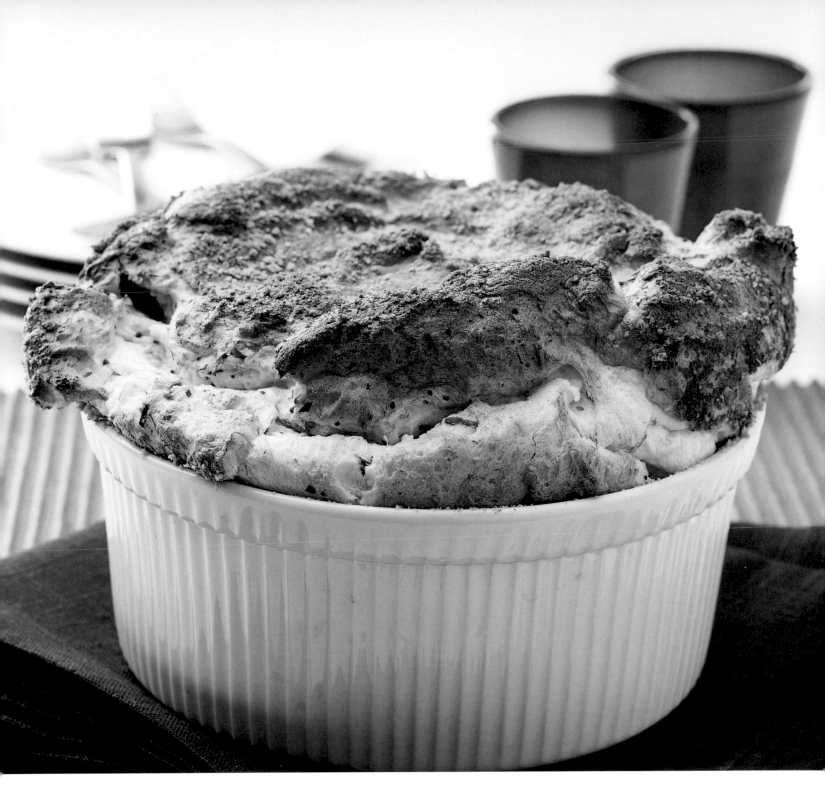

Another idea

• To make a Mediterranean-style goat's cheese soufflé, put 55 g (2 oz) dry-packed sun-dried tomatoes in a small bowl and pour over boiling water to cover. Leave to soak for 30 minutes, then drain and finely chop. In step 3, make the thick sauce base with 3 tbsp cornflour and 300 ml (10 fl oz) semi-skimmed milk. After beating in the egg yolks, add 100 g (3½ oz) creamy goat's cheese and beat until smooth. Stir in the sun-dried tomatoes and the herbs, and season with salt and pepper to taste. Fold in the stiffly whisked egg whites, then spoon the mixture into the soufflé dish. Finish and bake as in the main recipe.

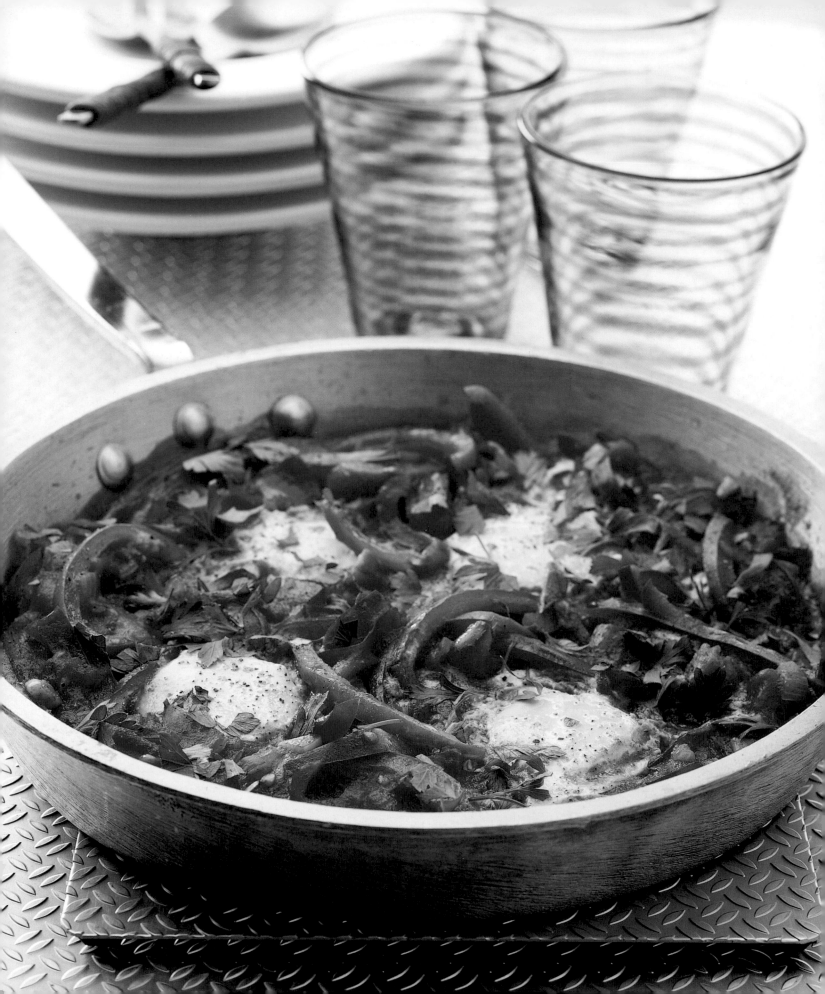

Chakchouka

This dish is popular all over the Mediterranean region and there are many different variations. Basically it is a tomato-based vegetable stew, like a ratatouille, with eggs poached right in the mixture. Serve it for a fast and sustaining lunch for 2 with garlic and rosemary focaccia or olive ciabatta, or as a snack for 4.

Serves 2

1 tbsp extra virgin olive oil
1 small onion, roughly chopped
2 garlic cloves, crushed
1 red pepper, seeded and thinly sliced
1 green pepper, seeded and thinly sliced
400 g (14 oz) large ripe tomatoes, roughly chopped
2 tbsp tomato purée
$\frac{1}{4}$ tsp crushed dried chillies (optional)
1 tsp ground cumin
pinch of sugar
4 eggs
salt
sprigs of fresh flat-leaf parsley to garnish

Preparation and cooking time: 30 minutes

Each serving provides

kcal 321, protein 19 g, fat 20 g (of which saturated fat 5 g), carbohydrate 18 g (of which sugars 17 g), fibre 6 g

✓✓✓	A, B$_{12}$, C, E, copper
✓✓	B$_1$, B$_2$, B$_6$, folate, niacin, iron, potassium, zinc
✓	calcium, selenium

1 Heat the oil in a deep, heavy-based frying pan. Add the onion, garlic, and red and green peppers, and cook gently for 5 minutes or until softened.

2 Stir in the tomatoes, tomato purée, chillies, if using, cumin, sugar, and salt to taste. Cover and cook gently for about 5 minutes or until the mixture is thick and well combined.

3 Make 4 hollows in the vegetable mixture using the back of a wooden spoon, then break an egg into each hollow. Cover the pan again and cook gently for 6–8 minutes or until the eggs are just set.

4 Serve immediately, straight from the pan, garnishing each plate with sprigs of parsley.

Some more ideas

• Add 55 g (2 oz) stoned black olives or chopped sun-dried tomatoes to the vegetable mixture.
• Instead of the chillies, add 1 tsp harissa sauce, or to taste.
• To make an omelette-like chakchouka, after breaking the eggs into the mixture, stir them gently to mix up the whites and yolks.
• For chakchouka with aubergine and mushrooms, replace the red and green peppers with 1 aubergine, cut into small chunks. In step 2, use 1 can chopped tomatoes, about 400 g, with the juice, instead of fresh tomatoes and add 170 g (6 oz) chopped button or chestnut mushrooms. Omit the chillies and cumin, and instead flavour with 1 tsp fennel or caraway seeds. Cover and cook gently for 15 minutes before breaking the eggs into the mixture.

Plus points

• Eggs are a useful source of vitamin A, but it is a myth that a darker-coloured yolk has a higher content of this vitamin (as carotene). The coloration is due to pigments found in grass and other food the chicken eats.
• Tomatoes are rich in the antioxidants vitamin C, beta-carotene and lycopene. Antioxidants help to protect the body's cells against the damaging effects of free radicals.
• The naturally waxy skin of peppers helps to protect against oxidation and thus against loss of vitamin C during storage. As a result, the vitamin C content remains high for several weeks after harvesting.

Mozzarella with grilled fennel and peppers on crostini

Here is a colourful, Mediterranean-style dish that is very easy to make. The vegetables can be prepared in advance if you like, and left to soak up the flavours in the dressing, then mixed with the mozzarella and piled onto freshly toasted, garlicky ciabatta bread. A perfect summer lunch.

Serves 4

1 large bulb of fennel, about 300 g (10½ oz)

3 tbsp extra virgin olive oil

1 small red onion, halved

1 red pepper, halved and seeded

1 yellow pepper, halved and seeded

2 tsp balsamic vinegar

150 g (5½ oz) mozzarella cheese, diced

85 g (3 oz) mixed salad leaves

15 g (½ oz) fresh basil leaves

1 ciabatta loaf, thickly sliced

1 garlic clove, halved

salt and pepper

Preparation and cooking time: about 45 minutes

Each serving provides

kcal 410, protein 19 g, fat 19 g (of which saturated fat 7 g), carbohydrate 42 g (of which sugars 8 g), fibre 5 g

✓✓✓	A, C
✓✓	B_{12}, calcium, selenium
✓	B_1, B_6, E, folate, niacin, copper, iron, potassium, zinc

1 Preheat the grill to high. Cut the fennel bulb in half lengthways, then cut each half lengthways into 1 cm (½ in) thick slices, not cutting all the way through the base so the layers remain attached. Place the halves cut side down on a baking tray and brush lightly with 1 tbsp of the oil.

2 Put the onion halves and peppers cut side down on the baking tray. Grill the vegetables for 10–15 minutes, turning once, until the fennel is golden brown and the peppers and onions are tender and blackened in places.

3 Transfer the vegetables to a chopping board (leave the grill on). Pour any juices from the baking tray into a small bowl and whisk in the remaining 2 tbsp oil and the balsamic vinegar. Season this dressing with salt and pepper to taste.

4 Thickly slice the peppers and onion. Cut through the base of the fennel halves to separate the slices. Put all the vegetables in a mixing bowl. Pour over the dressing and toss well to coat the vegetables evenly. Add the mozzarella, salad leaves and basil to the bowl, piling them on top of the vegetables (do not toss together yet).

5 Spread out the ciabatta slices on a clean baking sheet and toast under the grill for 2–3 minutes or until golden on both sides. Rub one side of each slice with the cut surface of the garlic clove; discard the garlic.

6 Toss the mozzarella, leaves and vegetables to mix them together, then pile on top of the ciabatta toasts. Serve immediately.

Plus points

- Mozzarella cheese is lower in fat than many other varieties of cheeses and so contains fewer calories.
- Fennel is believed to help digestion, particularly by relieving colic, stomach cramps and wind.
- Peppers are an excellent source of vitamin C and of beta-carotene. However, the beta-carotene content varies according to the colour of the pepper, with red peppers containing the most and green peppers the least.

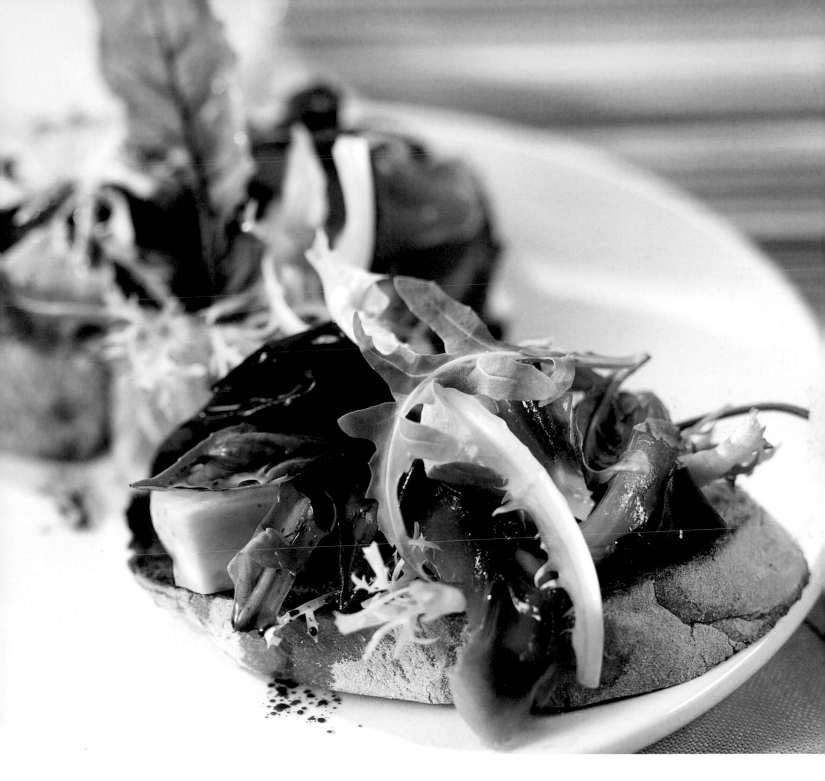

Some more ideas

• For a rich, nutty flavour, replace the olive oil with hazelnut or walnut oil.

• To make mozzarella and vegetable pitta pockets, cut 4 pitta breads across in half and warm under the grill. Open the pockets and spoon in the mozzarella and grilled vegetables.

• Make the classic Italian mozzarella, avocado and tomato salad and serve on toasted ciabatta. Peel a large avocado and cut across into slices. Slice 2 large, ripe tomatoes and 150 g (5½ oz) mozzarella. Mix together 2 tbsp extra virgin olive oil, 2 tsp balsamic vinegar, and seasoning to taste in a bowl. Add the avocado, tomatoes and mozzarella, together with a handful of torn fresh basil leaves, and mix gently with the dressing. Toast the ciabatta and rub with garlic as in the main recipe, then top with the salad and serve.

Stuffed Thai omelette

For these delectable chilli-flavoured omelettes, the eggs are whisked with cornflour to give them a slightly firmer texture, suitable for folding round a colourful filling of stir-fried vegetables and rice noodles.

Serves 4

4 tsp cornflour

8 eggs

¼–½ tsp crushed dried chillies, to taste

2 tbsp sunflower oil

125 g (4½ oz) fine rice noodles

1 tsp toasted sesame oil

115 g (4 oz) chestnut mushrooms, sliced

2 carrots, cut into 5 cm (2 in) matchstick strips

1 small green pepper, seeded and cut into thin strips

170 g (6 oz) white cabbage, finely shredded

2 tbsp light soy sauce

2 tsp white wine vinegar

2 tsp chopped root ginger bottled in oil

salt and pepper

1 tbsp toasted sesame seeds to garnish (optional)

Preparation and cooking time: 30 minutes

Each serving provides

kcal 401, protein 18.5 g, fat 20 g (of which saturated fat 4 g), carbohydrate 38 g (of which sugars 7 g), fibre 3 g

✓✓✓	A, B₁₂, C
✓✓	B₂, E, folate, niacin, copper, selenium, zinc
✓	B₁, B₆, calcium, iron, potassium

1 Mix the cornflour with 3 tbsp cold water in a mixing bowl. Add the eggs and whisk together until mixed. Stir in the chillies and season with salt and pepper to taste.

2 Heat 1 tsp of the sunflower oil in a 20 cm (8 in) non-stick frying pan over a moderate heat. Pour in one-quarter of the egg mixture, tipping the pan to spread out the egg in a thin, even layer. Cook for 2 minutes or until set and golden brown underneath.

3 Slide the omelette out of the pan onto a plate. Make 3 more omelettes in the same way, stacking them up interleaved with greaseproof paper. Keep warm.

4 While making the omelettes, soak the rice noodles in boiling water to cover for 4 minutes, or according to the packet instructions, then drain.

5 Heat the remaining 2 tsp sunflower oil with the toasted sesame oil in a wok or large frying pan. Add the mushrooms, carrots, green pepper and cabbage, and stir-fry for 4–5 minutes or until just tender. Add the soy sauce, vinegar, ginger and softened rice noodles. Gently toss together until piping hot.

6 Divide the vegetable and noodle mixture among the omelettes and fold them over in half. Sprinkle with the sesame seeds and serve immediately.

Another idea

• For a folded salad omelette, grill 2 rashers of lean back bacon until crisp, then crumble or chop. Whisk the eggs with the cornflour and water as in the main recipe, but leave out the chillies. For each omelette, heat 1 tsp sunflower oil in a 20 cm (8 in) non-stick frying pan, sprinkle one-quarter of the bacon pieces evenly over the bottom of the pan and then pour in one-quarter of the egg mixture. Cook the omelettes as in the main recipe, then slide onto serving plates and leave to cool. Finely shred ½ small iceberg lettuce and mix with 2 chopped celery sticks, 1 seeded and thinly sliced red pepper and 6 chopped spring onions. Season to taste. Spread half of each omelette with 2 tbsp hummus and top with the salad mixture. Fold the omelettes over in half and serve.

Plus points

• Rice noodles contain no gluten and are therefore suitable for people with coeliac disease who are unable to tolerate gluten-containing food.
• White cabbage contains beneficial phytochemicals including glucosinolates, which have strong anti-cancer effects.

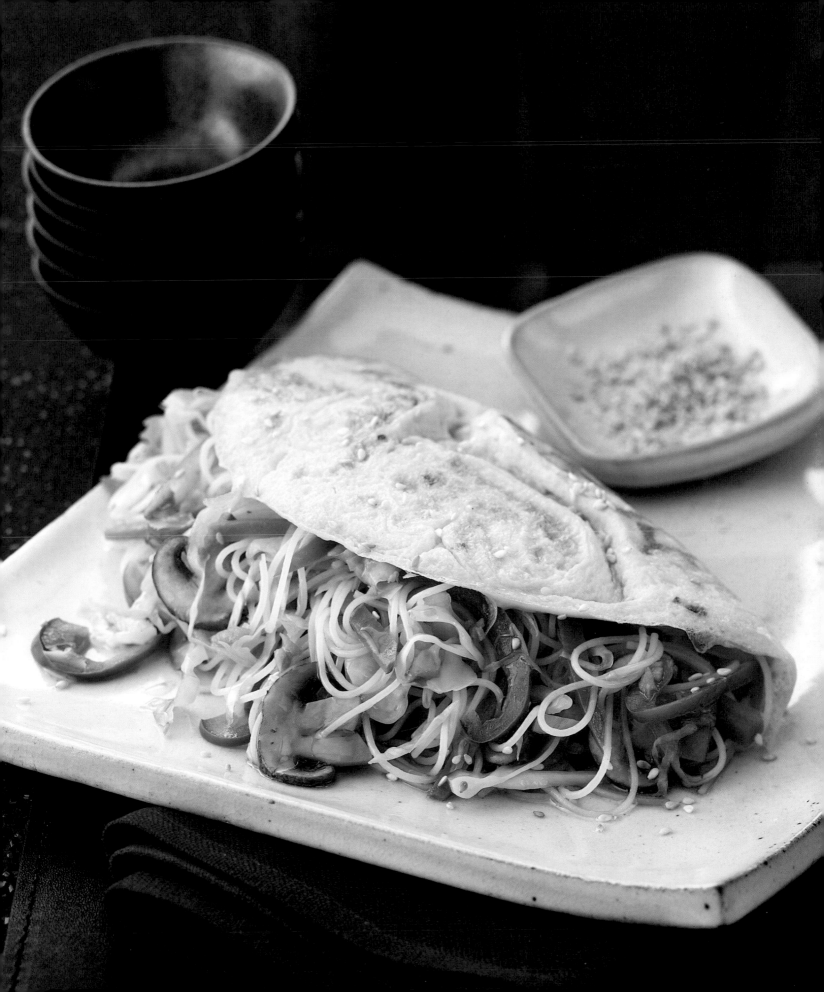

Camembert and broccoli pancakes

Lacy, thin pancakes rolled around a tasty filling make a delightful main course. The beauty of this dish is that the pancakes, filling and tomato sauce topping can all be made in advance, then assembled and baked later. Serve with some crusty multigrain bread or boiled new potatoes, to boost the carbohydrate content.

Serves 4 (makes 8 pancakes)

115 g (4 oz) plain flour
2 eggs, beaten
250 ml (8½ fl oz) semi-skimmed milk
4 tsp sunflower oil
15 g (½ oz) Parmesan cheese, freshly grated
sprigs of fresh flat-leaf parsley to garnish

Tomato sauce
1 onion, chopped
1 garlic clove, chopped
1 can chopped tomatoes, about 400 g
pinch of sugar
2 tbsp chopped fresh flat-leaf parsley

Camembert and broccoli filling
250 g (8½ oz) broccoli, broken into
   tiny florets
150 g (5½ oz) Camembert cheese, diced
4 tbsp quark cheese
salt and pepper

Preparation time: 45 minutes
Cooking time: 25 minutes

Each serving provides

kcal 399, protein 27 g, fat 19 g (of which saturated fat 8 g), carbohydrate 34 g (of which sugars 10 g), fibre 4 g

✓✓✓	B_{12}, C, calcium
✓✓	B_2, E, folate, niacin, zinc
✓	A, B_1, B_6, copper, iron, potassium

1 First make the pancakes. Sift the flour into a bowl, add the eggs and a pinch of salt, and gradually whisk in the milk to form a smooth batter.

2 Brush an 18 cm (7 in) non-stick frying pan with a little of the oil, then heat. Add about one-eighth of the batter and tilt the pan so the batter coats the bottom thinly and evenly. Cook for about 45 seconds or until the pancake has set and the underside is lightly browned. Use a palette knife to loosen the edge of the pancake, then carefully turn it over and cook the other side for 30 seconds. Slide onto a plate.

3 Use the remaining batter to make 7 more pancakes, brushing the pan with more oil as necessary. Stack the cooked pancakes on the plate as they are made, interleaving them with greaseproof paper.

4 To make the tomato sauce, put the onion, garlic and tomatoes with their juice in a saucepan, and add the sugar, and salt and pepper to taste. Simmer for 10–15 minutes, stirring occasionally, until slightly thickened.

5 Meanwhile, make the filling. Cook the broccoli florets in boiling water for 4–5 minutes or until tender, then drain well. Tip into a bowl and add the Camembert, quark, and salt and pepper to taste. Fold together gently.

6 When the tomato sauce is cooked, remove from the heat and purée using a hand-held blender. Alternatively, leave to cool for 1–2 minutes, then pour into a food processor or blender to purée. Stir in the chopped parsley.

7 Preheat the oven to 200ºC (400ºF, gas mark 6). Divide the filling among the pancakes, roll them up and arrange side by side in an ovenproof dish. Pour over the tomato sauce to cover evenly and sprinkle with the Parmesan cheese. Bake for 25 minutes or until bubbling and golden brown. Garnish with parsley sprigs and serve.

Plus points

• Camembert and Brie are similar cheeses – both have a downy white rind and a soft, unctuous texture – but Camembert is smaller, and it is slightly lower in fat.
• Broccoli contains a number of disease-fighting phytochemicals, including indoles, which may help to protect against breast cancer. Indoles appear to inhibit the action of oestrogens that initiate tumour growth.
• Quark is a curd cheese from Germany. It is low in both fat and sodium.

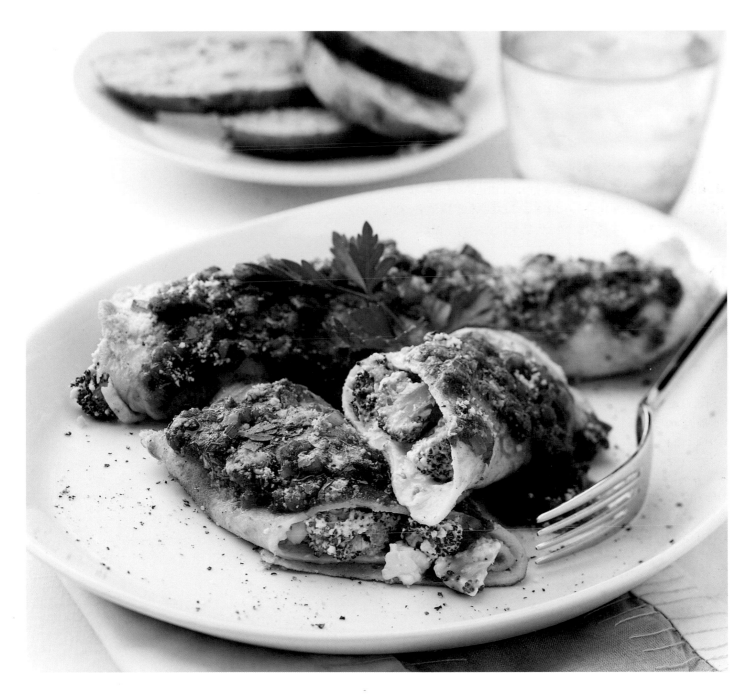

Some more ideas

• The pancake batter can also be made in a food processor. Just put all the ingredients in the container and blend until smooth.

• Make up a double quantity of batter and prepare 16 pancakes, then freeze half for a later date. They will thaw at room temperature in about 2 hours.

• For Parma ham and broccoli pancakes, cook the broccoli as in the main recipe, then mix with 100 g (3½ oz) curd cheese. Trim all fat from 4 thin slices of Parma ham, about 50 g (1¾ oz) in total, and cut each slice in half. Place a piece of ham on each pancake, add the broccoli mixture and roll up. Arrange in an ovenproof dish and cover with a white sauce. To make the sauce, mix 1½ tbsp cornflour with a little semi-skimmed milk taken from 300 ml (10 fl oz). Heat the rest of the milk to boiling point. Stir into the cornflour mixture, then return to the pan and heat gently, stirring, until thickened. Simmer for 2 minutes. Add 1 tsp Dijon mustard, and salt and pepper to taste. Pour evenly over the pancakes and sprinkle with 55 g (2 oz) grated mature Gouda or other well-flavoured cheese. Bake as in the main recipe.

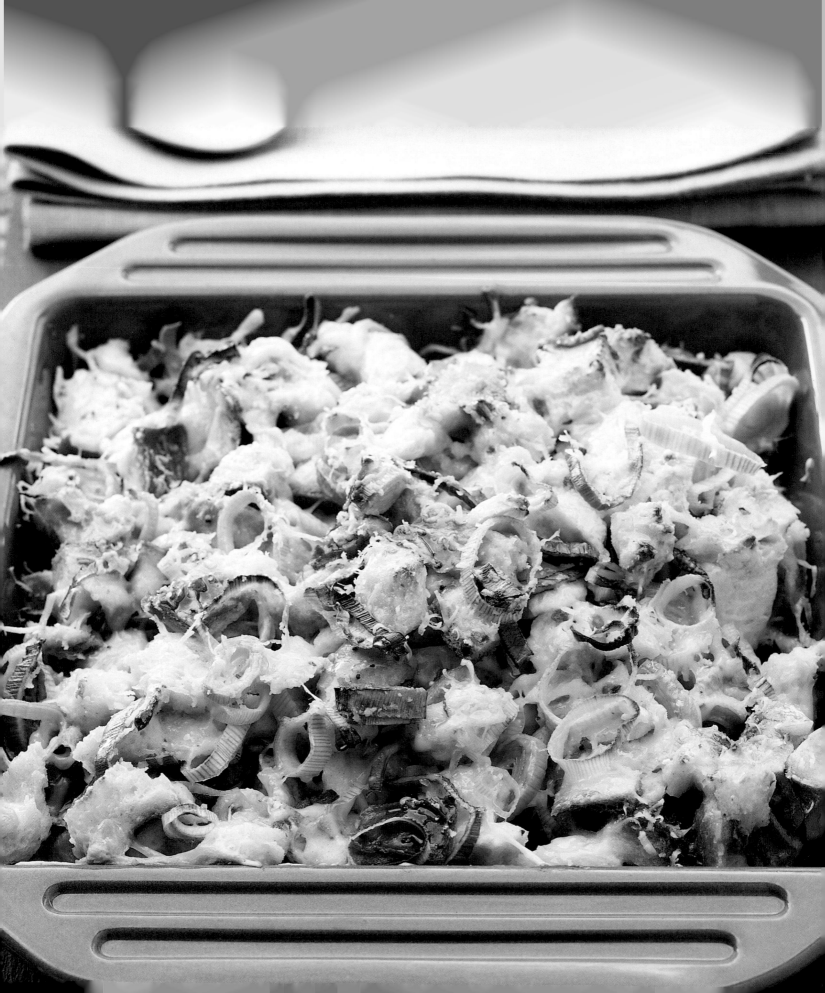

Cheese and onion bread pudding

A simple, homely dish of diced challah bread baked in a cheesy custard with leeks and spring onions makes great comfort food, and is an excellent way to use up slightly stale bread. Serve with a crisp salad of cos or Little Gem lettuce leaves tossed with sliced cucumber and halved cherry tomatoes.

Serves 4

340 g (12 oz) day-old challah bread

600 ml (1 pint) semi-skimmed milk

3 eggs

pinch of crushed dried chillies

100 g (3½ oz) Emmenthal cheese, grated

2 leeks, thinly sliced

4 spring onions, thinly sliced

2 tbsp freshly grated Parmesan cheese

salt and pepper

Preparation time: 20 minutes

Cooking time: 30 minutes

1 Cut the bread into small cubes about 1 cm (½ in) square. Put the bread into a large mixing bowl, pour over the milk and leave to soak for 15 minutes.

2 Meanwhile, preheat the oven to 180°C (350°F, gas mark 4). Break the eggs into a small mixing bowl and add the chillies, and salt and pepper to taste. Beat lightly together with a fork. Add the Emmenthal cheese, leeks and spring onions, and stir to combine.

3 Add the egg mixture to the soaked bread cubes. Fold together gently but thoroughly, then pour into a lightly greased 2 litre (3½ pint) shallow ovenproof dish.

4 Sprinkle the grated Parmesan evenly over the surface, then bake for 30 minutes or until puffed and just set, and the top is crisp and golden. Serve hot.

Some more ideas

• Make sun-dried tomato bread pudding with peppers. Thickly slice 340 g (12 oz) day-old sun-dried tomato-flavoured bread. Cut 100 g (3½ oz) Emmenthal cheese into thin slices and use to make sandwiches with the bread. Cut the sandwiches in half, then arrange in a single layer in a lightly greased 2 litre (3½ pint) shallow ovenproof dish. Scatter over 3 seeded and finely diced peppers (1 green, 1 yellow and 1 red). Beat 3 eggs with 600 ml (1 pint) semi-skimmed milk, 2 tbsp sun-dried tomato paste, and salt and pepper to taste. Pour over the sandwiches and leave to soak for 15 minutes. Sprinkle the surface with 2 tbsp freshly grated Parmesan cheese and bake as in the main recipe.

• For olive bread pudding, in the sun-dried tomato bread pudding above, use olive bread instead of sun-dried tomato bread and replace the sun-dried tomato paste with tapenade (black olive paste).

Each serving provides Ⓥ

kcal 469, protein 28 g, fat 18 g (of which saturated fat 9 g), carbohydrate 52 g (of which sugars 11 g), fibre 3 g

✓✓✓	A, B₁₂, calcium, copper, selenium
✓✓	B₁, B₂, B₆, C, folate, niacin, zinc
✓	E, iron, potassium

Plus points

• Emmenthal, a Swiss cheese made from cow's milk, has a sweet and nutty flavour. With the other dairy products used here, it makes a significant contribution to the total protein and calcium content of the dish.

• Challah bread, which is enriched with egg, is a good source of starchy carbohydrate. At least half the calories in a healthy diet should come from starchy foods.

• Both the white bulb and green leaves of spring onions are edible, and using the leaves increases the amount of carotene in this dish.

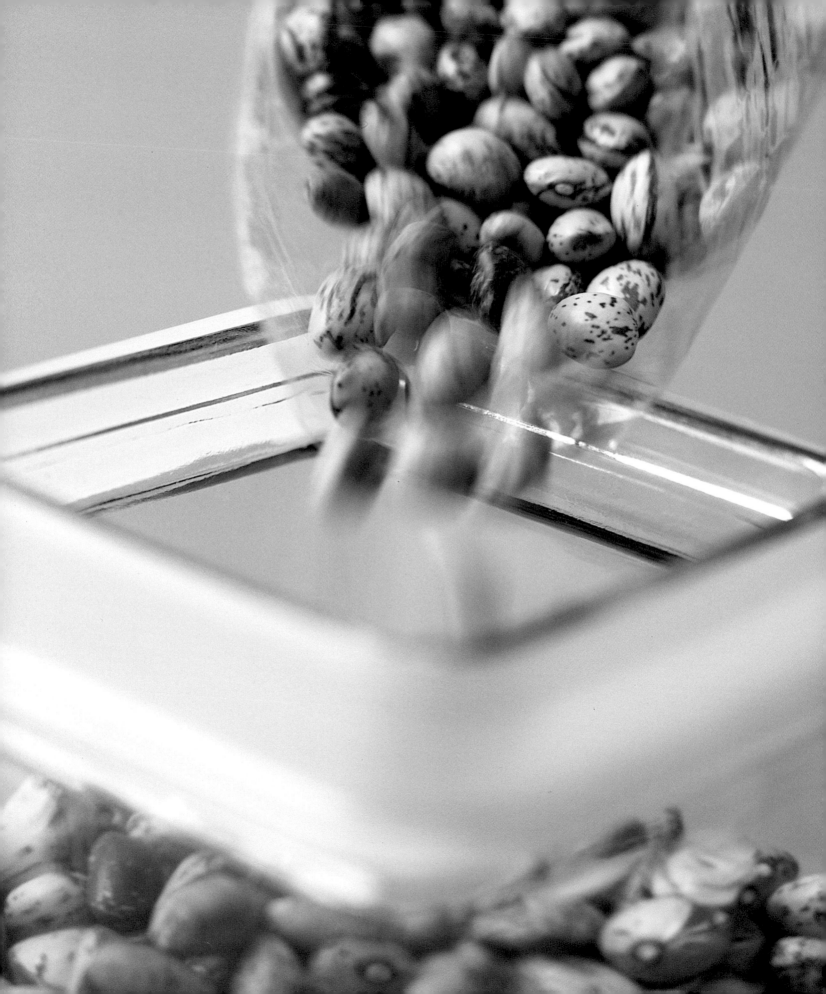

Rice, Beans and Grains

Here are the new stars of good cooking – cereal grains and pulses. Today, they are found on all the most fashionable restaurant menus and in recipe books galore. It's no wonder, with such a wide array of colourful varieties to choose from, and the amazing range of delicious breads and dishes that can be created with them. The fact that they are also among the most nutritious foods you can eat is a fantastic bonus. So if you haven't cooked much with rice, grains and pulses in the past, now is the time to join the growing army of fans.

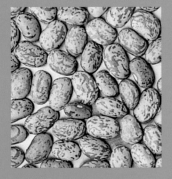

Versatile rice, beans and grains

These wonder foods are high in nutrients and fibre and low in fats and sodium, as well as being one of the cheapest food groups.

Why eat rice, beans and grains?

Most of the calories in grains and pulses are in the form of starchy carbohydrate, which should contribute at least 50% of the calories in our daily diet. In addition, wholegrains (those that are unrefined) and all pulses are high in natural fibre. Beans also contain protein, which makes them especially useful for vegetarians. Indeed, for thousands of years they have been a main source of protein in many parts of the world. Grains and pulses also provide a a variety of phytochemicals – compounds that are believed to have many health benefits.

Divine rice

Originating in China and India, rice has been a staple of the diet there for thousands of years, as well as in other parts of Asia, Africa and South America. Today, it is estimated that more rice is eaten than any other cereal crop. Indeed, rice is revered as divine in many communities, and when it was first introduced into ancient Greece it was more highly prized than Beluga caviar is today!

Like other cereals, rice is low in fat. It contains some protein although less than other cereals. Because it contains no gluten, it is an ideal alternative to grains such as wheat, barley and oats for people with coeliac disease (gluten intolerance).

- Brown rice is often called wholegrain rice, a term that isn't strictly true as the outer, inedible husk is removed. But all the rest of the grain remains intact, including the outer bran layers and the germ in the centre. Brown rice is a good source of most B vitamins, except B_{12}. It also contains a good range of minerals, such as magnesium and copper.
- White (polished) rice has had the husk and germ removed. It keeps longer than brown rice because when the husk and germ are removed, rice becomes harder, with less tendency to spoil. Polishing the grain to achieve white rice removes most of the fibre and B vitamins and a high proportion of the minerals.

Pulses for cheap protein

The generic (family) name for all dried beans, lentils and dried peas is pulses. Although their individual nutrient content varies, pulses are, as a family, an important source of non-animal protein as well as starchy carbohydrate and fibre. Pulses are highly adaptable, able to be used as the protein, starchy carbohydrate or vegetable element in a meal.

Most pulses are rich in folate and other B vitamins, and some are good sources of vitamin E, as well as a wide range of minerals, including magnesium and iron. The nutritional content of pulses increases dramatically when they are sprouted – there is 60% more vitamin C and almost 30% more B vitamins in the sprout than in the original bean.

Bran and minerals

It has been thought that the bran in brown rice and wholegrains might hinder the body's uptake of minerals such as iron and calcium. This is because bran contains phytic acid, which binds with the minerals, rendering them indigestible. However, studies show that bran eaten as part of a wholegrain is less likely to have this effect than bran extracted from a grain and used separately – wheat bran sprinkled onto cereals, for example. There is also some evidence to show that eating foods rich in essential fatty acids (e.g. oily fish and nuts) at the same time may counteract the possible adverse effect of the bran and aid absorption of the minerals. Until we know more, the sensible solution is to enjoy brown rice and wholegrains, and to eat plenty of calcium and iron-rich foods at other times. And to remember that wholegrains have positive effects on health in all other respects.

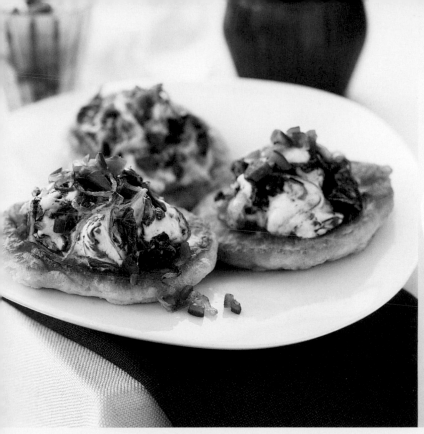

▲ Rice can be used in lots of imaginative and nutritious ways, such as in these tasty rice pancakes with an onion and spinach topping.

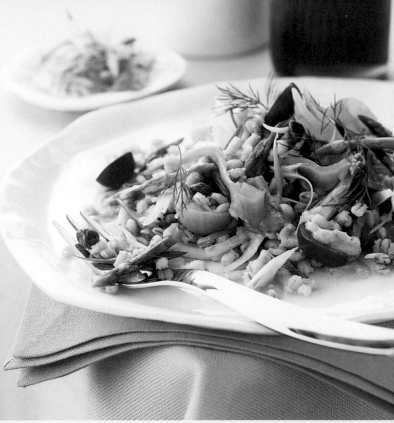

▲ Try a grain dish such as dilled barley and smoked salmon salad for a delicious lunch or supper.

▼ Make a hearty roast vegetable and bean stew with butternut squash, and serve with jacket baked potatoes

Grains make good eating

In many regions of the world, grains make up a large part of every meal, and cereal crops such as wheat, barley and oats are the most important plant food available. In the West, wheat is the most-grown cereal crop, used to make bread, pasta and many other popular foods.

Wholegrains (those that still retain all of their layers, including the bran and germ) contain considerably more dietary fibre than grains that have been highly milled (such as white flour). As such, wholegrains have been linked with lowered risk of bowel cancer and diverticular disease, and can help to prevent constipation. Wholegrains also contain several of the B-group vitamins, including folate, which may help to protect against heart disease. When grains are refined they lose a large percentage of their vitamins and minerals.

All grains contribute valuable starchy carbohydrate as well as some protein.

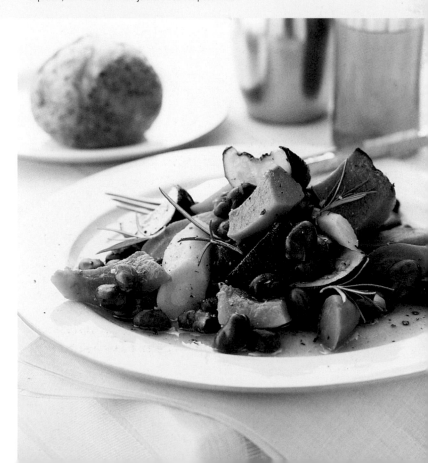

Wild about rice

Rice makes a delicious, versatile alternative to potatoes and pasta, and there are lots of varieties to choose from. Mixed with other ingredients, it makes a great meal.

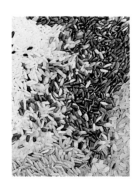

Different types of rice

Rice is classified by the size of its grain – long, medium and short – and varieties range in texture from fluffy to creamy to sticky. Colour varies from brown to white to red. The shape, size, texture and other characteristics of the different varieties affect the way the rice is used in recipes – what types of dish it is suitable for and the way it is cooked. Each country favours particular varieties for its cuisine.

Long-grain rices

Long-grain rice, as the name suggests, has grains that are long and slim. When cooked, the grains tend to remain separate, and the finished result is usually fairly dry and firm.

Basmati rice With very long, slim grains, basmati is often called the 'king' of rices, as it has excellent cooking qualities and a full flavour. It is grown only in northern India and Pakistan, and no other rice can be labelled as basmati. It also comes in a wholegrain form, which tends to be lighter and quicker to cook than other brown rices. The extra nutritional advantage of basmati rice is that it scores low on the Glycaemic Index – its carbohydrate content is absorbed less quickly into the bloodstream than other types of rice, and thus it helps to keep blood sugar levels stable. Basmati rice should be rinsed before cooking to get rid of the starchy powder left over from milling.

Long-grain rice This is usually the patna or Carolina varieties of rice (sometimes it will be labelled as such). Most is in a polished white form, although brown long-grain rice is also available. Patna rice comes from Asia; Carolina rice, which is slightly chunkier in appearance, is from North America.

Parboiled rice Sometimes called 'converted' rice or 'processed' rice, this is wholegrain rice that is soaked, steamed and dried before milling and polishing. The process forces the vitamins and minerals into the centre of the grain so that more are retained than in ordinary white rice. The colour of this rice is more golden than other white rice and it takes a little longer to cook. Even with over-cooking, the grains will remain separate.

Quick-cook rice Also called easy-cook rice, this shouldn't be confused with parboiled rice. Quick-cook rice is part-cooked after milling and then dried, so that when you cook it, it takes about half the time of ordinary long-grain rice. Quick-cook rice has lost most of its nutrients, especially the water-soluble B vitamins, because of this 'double-cook' process.

Red rice A wholegrain rice with a red outer skin, this has a nutty flavour and slightly chewy texture. The best quality red rice comes from the Camargue region of France; other red rices, produced in North America, are also available.

Thai fragrant rice Also known as jasmine rice, this is grown in eastern Asia. It has a slight perfume and when cooked is slightly more sticky than other long-grain rices. It marries well with other Asian foods and is the rice to use in Thai cookery.

New strains of long-grain rice

New types of rice are being produced in North America, Australia and other parts of the world. Texmati is the USA's version of basmati, created to satisfy the huge world demand for this type of rice – true basmati can only be produced in relatively small amounts in India and Pakistan. Two other new American long-grain rices are wahani, suitable for Asian cooking, and wild pecan rice, which has a mild nutty flavour. Doongara is a new Australian rice, similar to basmati.

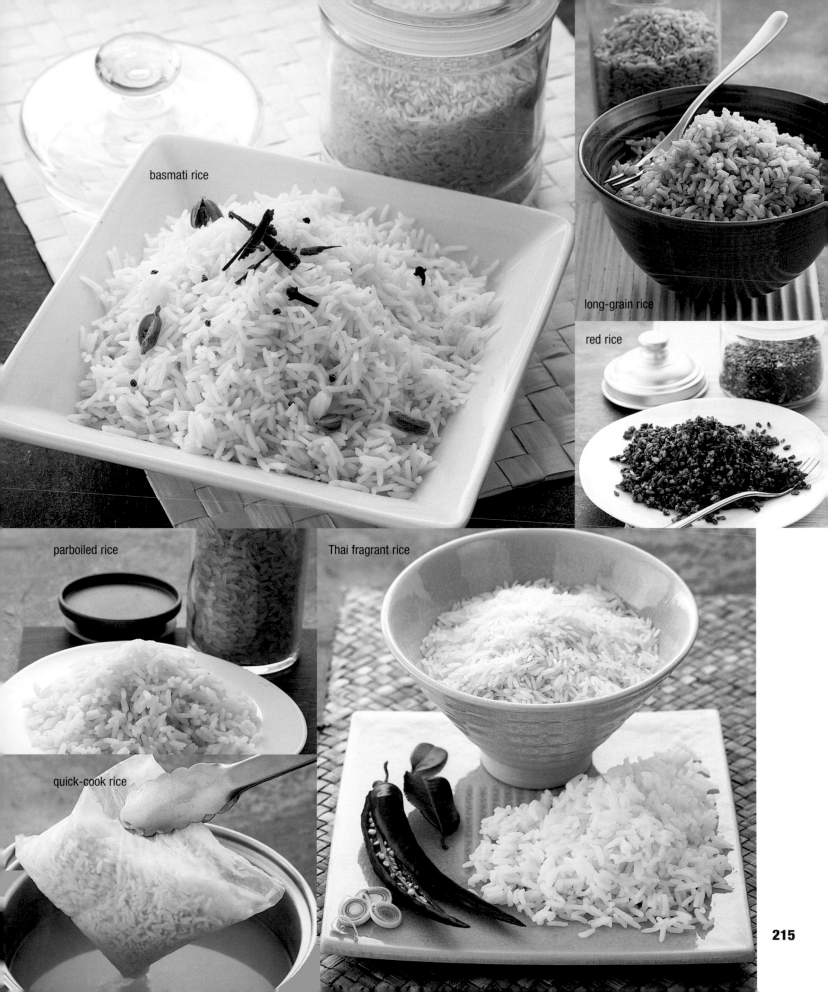

basmati rice

long-grain rice

red rice

parboiled rice

Thai fragrant rice

quick-cook rice

215

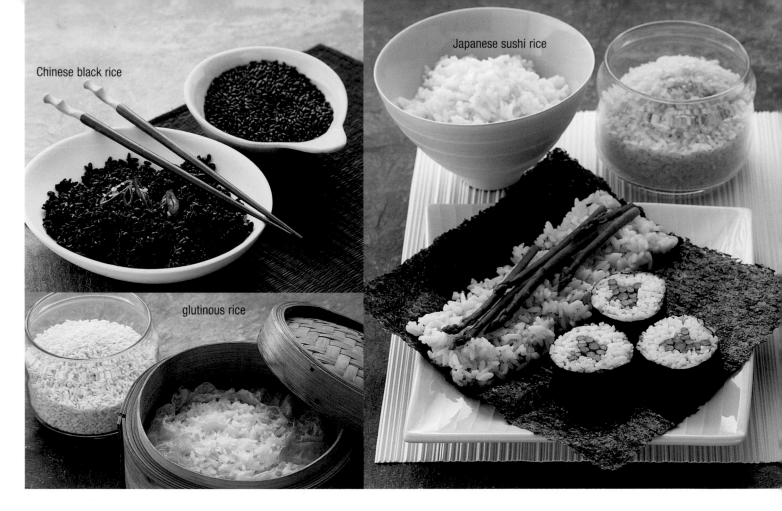

Chinese black rice

Japanese sushi rice

glutinous rice

Wild rice

Wild rice is not, in fact, a member of the rice family but a type of grass. It is native to the Minnesota Lakes area of the USA and was first harvested by the North American Indians. Most of the wild rice now sold is grown commercially in artificial ponds. Dark brown in colour, with very long, thin, pointed grains, it has a distinctive, strong flavour. Its protein content is higher than other rices and it contains twice as much folate as ordinary brown rice. It can be used on its own, when its cooking time is quite long, but it is more usually mixed with white or brown long-grain rice. When sold mixed with white rice, the outer skin has been broken to shorten the cooking time.

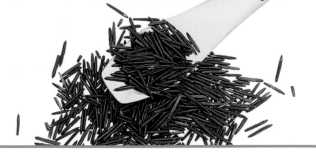

Short and medium-grain rices

These rices contain a starchy substance called amylopectin, which causes stickiness (long-grain rice has much less of this starch). After cooking, the individual grains cling together, which is why these rices are used in dishes where a creamy or sticky texture is wanted, such as risottos, puddings and sushi.

Chinese black rice An unrefined rice, this has a brownish-black skin and flattish, wide grains. It is usually soaked and then steamed. In Asia it is also used to make a dessert with coconut milk and palm sugar.

Glutinous rice Sometimes referred to as 'Chinese rice' or 'sticky rice', this is widely used in South-east Asia for both sweet and savoury dishes. Its grains are almost round and chalky-white. Ironically, the name is misleading as, like all other rices, it contains no gluten. The normal cooking method is to soak and then steam it, after which the grains stick together as if with glue. This means it can be eaten in small balls picked up with the fingers or chopsticks.

Japanese sushi rice A short-grain rice, this is usually soaked and then cooked by the absorption method. Once cooled, it is

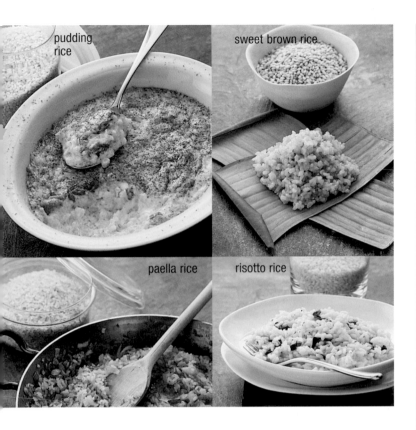

pudding rice

sweet brown rice

paella rice

risotto rice

flavoured with sweetened rice vinegar and rolled up in nori seaweed with other ingredients such as raw fish or vegetables to make sushi. It is the stickiness of the rice which holds the sushi rolls together.

Paella rice From the Spanish region of Valencia, this is used in the traditional dish of Spain, paella. It is a plump, short-grain rice similar to risotto rice, but with a less creamy texture.

Pudding rice This short-grain rice is very similar to risotto rice, but with sweeter-tasting grains. It needs long, slow cooking and produces a silky, creamy texture, which is why it is used to make rice puddings. It should not be used for savoury dishes, even risottos, as the taste will be disappointing.

Risotto rice The famous medium-grain rice of Italy, this has plump, white, oval grains. When cooked with liquid stirred in slowly, the grains retain their individual shape yet become creamy. Arborio is the best-known of the risotto rices, but of even better quality are Carnaroli and Vialone Nano.

Sweet brown rice Called mochi in Japan, this is a sweet-flavoured, very glutinous rice with a high starch content. It is used to make rice cakes and sweet confections.

Rice in other forms

Being gluten-free, rice products are suitable for people with a wheat or gluten intolerance.

Ground rice is white rice coarsely milled to the consistency of semolina. It can be used in puddings and baby food.

Rice cakes are discs of rice that have been baked. They are low in fat and calories, and can be a tasty substitute for bread, wheat crackers or crispbreads.

Rice flakes are produced by parboiling and then flattening rice between rollers before drying. They are quick to cook and can be used in puddings, or added to stews as a thickener.

Rice flour is a fine-milled flour (with a finer texture than ground rice), which can either be wholegrain or white. It is useful for baking and bread-making.

Rice noodles are fine, translucent noodles made from rice flour, used in South-east Asian cooking. They come in several shapes and sizes, and are quick to cook.

Rice vinegar is made from fermented rice.

Rice wine, also called sake (or saki), is, in fact, a flat beer made from fermented steamed rice and water. It is pale in colour, with a sweet taste and a slightly bitter aftertaste. Mirin is a golden wine made from glutinous rice.

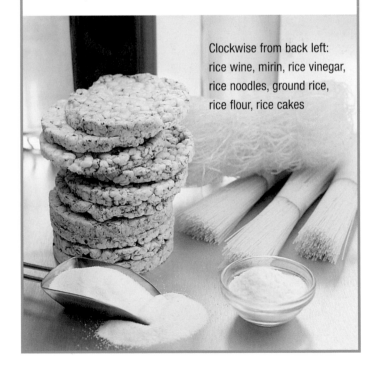

Clockwise from back left: rice wine, mirin, rice vinegar, rice noodles, ground rice, rice flour, rice cakes

Basic rice cookery

However you cook it, rice is good for you. Some methods minimise the loss of valuable water-soluble B-vitamins, by allowing the rice to absorb all the cooking water.

Cooking long-grain rice

Long-grain rice is usually cooked by boiling, which can either be open boiling or the absorption method. The latter produces very tasty rice with a good texture, and it retains a high proportion of the nutrients because all the water used is absorbed into the rice. Long-grain rice can also be steamed and microwaved.

The absorption method

To cook one of the white long-grain rices by this method, first weigh out the quantity specified in a recipe. Then, if no liquid quantity is specified, tip the rice into a measuring jug – you need about twice the volume of water to rice.

Put the rice and water in a heavy-based saucepan that has a tight-fitting lid and bring to the boil. When the water is boiling, turn the heat down to low so the water is very gently simmering. Give the pan's contents a good stir with a fork, and put the lid on. Leave to cook, covered, for 10–15 minutes (or according to the packet instructions).

To test if the rice is ready, lift out a few grains on a fork. If the rice still seems too firm but all the water has been absorbed, add a little more boiling water and simmer for a few more minutes. When the rice is tender, remove the pan from the heat and set aside to rest for a few minutes. This will allow the rice to absorb any last traces of water. (The rice will retain its heat if you keep the lid on, and you can slip a clean teatowel between the pan and the lid to help dry out the rice.) Finally, fluff up the rice lightly with a fork to separate the grains, and serve.

Wholegrain long-grain rices (brown rice, wild rice and red rice) can also be cooked by the absorption method, but need more water – $2\frac{1}{2}$ times the volume of water to rice – and longer cooking. Brown basmati rice takes about 25 minutes; other long-grain brown rices, wild rice and red rice need 30–40 minutes cooking.

Boiling

Long-grain rice can simply be cooked in a large volume of fast-boiling water, in which case it will take 10–15 minutes for white rice or 30–35 minutes for wholegrain. When tender, it should be drained in a sieve. This method can result in soft, mushy, tasteless rice if you overcook it.

Steaming

The aborption method is, in fact, a type of steaming, but rice can also be cooked in a steamer over boiling water. In China, a traditional bamboo steamer is used lined with muslin. The rice is soaked for up to 1 hour, then drained, put into the muslin-lined steamer and steamed for 20 minutes or until tender. This method is used for both long-grain rices and glutinous rice.

Microwaving

Long-grain rice can be cooked very successfully in the microwave, using the absorption method. Measure 1 part rice to 2 parts water and cook in a microwavable basin, with a lid lightly resting on the top, for 12 minutes. Leave to stand for 5 minutes, still covered, then stir before serving.

Using an electric rice cooker

If you eat a lot of rice, you might want to invest in an electric rice cooker. Rice cooked in a rice cooker has a slightly different texture from that cooked in a pan, but the finished result is always acceptable if the manufacturer's instructions are followed.

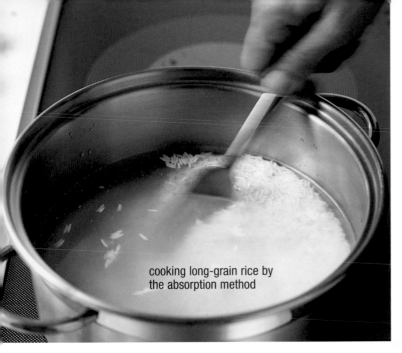
cooking long-grain rice by
the absorption method

Cooking other rices

Short-grain and medium-grain rices tend to be cooked by longer, slower techniques than those used for long-grain rice. Sometimes a combination of methods is used.

- **Glutinous rice and sushi rice** These sticky rices are usually soaked for 30 minutes before steaming or cooking by the absorption method.
- **Paella and risotto rices** These are an integral part of a recipe, not cooked separately. For a risotto, the normal method is to 'toast' the uncooked rice in hot oil, then to gradually add hot liquid such as stock or water. Each addition of liquid should be almost all absorbed before the next is added, and the rice is stirred almost constantly. At the end of cooking, the rice will be creamy and tender but with a firm centre. Paella rice is cooked by a similar method, but the liquid may be added all at once and it is not usually stirred during cooking.

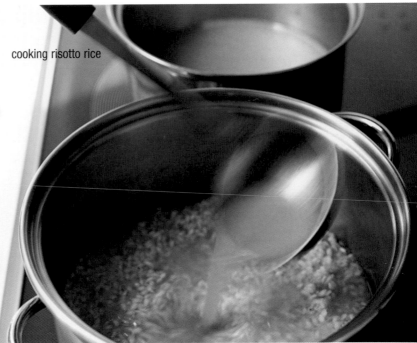
cooking risotto rice

- **Pudding rice** White pudding rice needs long, slow cooking in liquid (usually milk) to produce a traditional rice pudding.

Storing and reheating cooked rice

Cooked rice can be stored overnight in a covered container in the fridge. It should always be kept cool, as otherwise it could develop toxins that can cause food poisoning.

Rice can be reheated in a steamer, or in the microwave, loosely covered, for 1–2 minutes or until piping hot. Another way to reheat cooked rice is by using it in a stir-fry.

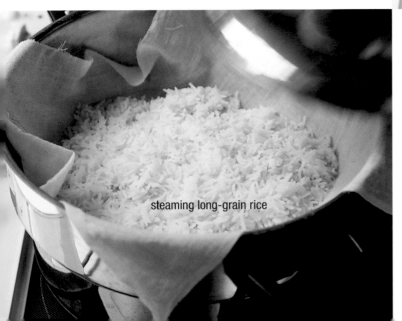
steaming long-grain rice

Getting to know pulses

Dried beans, lentils and peas are wonderfully nutritious, being low in fat and high in dietary fibre. The goodness they provide is not often found in modern diets.

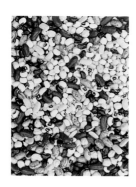

Why are pulses important?

Almost all of the pulses contain a near-perfect balance of starchy carbohydrate and protein – roughly 50% of their calorie content comes from carbohydrate, which is almost all starchy, or complex, rather than simple carbohydrate or sugars, and 20–30% from protein.

- Pulses are an important source of protein for people trying to cut down their animal and dairy intake, and for vegetarians and vegans. The protein provided by most pulses does not contain all 8 of the essential amino acids – the building blocks of protein (soya beans are the one exception) – but the nutritional value of pulse protein is easily enhanced by eating them with pasta, rice or other grains, or with small quantities of lean meat, which contain the 'missing' amino acids.
- Most pulses are excellent sources of both soluble and insoluble fibre. Soluble fibre has been shown to lower blood cholesterol as part of an overall diet low in fat. Insoluble fibre is important for digestive health and may help to prevent colon cancer and diverticular disease.
- Pulses in general are very low in fat and only a small percentage of the fat is saturated; much of the remainder is in the form of the essential fatty acids, omega-3 and omega-6, which have many health benefits.
- Many pulses are good sources of B vitamins, including folate, and vitamin E. They are also good sources of iron, zinc and magnesium, all of which may be in short supply in a modern, fast-food diet, as well as in vegetarian and vegan diets where meat – normally a main source of supply – is excluded. To aid absorption of these minerals, try to eat pulses with a vitamin C-rich food, such as fresh vegetables, potatoes or fruit. Many types of beans contain some calcium too.

An ABC of beans

There are hundreds of different varieties of dried beans throughout the world. Here is a selection of those that you are most likely to come across (numbers refer to the picture on the opposite page).

1 Aduki bean This is a very small, roundish, dark red bean with a slightly sweet taste. Popular in Japan and the Far East, it is used in a variety of dishes, both savoury and sweet. Aduki beans are higher in protein than many other pulses.

2 Black bean (Chinese) A variety of soya bean, this is a medium-small, round, shiny black bean. It is normally fermented and salted, which gives it a rich savoury flavour. In Chinese cookery, fermented black beans are often mashed with a little sugar and water and added to dishes as a paste.

3 Black kidney bean Similar in shape and size to the red kidney bean, this has a black skin and a white flesh; it turns brown on cooking. Popular in Central and South America, black kidney beans are used to make the Brazilian national dish, feijoada.

4 Black-eyed bean Popular in Caribbean cookery as well as in India and the Mediterranean, this is a pale, oval bean with a black 'eye'. It has a creamy texture with a slightly sweet flavour, and is good used in soups and casseroles.

5 Broad bean Also called fava or faba bean, this is the dried form of our garden broad bean. Large, flat and pale brown, with an earthy flavour, it is most often added to casseroles.

6 Borlotti bean This attractive, medium-sized bean, pale pink speckled with brown, comes from Italy. Being soft-textured it makes a creamy purée and is delicious in soups and salads.

7 Cannellini bean A variety of haricot bean grown widely in Italy, the cannellini is medium-large, cream-coloured and mild but pleasant in taste. Cannellini beans are good in soups, salads and casseroles, and go well in fish dishes, particularly those made with tuna.

8 Butter bean Originating from South America, this is a very large, flattish bean with an attractive deep cream colour. There is a hint of potato in the flavour. Butter beans purée well and can be used as a side dish or dip; they also make good soup. Lima beans are a close relation but slightly smaller.

9 Ful medames (Egyptian brown bean) Small, round and mid-brown, with a full flavour, this is a variety of broad bean. It is native to Egypt where, combined with eggs, garlic and spices, it is made into the national dish of the same name. Ful medames are widely used in the Eastern Mediterranean.

10 Flageolet Popular in France and Italy, this is a medium-sized, pale green bean with a delicate yet distinctive flavour. It keeps its attractive colour when cooked, and is ideal in salads.

11 Pinto bean Looking like a borlotti bean but a little smaller, the pinto bean comes from Central and South America. With its creamy texture, it is good in soups.

12 Haricot bean This is the bean used for 'baked beans', so popular throughout the Western world – no wonder it is one of the most widely grown of all beans. Medium-sized and pale cream in colour, it is also the classic bean to use in a French cassoulet. Haricot beans contain more soluble fibre than any other pulse.

13 Soya bean Much harder than other beans, the soya bean needs very long soaking and cooking. It is also quite bland, so needs to be cooked with strongly flavoured ingredients, such as onion, tomato, spices or herbs. One of the world's biggest crops, soya beans are converted into many other kinds of food.

14 Red kidney bean This red-skinned bean, with meaty white flesh, keeps its colour on cooking and absorbs other flavours well. Its robust taste and texture means it works well in hot, spicy dishes, such as chilli con carne.

A word about soya beans

The soya is the only bean that contains all 8 amino acids. Soya beans are unique in other ways too. For example, the iron they provide is better absorbed by the body than the iron in other pulses. Soya beans are also a good source of calcium – an important point for vegans who don't eat dairy products. They contain more omega-3 and omega-6 fatty acids than other pulses, and offer more soluble fibre than most.

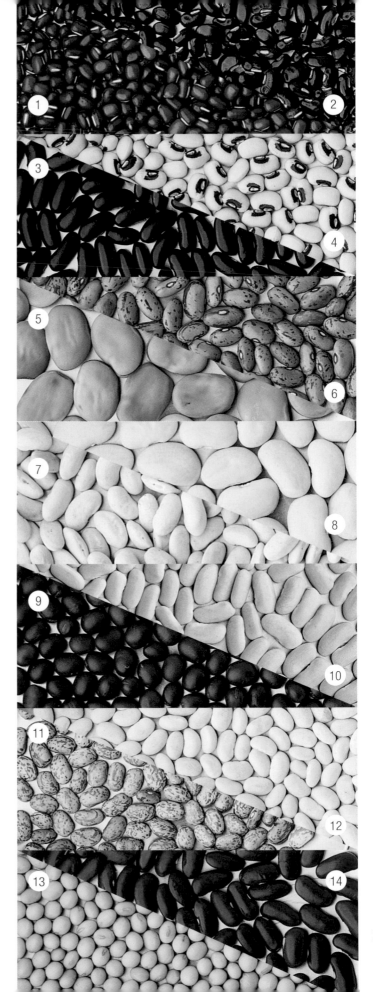

An ABC of lentils and peas

These seeds of leguminous plants make up the rest of the family of pulses.

Chana dal A small, brown relation of the chickpea, this is usually sold split – it looks similar to yellow split peas. Chana dal have a slightly sweet flavour and are widely used in Indian and Middle Eastern cookery for dal or as part of a pilau. They are usually only available from Indian grocers. In India, it is chana dal that is used to make chickpea flour, rather than the larger chickpea from the Mediterranean region.

Chickpea Despite the name, this is not really a pea but a seed. Medium-sized, round and beige, it is widely used in North Africa and the Eastern Mediterranean as well as in India. Chickpeas are the main ingredient of hummus and of falafel. They are richer in vitamin E than most other pulses.

Gunga pea (pigeon pea) Round, smooth, medium-sized and usually brown, this pea comes from Africa. It is much used in Indian cookery for dal.

Lentil Grown mainly around the eastern Mediterranean and in India, the lentil is one of the world's oldest crops. Brown or green 'continental' lentils are very tasty, and retain their shape well after cooking, so are ideal in salads or as a vegetable accompaniment. They also purée well and add richness and texture to soups and casseroles. Grey-green Puy lentils are a small variety grown only in the Puy region of France. They have an excellent flavour. Red and yellow lentils are normally available split in half. They cook very quickly and can be easily puréed. All brown and green lentils are good sources of vitamin B_6, folate and iron; split lentils are less nutritious because the outer layer of the lentil has been removed.

Mung bean Native to Asia, this small, cylindrical-shaped green seed is most often used for sprouting, and is the familiar 'bean sprout'. It can also be used as a vegetable in a variety of dishes, and marries very well with rice and Indian spices.

Split pea Usually green or yellow in colour, this is a dried pea that has had its outer skin removed and has then been split in half. Split peas can be cooked to serve as a side vegetable, used in casseroles and soups, or puréed. They have less fibre, vitamins and minerals than most other pulses, but are a useful source of protein.

Urd (gram) This very small pea looks a little like a darker version of a mung bean. Available whole or split, it can be used like mung beans, or puréed.

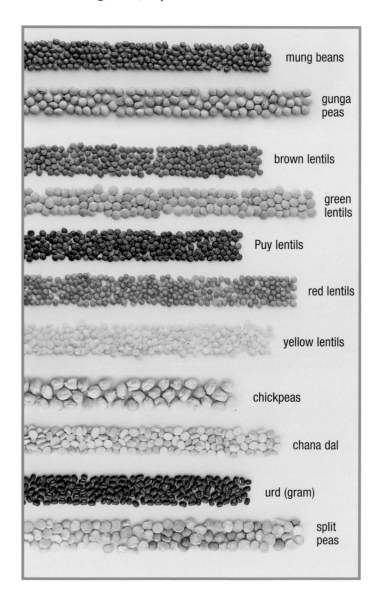

mung beans

gunga peas

brown lentils

green lentils

Puy lentils

red lentils

yellow lentils

chickpeas

chana dal

urd (gram)

split peas

Bean products

The humble bean – particularly the soya bean – can be transformed into a wide variety of other foods. Here are a few of them.

Black and yellow bean sauces are made from crushed or puréed, fermented black or cream-coloured soya beans. They are sold in cans, jars or sachets, usually with additions such as vinegar, oil, sugar or garlic.

Cellophone noodles, also called transparent or bean thread noodles, are made from the starch of the mung bean. Fine and white, they are soaked in water or stock before use, which makes them slippery and translucent. They are used in soups and stir-fries. In Chinese cooking they are also often deep-fried in hot oil.

Chickpea flour (besan, gram flour) is made by grinding dried chickpeas (or, in India, chana dal) until fine. It is used in Indian cookery for thickening and to make batters.

Miso is a thick paste made from fermented soya beans. It is useful for flavouring casseroles and stews, but is quite salty.

Soya milk is a useful alternative to cow's milk for vegans and people allergic to dairy products. It is high in protein, with a similar fat content to semi-skimmed milk, and is often fortified with calcium.

Soy sauce is a thin, dark brown sauce made from soya beans fermented with barley or wheat. Naturally fermented soy sauce, called shoyu or tamari, is considered to be superior to the less expensive, commercial soy sauces which usually contain sugar and other additives.

Tofu is a pale cream, high-protein food manufactured from soya beans. Firm tofu, sold in blocks (often vacuum-packed or in water), has a texture similar to that of feta cheese. It can be sliced and used in stir-fries, casseroles and many other dishes as a substitute for meat; although very bland, it soaks up other flavours well. Silken tofu has a creamier texture and is useful for making non-dairy, low-fat dips and a mayonnaise-like salad dressing.

TVP (textured vegetable protein) is soya that has been manufactured to look like mince or small chunks of meat, and can be used in recipes in the same way that you would use minced beef or lamb. TVP is usually sold dry, in bags, although it also comes in cans and frozen.

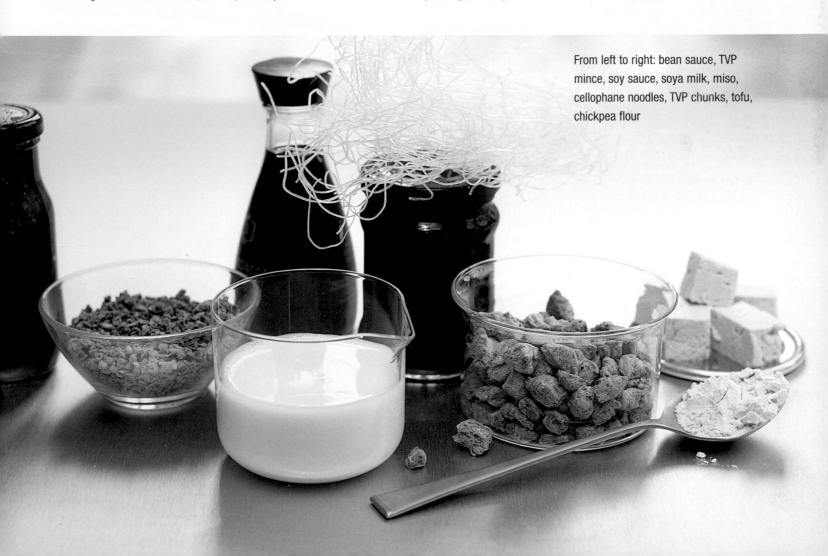

From left to right: bean sauce, TVP mince, soy sauce, soya milk, miso, cellophane noodles, TVP chunks, tofu, chickpea flour

Basic pulse cookery

Most dried pulses need to be soaked before cooking, to release their flavour and protein content. Canned pulses are already cooked and need only be rinsed.

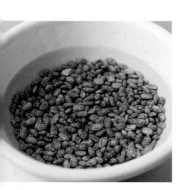

A soak to rehydrate

Soaking pulses ensures that they will cook evenly and relatively quickly. It may also help to get rid of some of the substances called oligosaccharides that cause flatulence, although most of these are lost during cooking. How long a dried pulse needs to be soaked depends on the variety and on how long it has been stored.

Lentils and split peas need no soaking at all, whereas most dried beans, chickpeas and other whole peas should be soaked for at least 8 hours. Soya beans are notorious for needing longer-than-average soaking and are best left overnight. In hot weather, it's a good idea to soak pulses in the refrigerator.

Recently-dried pulses – such as the dried flageolets you see in France in the autumn, labelled 'new season' – tend not to need such a long soak, whereas pulses that have been stored a long time, and are thus even more dried out, may need longer soaking than is normally recommended.

A good rule-of-thumb for telling when a pulse has been soaked long enough is that there will be no wrinkling remaining on the skin. The pulse will look plump and have increased in size, sometimes up to 3 times the original size.

Pulses can be soaked longer than 8–12 hours, although if they are left for more than 1–2 days, they will begin to sprout and ferment. (If you want to sprout them, you need to rinse them and refresh the water regularly – see the box opposite for instructions.)

After soaking, drain and rinse the pulses. Discard the soaking water and use fresh water for cooking.

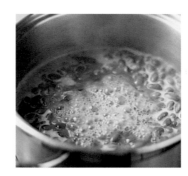

Fast boiling

There are toxic proteins (lectins or haemoglutigens) contained in the outer layers of most pulses, which cannot be digested in the stomach, and which may cause symptoms of severe food poisoning such as diarrhoea and vomiting. This is of special concern for people with poor digestion, the elderly and those convalescing from illness. Red kidney beans and soya beans are particularly high in these toxins.

A short period of rapid boiling will destroy the toxins, so a 10–15 minute fast boil at the start of cooking has always been recommended for red kidney beans and soya beans. However, current advice is that all pulses – with the exception of chickpeas, gunga peas, lentils and split peas – should be boiled before cooking begins.

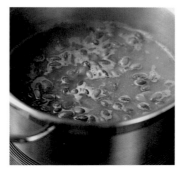

Cooking

Once pulses have been given their fast boil, reduce the heat so the liquid is just simmering. Skim the froth from the surface, then partly cover the pan and leave to cook gently until the pulses are tender, topping up with more boiling water as necessary. The length of the simmering time depends on the variety of pulse and how dry it is.

For example, dried haricot beans can take 50 minutes to 1½ hours, and chickpeas from 1 to 3 hours. Soya beans take the longest time to cook – 2½ to 4 hours. Recipes in the book give tested cooking times, but you may prefer to follow the instructions on the packet. Do not salt the cooking water, because this may toughen the pulses and prolong the cooking time – instead, add salt and other seasonings at the end of cooking.

Pulses are sometimes cooked in water before being added to a casserole that will be cooked further (such as when making baked beans or chilli con carne). If the sauce mixture contains an acidic ingredient such as tomatoes, the pulses will not become any softer. So they must be thoroughly cooked and tender before they are added to the casserole.

Canned pulses, which are already cooked, can be used cold or reheated gently to serve hot.

Sprouting pulses

Bean and other pulse sprouts make a crisp and nutritious addition to salads and stir-fries, providing useful amounts of B vitamins, especially folate, and vitamin C. The bean sprouts you are most likely to find in the shops are from mung and aduki beans, but many other pulses can be sprouted successfully. Whole green and brown lentils and chickpeas are particularly good.

You can buy special layered sprouting containers, which are useful if you want to sprout different varieties at the same time. Here's how to do it the simple way.

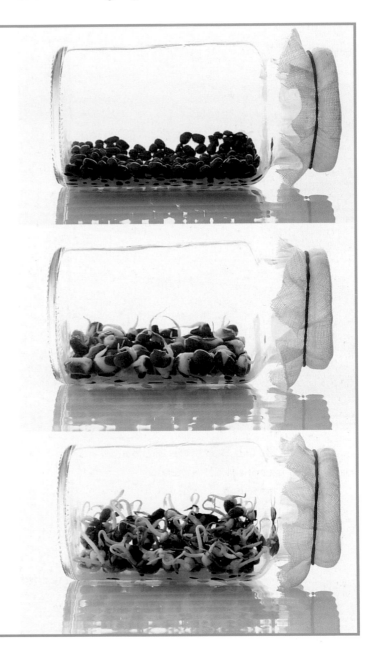

• Rinse the pulses, then place in a large jar (a kilner-type jar is ideal). Fill the jar with water, then cover with a piece of muslin secured with an elastic band. Leave to soak in a warm place overnight.

• The next day, pour off the water through the muslin, then refill the jar with water through the muslin. Shake gently, then drain off the water and leave the jar on its side (**top right**), away from direct sunlight.

• Twice a day, rinse the pulses well with water and drain. After a few days they will begin to sprout (**middle right**).

• When the shoots are 1–2 cm (½–¾ in) long, place the jar in a sunny but not too hot place. Leave for a few more days, still rinsing regularly, until they have grown to the desired size (**bottom right**).

• Rinse well and remove any ungerminated beans before using. The sprouts can be kept in a plastic bag in the fridge for 1–2 days.

• Eat the sprouts as fresh as possible and before their seed leaves form.

Going for grains

Grains have been grown for food since the Stone Age. Then, as now, they were the major source of starchy carbohydrate in the everyday diet.

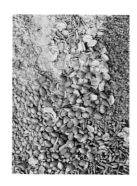

An ABC of grains

Every great civilisation has been founded on agriculture – the growing of wheat, barley, rye, rice, oats and corn – with the staple grain varying according to the geographic location and growing conditions. Wheat and rye were most important in the West, and rice and millet were the staples of the East, with maize being the primary crop of Africa and central and south America. Nowadays, these divisions are much less noticeable, with different grains being grown all over the world, for export to almost anywhere. The wide and exciting range of grains can be used to bring variety, flavour and good nutrition to your table.

Those grains that are gluten-free – buckwheat, maize, millet and quinoa – are ideal for people who are gluten-intolerant.

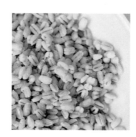

Barley

In early times, barley was used to make bread. Now that is rare, but barley is regaining popularity as a versatile grain that is rich in nutrients, in particular vitamin B_6, niacin, potassium and iron. Like other grains, when barley is refined, it loses much of its vitamin and mineral content – for example, the vitamin B_1 content is depleted by 60% in its pearl barley form.

Barley flakes are made from whole grains of barley, which are processed into flakes and dried. They are suitable for use in muesli (and make a good alternative for people with a wheat allergy). They can also be cooked as a porridge.

Barley meal is produced by grinding barley grains into a meal or flour, which can be used in breads and bakes or stirred into soups and casseroles to thicken them.

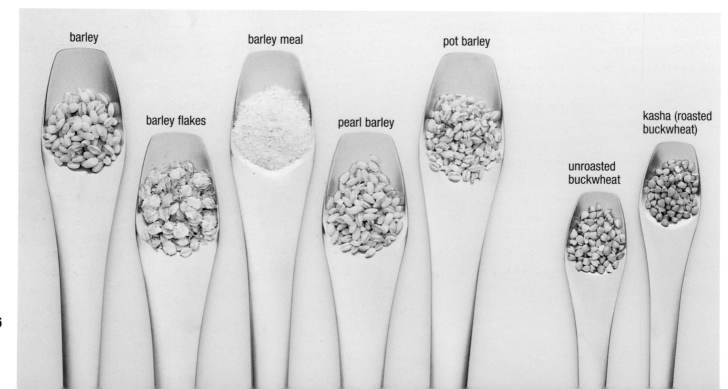

barley

barley flakes

barley meal

pearl barley

pot barley

unroasted buckwheat

kasha (roasted buckwheat)

Pearl barley is made by milling the whole barley grain to remove the outer layers, leaving the pale interior. Pearl barley is a good source of low-fat, easily digested complex (starchy) carbohydrate and is most often used in soups and casseroles, although it also works well in salads. The starch in the grains is easily released and acts as a thickener.

Pot barley is the whole grain of barley, rich in starchy carbohydrate, and containing much more dietary fibre, particularly soluble fibre, than any other cereal. Pot barley can be cooked in a similar way to rice as a side dish or to use in salads and pilafs. It has a nutty flavour, similar to brown rice.

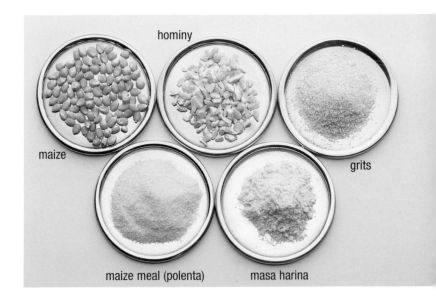
hominy
maize
grits
maize meal (polenta)
masa harina

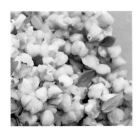

Buckwheat

This isn't really a cereal grain, but the seed of a plant that is a member of the rhubarb family. However, the seeds are grain-like, and it is cooked like a grain. Buckwheat is higher in protein than many other grains, and also contains excellent amounts of iron, calcium, vitamin E and B vitamins.

Kasha is the name frequently given to whole buckwheat grains (often cracked) that have been toasted or roasted. It is also the name of a porridge-like dish popular in Asia and Eastern Europe. Kasha makes an excellent and tasty substitute for rice and is good in spicy risotto-like dishes because the grains tend to break down when cooked.

Unroasted buckwheat grains are crushed and hulled grains, pale green-grey in colour, which can be cooked like rice. They are good with any savoury dish or for stuffing vegetables. You can toast or roast (both terms are used) your own buckwheat for an even better flavour and texture – spread the grains on a baking tray and cook in a preheated 180°C (350°F, gas mark 4) oven until they turn golden brown.

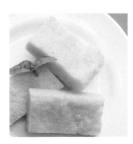

Maize

Maize is one of the world's most versatile crops. It can be harvested before the grains have matured for sweetcorn cobs, to be eaten as a vegetable. Left to mature, the maize grains can be harvested to be milled or left whole for a variety of uses (depending upon the type of maize), for example as breakfast cornflakes and popcorn. Others are ground into fine or coarse meals and flours. Maize is a good source of iron, but lower in the other nutrients typical of most grains. Yellow maize contains antioxidant carotenes, but white forms don't.

Hominy is dried white or yellow corn kernels, whole or broken into particles, from which the husk and germ have been removed. Hominy is sold canned, ready-to eat or dried; if dried, it needs to be softened by boiling in water or milk. It can be fried, baked or added to a casserole. Grits are ground hominy and may be fine, medium or coarse. They are generally simmered in water or milk until very thick, to make a breakfast dish or an accompaniment to meat dishes. Because hominy and hominy grits have had the germ and outer husk removed, their nutrient content is reduced. In the USA, where hominy and grits are popular, they are usually enriched with B vitamins and iron.

Maize meal (cornmeal, polenta) is ground corn, which comes in various textures from a powder to a coarse meal. It contains about 95% of the whole grain and is a good source of iron. Dishes made from maize meal, such as porridge, pancakes and bread, are an easily digested form of starchy carbohydrate. One of the most popular ways of using cornmeal is in the traditional Northern Italian dish polenta, when the meal is cooked with water or stock until it thickens; it can then either

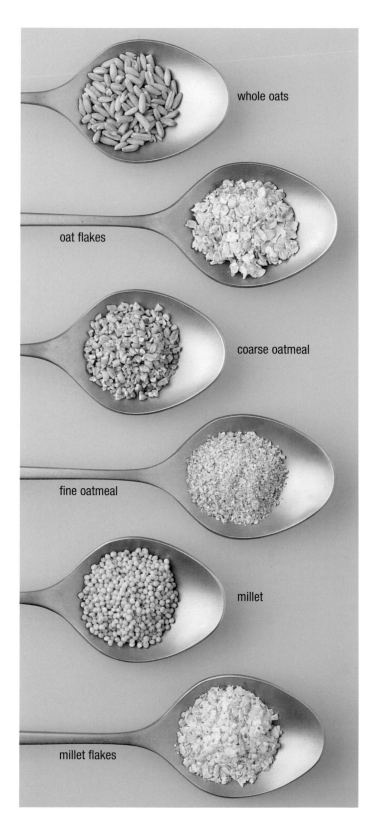

whole oats

oat flakes

coarse oatmeal

fine oatmeal

millet

millet flakes

be eaten soft, like a purée, or set. Special polenta cornmeal can be bought, which is bright yellow with a granular texture similar to semolina.

Masa harina, or tamale flour, is the flour used to make corn tortillas. Dried corn kernels are soaked and then cooked in limewater (water mixed with calcium oxide), before they are ground to a meal and dried.

Millet

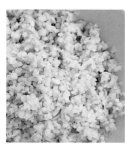

This very small, golden cereal grain, native to Asia and Africa, has a delicate, slightly nutty flavour. It contains useful amounts of many of the B vitamins, as well as more iron than other cereals and higher levels of protein than some.

Millet, in its wholegrain form, can be cooked in a similar way to other wholegrains – it absorbs up to 4 times its own weight in water. It can be used to stuff vegetables, as part of a burger mix.

Millet flakes can be added to casseroles, soups and stews. Sorghum is a larger relative of millet and can be used in similar ways.

Oats

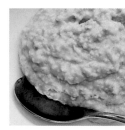

Oats are native to Eastern Europe but are probably best known as the main ingredient in porridge. Oats contain approximately twice as much fat as most other cereals, and they tend to go rancid quickly unless they have been through a steaming process before packaging, so they are best stored in a cool, dark place (preferably the fridge).

Oats can help to reduce blood cholesterol levels when eaten regularly, particularly if consumed with a low-fat diet, and thus may help to prevent coronary heart disease. They can also help to keep blood sugar levels stable, as they score low on the Glycaemic Index.

Oat flakes/rolled oats are whole oat grains that have simply been husked, then flattened or rolled, and thus contain virtually all of the vitamins and minerals in the whole grain.

'Steelcut' oats may retain more of the essential fats in the oat because this process does not use heat, which destroys these fats. Oats can be cooked with water and/or milk to make porridge, eaten raw, or used in baking.

Oatmeal, which is milled oat grains, comes in varying degrees of coarseness. The fine variety can be used in biscuits, bread and oatcakes, while coarser varieties can be used to make porridge. Instant oatmeal is a quick breakast cereal, but contains fewer nutrients than oat flakes/rolled oats.

Whole oats are whole oat grains (also known as kernels or groats). They can be bought in healthfood shops and used like brown rice or pot barley.

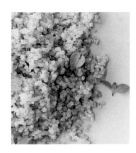

Quinoa

Quinoa (pronounced 'keen-wah') is a small, yellowy-brown, South American grain that is becoming more widely available elsewhere. It should be rinsed well before cooking, to remove the slightly bitter natural outer coating, and then cooked like the other wholegrains. It can be used like brown rice but has a slightly sweeter taste. The dried grains can be made into flour.

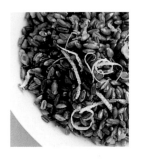

Rye

Rye is perhaps the most important cereal crop in Scandinavia and parts of Central Europe, such as Russia and Germany, and is a hardy alternative to wheat. Rye grains contain relatively little gluten, which is why rye flour doesn't make very good risen yeast bread. However, it does make excellent pumpernickel-type bread and crispbreads that have a good, strong, nutty flavour.

Cracked rye, whole grains of rye cracked so they cook more quickly, is often used in rye bread to add texture.

Rye flakes are similar in appearance to oat flakes. They are wholegrains that have been flattened and often toasted. They can be used in muesli.

Whole rye grains can be cooked like rice, but, as they are very tough when raw, they need to be soaked overnight and then drained before cooking.

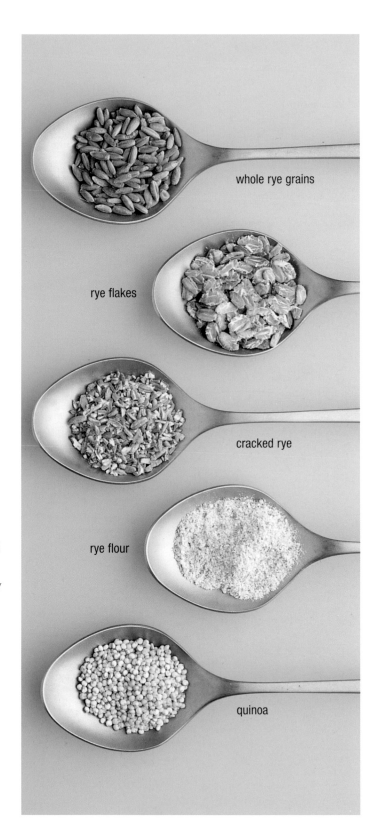

whole rye grains

rye flakes

cracked rye

rye flour

quinoa

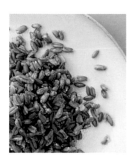

Spelt

This is an ancient variety of wheat, from which our modern wheat was developed. Wholegrains of spelt can be cooked and used like rice. Spelt flour and spelt pasta are also available. Spelt is higher in iron and B vitamins than modern wheat.

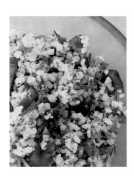

Wheat

Half the world's population relies on wheat as its staple food. First grown as a crop 12,000 years ago in the plains of Mesopotamia, it arrived in Italy around the time of Julius Caesar, in Britain at the time of the Roman invasion, and in the West Indies with Columbus in 1493.

Ground into flour, it is the most popular grain for bread-making, but it also has other forms and uses. Wheat contains gluten and is unsuitable for coeliacs.

Bran is the tough outer layer of the grain which is removed in the milling of white flour. The bran contains much of the grain's fibre and is often used as an additive in commercial products to increase a food's overall fibre content.

Bulghur wheat is often referred to as cracked wheat, but is actually a more refined version. It is produced by cooking grains of wheat, which contain all the grain except the bran, until they crack. They are then dried and ground between rollers to either a fine, medium or coarse consistency. Bulghur wheat needs only a few minutes cooking or can be soaked for 15–30 minutes. With its attractive golden appearance and nutty flavour, it is delicious in salads such as tabbouleh and for stuffing aubergines, beef tomatoes and other vegetables.

Cracked wheat is also known as kibbled wheat. Grains of wheat are cut by steel blades or roughly milled to crack the wheat into coarse, medium or fine pieces. It is not pre-cooked so it takes longer to cook than bulghur wheat (and cooks to a stickier texture), but takes less time than wholewheat.

Wheat flakes are whole grains of wheat flattened under rollers to make flakes for adding to muesli, or use in vegetarian burgers, or as part of a savoury crumble topping.

Wheatgerm, the tiny embryo within the seed of wheat that contains much of the nutrient profile of the grain, can be sprinkled on foods such as breakfast cereal or salads. Untreated wheatgerm can quickly go rancid because of its high fat content, and should be kept in the fridge.

Wholewheat grains, or 'berries', can be boiled and used in the same way as brown rice and other wholegrains. Pre-cooked wholewheat is available in many supermarkets.

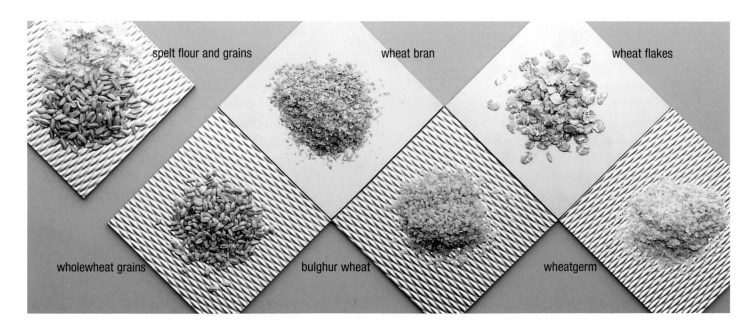

spelt flour and grains   wheat bran   wheat flakes

wholewheat grains   bulghur wheat   wheatgerm

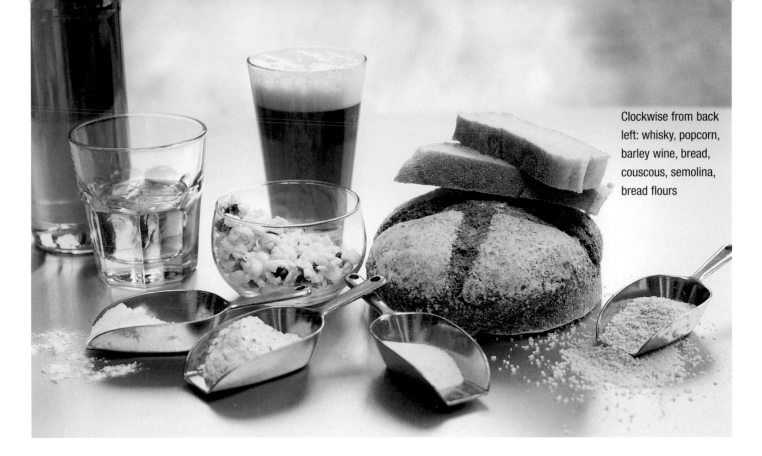

Clockwise from back left: whisky, popcorn, barley wine, bread, couscous, semolina, bread flours

Cooking whole grains

Whole grains – pot barley, whole oats, quinoa, whole rye, spelt and wholewheat – can be cooked like rice, and served as part of a main course or as an accompaniment. Whole rye grains need to be soaked in cold water overnight before cooking. Wholewheat grains, if not pre-cooked, can be soaked overnight to shorten the cooking time.

● Weigh out the grains, allowing about 75 g (2½ oz) per person for part of a main course.

● If the quantity of liquid needed for cooking is not specified on the packet, pour the grains into a measuring jug to check the volume. Then measure out 3 parts water to one part grains (with the exception of millet, which needs 4 parts water).

● Pour the water into a saucepan with a tight-fitting lid and bring to the boil, then add the grains and return to the boil. (Or, add the grains to the water and bring to the boil, according to the recipe or packet instructions.) For extra flavour, stir the grains in a little hot oil or melted butter in the saucepan, to toast them lightly, before adding the water.

● Lower the heat and simmer very gently until all the water has been absorbed, without stirring. Cooking time will vary from grain to grain: millet and quinoa will usually be tender in about 20 minutes; tougher grains may take an hour or more.

● Remove from the heat and leave, with lid on, for a further 10 minutes. By this time the grains should be separate and tender but not mushy. Fork through the grains and serve.

Favourite foods from grains

Grains are used to make many of our favourite foods. Flours and bread are the most commonly known form of processed grains and both are staple foods throughout the world. Flour and bread can be made from almost any grain – cornbread is popular in the Americas, and dark and light rye breads in Eastern Europe. Grains can also be used to make alcoholic beverages such as whisky and barley wine.

● **Semolina** is a processed form of durum wheat, made from the starchy part (endosperm) of the grain. It can be used in milk puddings. Semolina flour is mixed with water, and sometimes egg, to make pasta.

● **Couscous** is made from a mixture of semolina flour and water that is rolled in flour to produce tiny, round, yellow pieces. It is simply soaked or steamed, and then used as an accompaniment or part of a salad or other dish.

● **Popcorn** is made from whole grains of an especially hard variety of corn, which when heated make a popping sound and puff up to quadruple their size.

Flours for good baking

Flour is the basis of every loaf of bread and virtually every cake. Choosing the right type is vital for successful home baking.

Wheat flours

A huge percentage of the flours used in baking is made from wheat, the staple grain of Europe and, indeed, much of the Western world.

Brown flour (also called wheatmeal flour) contains about 85% of the whole grain, and therefore a similar percentage of its nutrients. It produces a lighter bread than wholemeal flour.

Granary flour is a wheatmeal (brown) flour made from malted wheat (grains that have been allowed to start germinating). It contains cracked (kibbled) and whole wheat grains, and sometimes rye flour. Its nutritional benefits are similar to those of brown flour.

Plain (white) flour became available as a consequence of the modern milling methods invented over 100 years ago, whereby the starchy endosperm of the grain can be separated from the bran and the germ, which are discarded, leaving 72–74% of the whole grain. In the UK, by law, some of the nutrients that are removed in this milling process (vitamin B_1, niacin, iron and calcium) are artificially returned to the flour before it is sold. However, the fibre and protein content of white flour will be lower than that of wholemeal flour. If you want to avoid the heaviness of wholemeal bread and cakes, a good compromise is to use a mixture of white and wholemeal flours.

Plain white flour usually has a low gluten content, resulting in a crumbly texture that is good for baking cakes and biscuits but not suitable for bread. There are some even finer flours for cake-making, which contains only 50–65% of the wheat grain.

Self-raising flour has raising agents added to it after the milling process – usually a mixture of bicarbonate of soda and cream of tartar (tartaric acid). Both white and wholemeal self-raising flours are available.

Spelt is an ancient ancestor of wheat, containing more protein, B vitamins and iron than normal wheat, but less gluten.

Stoneground flour (usually wholemeal) is milled by traditional methods rather than modern factory roller-mills. Milling with modern metal rollers creates heat, which spoils some of the nutrients – particularly the B vitamins and the essential fats. Stonegrinding keeps the grain cool and preserves almost all of the nutrients. Stoneground flour is usually coarser and heavier

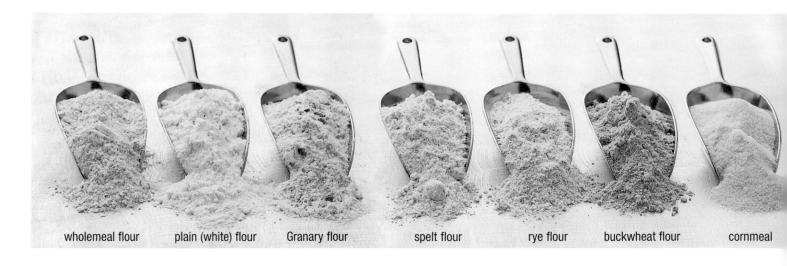

wholemeal flour   plain (white) flour   Granary flour   spelt flour   rye flour   buckwheat flour   cornmeal than factory-milled flour, so bread made from it may need a longer rising time or a little extra yeast to leaven it.

Strong flour, sometimes labelled 'bread' flour, is milled from hard wheat, which is high in gluten. It is gluten that helps dough to stretch and expand, and therefore to rise, so strong flour is ideal for bread-making. Both white and wholemeal bread flours are available.

Wholemeal flour (also called wholewheat flour) contains the whole of the grain – the bran (outer layers), the endosperm (starch middle part) and the germ (the embryo plant at the base of the grain) – and therefore retains most of its nutrients. It is high in B vitamins and a range of nutritionally important minerals, including magnesium, iron and selenium. It is also high in fibre and is a reasonable source of protein (12.7 g in each 100 g/3½ oz), as well as containing some essential fats. Breads and cakes made with 100% wholemeal flour will be heavier than those made with refined flours, and their keeping properties may be reduced because of their higher fat content.

Non-wheat flours

Baking with flours milled from grains and cereals other than wheat, and from vegetables and nuts, will bring variety to your breads and other baked goods, and may offer different nutritional benefits. When using these flours you need to consider their baking properties, as they all contain less gluten than wheat flour and some contain no gluten at all. So they usually need to be mixed with wheat flour to prevent the finished bread from being too dense and heavy.

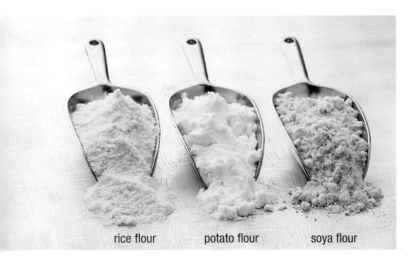

rice flour   potato flour   soya flour

Gluten-free and wheat-free baking

Gluten is a protein found in wheat and rye; a similar type of protein is found in barley and oats. Gluten intolerance causes coeliac disease, an inflammatory condition of the gastrointestinal tract. Another intolerance is to the wheat grain, which can then cause an allergic reaction.

Specially produced gluten-free and wheat-free commercial breads and baked goods are available now, as are specially blended gluten and wheat-free flour mixtures. However, there are various types of flour that you can use in breads and baking that are naturally gluten-free (see Non-wheat flours, below) and wheat-free. Although these tend to produce denser, heavier breads and baked goods than those made with wheat flours, they can be full of flavour and very satisfying. Most gluten-free breads are risen with bicarbonate of soda or baking powder, as yeast needs gluten to make bread dough rise.

Buckwheat flour, milled from a nutty-tasting grain, is rich in protein and offers useful amounts of iron. It is gluten-free.

Cornmeal (also called maizemeal or polenta), usually rich yellow in colour, may be coarse or medium. Cornflour, a very fine white flour milled from the heart of the maize kernel, is used mainly as a thickener. Both cornmeal and cornflour are gluten-free but otherwise nutritionally similar to wheat flour.

Oat flour contains few vitamins and minerals in significant quantities, but it is high in soluble fibre, which can help to reduce high blood cholesterol levels.

Potato flour is high in starchy carbohydrate and gluten-free. Rice flour, which has a fairly bland flavour, can be used in many types of baked goods. It is gluten-free. It has slightly less protein and fibre than white wheat flour.

Rye flour makes well-flavoured bread with a chewy texture. It can be used alone to make an acceptably risen loaf, but is normally mixed with wheat flour. Dark rye flour is a useful source of B vitamins, vitamin E, iron, copper, zinc and fibre. Light rye flours contain proportionally fewer of these nutrients.

Soya flour is made from raw or toasted soya beans (toasted has a better flavour). It is high in protein and gluten-free.

In addition to these non-wheat flours, flour for baking is also milled from barley, millet, chickpeas and chestnuts.

Yeasts and other raising agents

Raising or leavening agents are essential to give breads and cakes their characteristic lightness and texture.

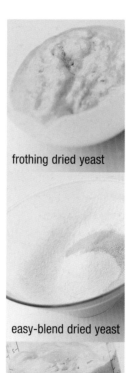

frothing dried yeast

easy-blend dried yeast

fresh yeast

Yeast

Yeast is a living organism. In a moist, warm environment and when fed with sugar and starch, yeast ferments to produce carbon dioxide, and it is this that makes bread doughs rise. Dried yeast is alive but dormant because of the lack of moisture. Yeast is a useful source of B vitamins.

Dried yeast is bought as granules, in individual sachets or tubs. It is usually mixed with a little tepid water, often with a pinch of sugar to help reactivate it, and then left in a warm place for 15 minutes or until a frothy head has formed. The mixture is then ready to add to the flour. Dried yeast can be kept in a cool, dry place for up to 6 months.

Easy-blend dried yeast (also called fast-action dried yeast) is quicker and more convenient to use than ordinary dried yeast, as it does not have to be dissolved in liquid but is sprinkled straight into the flour. In theory, only one rising is required with easy-blend yeast, saving even more time, but in practice a better result is obtained if you give the dough the traditional 2 risings. Easy-blend yeast can be kept as for dried yeast, or according to packet instructions.

Fresh yeast can be bought from bakers who bake bread on the premises, as well as from healthfood shops and supermarkets. Like ordinary dried yeast, it needs to be mixed with tepid liquid first and left to become frothy. Fresh yeast can be kept, loosely wrapped, in the fridge for up to 3 days, or it can be frozen in suitable-sized pieces for up to 4 months (leave it to thaw before using).

Wild yeasts are microscopic spores that are naturally present in flour and floating in the air. They have been used successfully to raise doughs for over 6000 years, and produce bread that has a delicious tangy, slightly sour flavour. A mixture of flour and tepid water (the 'starter') is left to ferment, at room temperature, for several days, being 'fed' regularly with more flour and water, until it is bubbling, which indicates that the wild yeasts have been activated. Once created, a starter can be kept going almost indefinitely and used for regular baking.

Other raising agents

The usual method of raising most cake mixtures, quick bread doughs and batters is by the inclusion of baking powder or bicarbonate of soda. Just as with yeast, these produce carbon dioxide gas bubbles, which expand during baking. Contact with moisture creates the carbon dioxide, so once mixed the cake or bread should be baked without delay. Both baking powder and bicarbonate of soda can be kept in an airtight container in a cool, dry place for up to 6 months.

Baking powder is a combination of bicarbonate of soda and and an acid such as cream of tartar. Self-raising flour contains baking powder as well as salt.

Bicarbonate of soda can be used as a raising agent on its own as long as the recipe includes an acidic ingredient, such as vinegar, soured cream, buttermilk or yogurt.

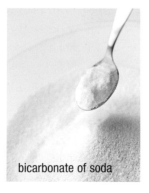

bicarbonate of soda

Flavourings for variety

Whether it is a sprinkling of herbs or chunks of chocolate, a little flavouring will give zest and variety to your baking.

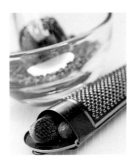

Alcohol

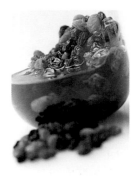

A spoonful or two of rum, brandy or sherry will enhance the flavour of fruit cakes or the dried fruit can be soaked in the alcohol first; simple sponge cakes can be made special by drizzling over a little fruit-flavoured liqueur. Alcohol is fat-free and the calories these tiny amounts contribute to your diet will be minimal.

Chocolate

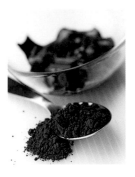

Chocolate is high in calories, sugar and fat (530 kcals, 56 g sugar and 30 g fat per 100 g/3½ oz), but it's not all bad news – dark chocolate also contains useful amounts of iron, plus an antioxidant that can help to prevent the build-up of harmful LDL cholesterol. Just a little good-quality chocolate is needed to add richness to sweet baking. When buying chocolate, always check the percentage of cocoa solids it contains. The higher the content (at least 70%), the better the chocolate, and the less added fat and sugar it will contain.

Cocoa powder is another, much healthier way to add a delicious chocolate flavour, and without the calories – 2 rounded tbsp contain 62 kcals and only 4.5 g fat.

Herbs and spices

Chopped fresh or dried herbs can be mixed into yeasted and quick bread doughs and mixtures for savoury muffins and scones for a flavoursome result, or the herbs can be sprinkled on top before baking. Basil, thyme, marjoram and chives are all delicious, as are rosemary and sage added more sparingly. Spices can be used in both sweet and savoury baking. Whole seeds, such as fennel, caraway and cumin, are good additions to savoury breads as well as some cakes and biscuits, mixed in or sprinkled over the top. Ground coriander and chilli can spice up breads, savoury muffins and tortillas, while ground cinnamon, nutmeg, ginger, allspice, cloves and mixed spice are traditional flavourings for cakes and biscuits and sweet breads.

Salt

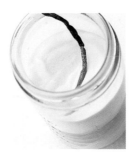

Salt is an indispensable ingredient in bread because it helps to toughen the gluten and make a good rise; it also improves the flavour – a loaf made without salt can taste quite bland. Surprisingly, salt brings out flavours in sweet baking too. Even a pinch can make a difference. The small quantity needed won't affect the total amount of salt in your diet. Home-baked breads and cakes contain less salt than commercial ones.

Vanilla

Vanilla adds a delicate flavour to plain sponges and biscuits as well as to icings. Always buy good-quality pure vanilla extract, which is distilled from vanilla pods, rather than vanilla essence or vanilla flavouring, both synthetic products that may not contain any vanilla at all. Using vanilla sugar is another way to add this flavouring to baked goods. To make your own vanilla sugar, push a vanilla pod into a container of sugar and leave for at least a week. The pod can be removed and reused, or left in the container, topping up the sugar as it is used.

Bread basics

Making bread is simple: measure ingredients carefully, use the correct size of tin and check your oven temperature.

Bread basics

If you are making a yeasted bread, you'll find that almost all recipes follow the same basic procedure: mixing in the yeast, kneading the dough, rising and shaping.

Kneading the dough

Once the yeast, flour and liquid (plus any other ingredients specified in the recipe) have been mixed together to make a dough that leaves the bowl clean, it is time for kneading. The kneading process gives a yeast dough elasticity, develops and strengthens the gluten, and ensures the bread will rise evenly.

Turn the dough out onto a lightly floured surface. Using the heel of your hand, push the dough away from you, to stretch it out, then fold the side farthest away back towards you, rolling the dough into a loose ball. Turn the dough slightly, then

> **Thinking of buying a bread-making machine?**
> Some people, especially beginners, find bread-making machines excellent, as they remove the 'need to knead'. However, they also remove some of the fun and sense of creativity that you get with traditional bread-making.

stretch it out again. Continue kneading like this for about 10 minutes. (Rather than kneading by hand, you can use a heavy-duty electric mixer fitted with a dough hook.)

The first rise

Shape the dough into a smooth ball and put it into a lightly oiled bowl. Cover to prevent a dry crust from forming, and leave to rise until doubled in size. This can be done in a warm place (about 30°C/86°F), which is the quickest, or in a cooler place such as at room temperature. The dough can even be left to rise in the fridge overnight.

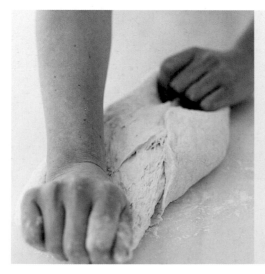
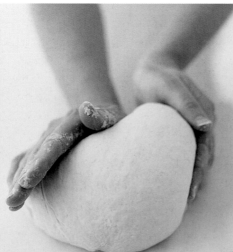

◄ Knead a yeasted dough by pushing and stretching it to develop the gluten; as you knead, the dough will gradually change in texture, becoming elastic, smooth and almost glossy

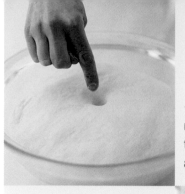

◀ To test if dough is properly risen, stick a finger into the centre; the indentation should remain after you pull your finger out

For a tin loaf, press or roll out the dough into an oblong, then roll it up like a Swiss roll; tuck the ends under and place it gently in the greased tin ▶

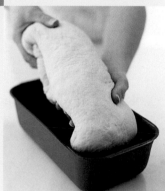

Shaping the loaf

Turn the risen dough out onto the lightly floured work surface again and 'knock it back' – punch it down with your fist to flatten it and expel excess air. Knead for 2–3 minutes to get it back to its original smooth texture, after which it is ready for shaping into loaves or rolls.

The simplest loaf shapes to make are balls, rounds and ovals, all of which are baked on a greased baking sheet. To shape dough to fit a loaf tin, flatten it to an oblong, making the short sides the same length as the tin, then roll up from a short side. Turn the roll so it is seam side down and tuck the ends under.

There are several more interesting shapes that are quite easy to make. For a spiral, shape the dough into a fat sausage, then curl it round itself, keeping it flat on the work surface. For a plait, divide the dough into 3 pieces and shape each one into a long, thin sausage. Press the top ends together, then plait together quite loosely. For shaping rolls, see Basic loaf, Some more ideas, page 255.

'Proving' and baking

Once shaped, most yeast doughs are left to rise again, or 'prove', before baking in a preheated oven. To test if a loaf is done, tap the base with your knuckle (if baked in a tin, tip the loaf out to test it). If the bread sounds hollow, like a drum, it is cooked. If it isn't ready, just return it to the oven (without the tin) and bake for a few more minutes, then test it again.

When the bread is done, leave it to cool on a wire rack for at least 2 hours before eating.

Freezing bread

Bread is very useful to have on hand in the freezer, and if you make your own it is well worth baking a large batch and then freezing some. Both yeasted breads and quick breads freeze extremely well, as long as they are tightly wrapped to prevent them from drying out. Plain loaves can be stored for up to 6 months, while enriched breads will keep for 3 months.

Most breads simply need thawing in their packaging at room temperature. Flat breads such as pittas, naan and tortillas benefit from being warmed after thawing: loosely wrap in foil and heat briefly in the oven before serving.

You can also freeze bread dough. The dough used for pizzas is a particularly handy standby. Make it but do not let it rise, then freeze in a sealed polythene bag; it can be kept for up to 1 month. Before use, re-seal the bag to allow space for rising, then leave in the fridge overnight. The next day, knock it back, shape and add the topping, then rise again briefly and bake.

Finishes for bread

Loaves and rolls can be glazed or sprinkled with a topping before baking to make them even more attractive and to add flavour.

• For a shiny, golden loaf, brush with beaten egg mixed with a pinch of salt.

• For a crusty top, brush with salt water.

• For a soft top, brush with milk.

• For a rustic loaf, dust lightly with wholemeal flour.

• Brush with beaten egg or oil, then top the loaf with seeds, such as poppy seeds (traditional for a plait), caraway or sesame seeds.

• Glaze with beaten egg, then sprinkle over a grain – oat flakes, cracked wheat and barley are all good.

• Sprinkle with grated hard cheese or chopped fresh herbs – a cheese-topped loaf is delicious with a vegetable soup.

Feta and chickpea salad

Made from ewe's milk, Greek feta cheese has a good tangy, slightly salty flavour. Cow's milk feta produced in other countries has a milder taste. Either type can be used in this classic Mediterranean salad, with ripe tomatoes, olives, cucumber and chickpeas. Serve with pitta bread warmed under the grill.

Serves 4

2 Little Gem lettuces, separated into leaves

4 ripe tomatoes, chopped

1 green pepper, seeded and cut into 1 cm (½ in) squares

1 small red onion, thinly sliced

1 cucumber, cut into quarters lengthways and then into chunks

1 can chickpeas, about 410 g, drained and rinsed

60 g (2¼ oz) stoned black olives, preferably Greek Kalamata olives

150 g (5½ oz) feta cheese, cut into small cubes

Parsley and mustard dressing

3 tbsp extra virgin olive oil

1½ tbsp lemon juice

1 tsp Dijon mustard

3 tbsp chopped fresh flat-leaf parsley

pepper

Preparation time: about 20 minutes

Each serving provides   Ⓥ

kcal 347, protein 16 g, fat 21 g (of which saturated fat 7 g), carbohydrate 24 g (of which sugars 8 g), fibre 8 g

✓✓✓ A, B₁, B₆, C, E, niacin

✓✓ B₁₂, folate, calcium, iron, potassium

✓ copper, zinc

1 Put all the dressing ingredients into a large salad bowl, adding pepper to taste (there is no need to add salt as the cheese is salty). Whisk together.

2 Add the lettuce leaves, tomatoes, green pepper, onion, cucumber, chickpeas and olives, and toss gently to combine and coat everything with the dressing.

3 Scatter the cubes of feta cheese over the salad, toss again gently and serve immediately.

Another idea

• Make a Middle Eastern-style goat's cheese and lentil salad. Cook 250 g (8½ oz) Puy lentils in boiling water for about 25 minutes, or according to the packet instructions, until tender. Drain thoroughly and leave to cool slightly, then add 6 tbsp Basic vinaigrette (see page 39) flavoured with ½ tsp ground cumin and 2 tbsp chopped fresh coriander. Toss well. Add 1 sliced red onion, 4 chopped plum tomatoes and 1 large grated carrot, and toss again until well mixed. Spoon onto Little Gem lettuce leaves in a salad bowl, and crumble over 150 g (5½ oz) goat's cheese.

Plus points

• Believing chickpeas to be a powerful aphrodisiac, the Romans fed them to their stallions to improve their performance. Although this reputation seems to be long forgotten, chickpeas do contribute valuable amounts of soluble fibre, iron, folate, vitamin E and manganese to the diet.

• The vitamin C from the lemon juice in the dressing will help to increase absorption of iron from the chickpeas.

• Although feta cheese is high in saturated fat and salt, it has a strong flavour so a little goes a long way.

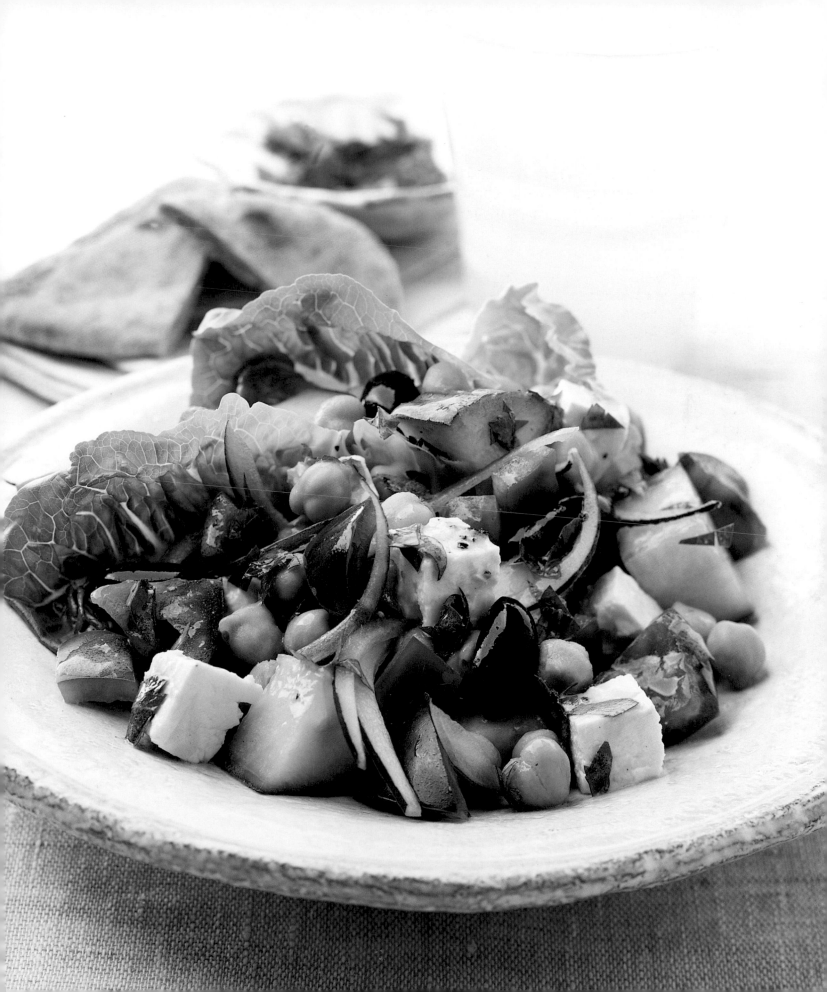

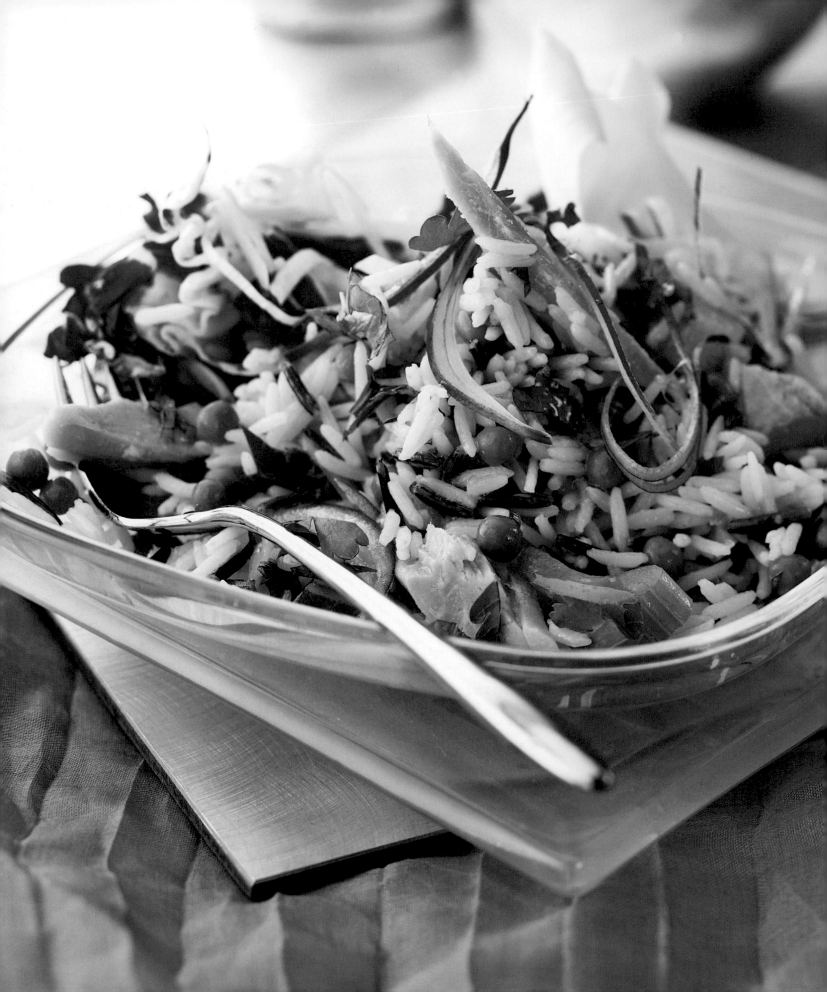

Risi bisi ham salad

Full of crisp crunchy vegetables, lean ham and plenty of fresh herbs, this wholesome rice salad is substantial enough to serve as a main meal on its own. It makes a refreshing and tasty dish, ideal for eating al fresco in the garden or packing for a picnic on a hot summer's day.

Serves 6

340 g (12 oz) mixed basmati and wild rice
600 ml (1 pint) boiling water
150 g (5½ oz) frozen petit pois
200 g (7 oz) piece lean cooked ham, trimmed of fat and cut into strips
3 celery sticks, sliced
1 red onion, thinly sliced
3 tbsp chopped parsley
2 tbsp chopped fresh mint
1 head chicory, leaves separated
100 g (3½ oz) radicchio, finely shredded
salt and pepper

Fresh orange dressing

6 tbsp orange juice
3 tbsp extra virgin olive oil
2 tsp Dijon mustard

Preparation time: 25 minutes, plus cooling

Each serving provides

kcal 327, protein 13 g, fat 8 g (of which saturated fat 1 g), carbohydrate 52 g (of which sugars 4 g), fibre 2 g

✓✓✓	B₁, B₆, B₁₂, E
✓✓	C, folate
✓	iron, potassium, zinc

1 Put the rice in a saucepan and pour over the boiling water. Bring back to the boil, then reduce the heat to low. Cover and simmer for about 15 minutes, or according to the packet instructions, until the rice is tender and all the water has been absorbed. Tip the rice into a large bowl and stir in the frozen petit pois, then leave to cool.

2 Add the ham, celery, onion, parsley and mint and toss well. Mix together the dressing ingredients, add to the bowl and toss until all the salad ingredients are evenly coated. Season with salt and pepper to taste.

3 Reserve a few whole chicory leaves for the garnish, then finely shred the rest. Serve the rice salad and shredded chicory and radicchio on individual plates, garnished with the reserved whole chicory leaves.

Another idea

• For a risi bisi sweetcorn salad, cook 250 g (8½ oz) brown rice in twice its volume of boiling vegetable stock for 35 minutes or until tender. Drain if necessary, then set aside. Heat 2 tsp extra virgin olive oil in a small saucepan and cook 1 seeded and finely diced red pepper over a high heat for 4 minutes or until it begins to char. Leave to cool. Cook 100 g (3½ oz) fine green beans, cut into short lengths, in boiling water for 4 minutes. Drain and refresh in cold water. Chop 6 spring onions and place in a bowl with the rice, red pepper and green beans and add a can of sweetcorn kernels, about 200 g, and a can of red kidney beans, about 400 g, both drained and rinsed. Mix together 2 tbsp balsamic vinegar, 2 tbsp extra virgin olive oil, 2 tsp wholegrain mustard, ½ tsp clear honey and salt and pepper to taste. Add this dressing to the salad together with 3 tbsp chopped parsley and toss well to mix.

Plus points

• Radicchio, a member of the chicory family, has deep red and white tightly packed leaves. The red pigment means this vegetable is high in beta-carotene and other cancer-fighting phytochemicals.
• Using orange juice as a base for the dressing rather than sharp vinegar means less oil is needed. It also increases the amount of vitamin C in the dish.
• The combination of lean ham, rice and peas provides almost half of the RNI of protein for an adult woman.

Bean pot with orange salad

Creole spices enliven this hearty mixed bean and vegetable casserole. Like the classic French cassoulet, it has a crisp crumb topping. With the accompanying refreshing salad, it makes a tasty, well-balanced meal.

Serves 4

1 tbsp sunflower oil

1 onion, finely chopped

3 garlic cloves, crushed

1 tsp freshly grated nutmeg

1 cinnamon stick

2 bay leaves

1 can chopped tomatoes, about 400 g

1 tbsp tomato purée

2 celery sticks, thinly sliced

150 g (5½ oz) chestnut mushrooms, thickly sliced

1 tbsp dark muscovado sugar

750 ml (1¼ pints) vegetable stock, preferably home-made light or rich (see page 28)

150 g (5½ oz) dried flageolet beans, soaked overnight and drained

150 g (5½ oz) dried pinto beans, soaked overnight and drained

3 tbsp chopped parsley

150 g (5½ oz) fresh breadcrumbs

30 g (1 oz) butter, melted

salt and pepper

To serve

1 Cos lettuce

2 oranges

1 tbsp sunflower oil

3 tbsp flaked almonds, toasted

Preparation time: 20 minutes, plus overnight soaking

Cooking time: 3½ hours

1 Preheat the oven to 160°C (325°F, gas mark 3). Heat the oil in a large flameproof casserole and add the onion and garlic. Cook for 5 minutes over a low heat to soften the onion slightly. Add the nutmeg, cinnamon stick, bay leaves, tomatoes with their juice, tomato purée, celery, mushrooms, sugar and plenty of pepper. (Do not add salt now as it will harden the beans.) Pour in the stock and stir in the flageolet and pinto beans, then bring to the boil. Cover the casserole and cook in the oven for 2½ hours or until the beans are tender.

2 Discard the cinnamon stick and bay leaves. Stir in 2 tbsp of the chopped parsley and add salt to taste. Increase the oven temperature to 180°C (350°F, gas mark 4). In a bowl, toss the breadcrumbs with the melted butter until it is evenly distributed. Spoon the breadcrumbs over the beans and return the casserole to the oven, uncovered. Cook for a further 45 minutes or until the liquid has thickened and the breadcrumbs are golden.

3 Just before the bean pot has finished cooking, make the salad. Shred the lettuce and place in a salad bowl. Cut all the peel and pith from the oranges. Holding the oranges over the salad bowl, use a small sharp knife to cut the segments from between the membranes, allowing the juice and segments to drop into the bowl with the lettuce. Drizzle the oil over, add the almonds and toss together gently.

4 Remove the bean pot from the oven, scatter on the remaining 1 tbsp of chopped parsley and serve with the salad on the side.

Plus points

• Oranges are an excellent source of vitamin C, which helps the body to absorb the iron provided by the beans.

• Beans and pulses are rich in soluble fibre and have a low glycaemic index. This means they are broken down slowly so they are more satisfying, making you feel full for longer and keeping blood sugar levels stable.

• Almonds contribute protein to the salad accompaniment plus some vitamin E.

Each serving provides

kcal 550, protein 25 g, fat 16 g (of which saturated fat 5 g), carbohydrate 80 g (of which sugars 17 g), fibre 14 g

✓✓✓	C, E, copper, iron
✓✓	B₁, folate, calcium, phosphorus, potassium, zinc
✓	A, niacin

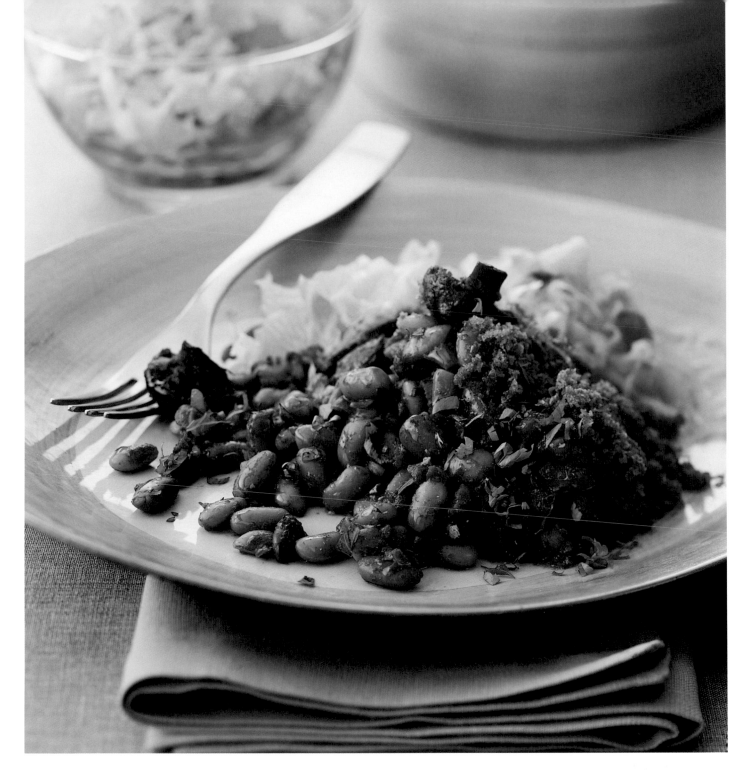

Some more ideas

• Instead of almonds, add 2 coarsely grated carrots to the salad with 2 tbsp poppy seeds. Soak 2 tbsp currants in 2 tbsp orange juice for several hours or overnight, then add them with the carrots and poppy seeds.

• Peppery rocket is delicious with the oranges and almonds in the salad. Use 85 g (3 oz) instead of the lettuce.

• Instead of breadcrumbs, top the casserole with slices of garlic bread. Cream 1 crushed garlic clove with 40 g (1½ oz) butter and spread over 8 slices of French bread. Cook for only 30 minutes.

• Use all flageolet beans instead of a mixture of pinto and flageolet, or a combination of haricot and flageolet. Haricot with black-eyed or red-kidney beans is also good.

Tabbouleh with goat's cheese

Tabbouleh is a classic Middle Eastern salad made with bulghur wheat. While the wheat is soaking, you have just enough time to chop the vegetables and herbs, and make the dressing. Serve with lavash or pitta bread.

Serves 4

280 g (10 oz) bulghur wheat

1 yellow pepper, seeded and chopped

20 cherry tomatoes, quartered

1 small red onion, finely chopped

10 cm (4 in) piece of cucumber, seeded and chopped

1 large carrot, grated

5 tbsp chopped parsley

2 tbsp chopped fresh coriander

2 tbsp chopped fresh mint

1 small fresh red chilli, seeded and finely chopped (optional)

200 g (7 oz) rindless soft goat's cheese, crumbled

salt and pepper

Lemon and cumin dressing

¼ tsp ground cumin

1 small garlic clove, very finely chopped

1 tbsp lemon juice

3 tbsp extra virgin olive oil

To serve

lettuce leaves

12 radishes, sliced

Preparation time: about 30 minutes

1 Put the bulghur wheat in a mixing bowl, pour over enough boiling water to cover and stir well. Leave to soak for 15–20 minutes.

2 Meanwhile, make the dressing. Whisk together the cumin, garlic and lemon juice in a small bowl, then whisk in the olive oil.

3 Drain the bulghur wheat in a sieve, pressing out excess water, then return it to the bowl. Add the pepper, tomatoes, onion, cucumber, carrot, parsley, coriander and mint, plus the chilli, if using. Pour the dressing over the top and season with salt and pepper to taste. Fold gently to mix well.

4 Arrange the lettuce leaves on 4 plates or a serving platter. Pile the bulghur salad on the leaves and sprinkle the goat's cheese over the top. Garnish with the radishes and serve.

Plus points

• Bulghur wheat is a good, low-fat source of starchy (complex) carbohydrate. Because it retains the particularly nutritious outer layers of the wheat grain, it contains useful amounts of B vitamins, particularly B_1.

• Goat's cheese is a tasty source of protein and calcium and lower in fat than cheeses such as Cheddar and Parmesan.

Some more ideas

• Use feta cheese instead of goat's cheese.

• For an apricot tabbouleh side salad, mix the soaked bulghur wheat with the yellow pepper and red onion, plus 4 chopped celery sticks and 115 g (4 oz) snipped, ready-to-eat dried apricots (omit the other vegetables and the herbs, as well as the goat's cheese). Add ½ tsp ground cinnamon to the dressing.

• For a spicy tabbouleh with chicken to serve 6, replace the goat's cheese with 2 cooked skinless boneless chicken breasts, about 280 g (10 oz) in total, cut into cubes. Mix the soaked bulghur wheat with the chicken, pepper, onion, carrot and parsley (omit the other vegetables and herbs). For the dressing, gently warm 3 tbsp extra virgin olive oil in a small frying pan with 1 finely chopped garlic clove. Add ½–1 tsp each of ground cumin, ground coriander, dry mustard and curry powder, and continue cooking for 1 minute. Stir in 2 tbsp lemon juice and seasoning to taste. Pour the dressing over the salad and stir gently to combine. Garnish with sliced cucumber rounds.

Each serving provides

kcal 473, protein 16 g, fat 18 g (of which saturated fat 7 g), carbohydrate 64 g (of which sugars 10 g), fibre 3 g

✓✓✓	B_1, B_6, B_{12}, E, niacin
✓✓	A, B_2, C, folate, calcium, copper, iron
✓	potassium

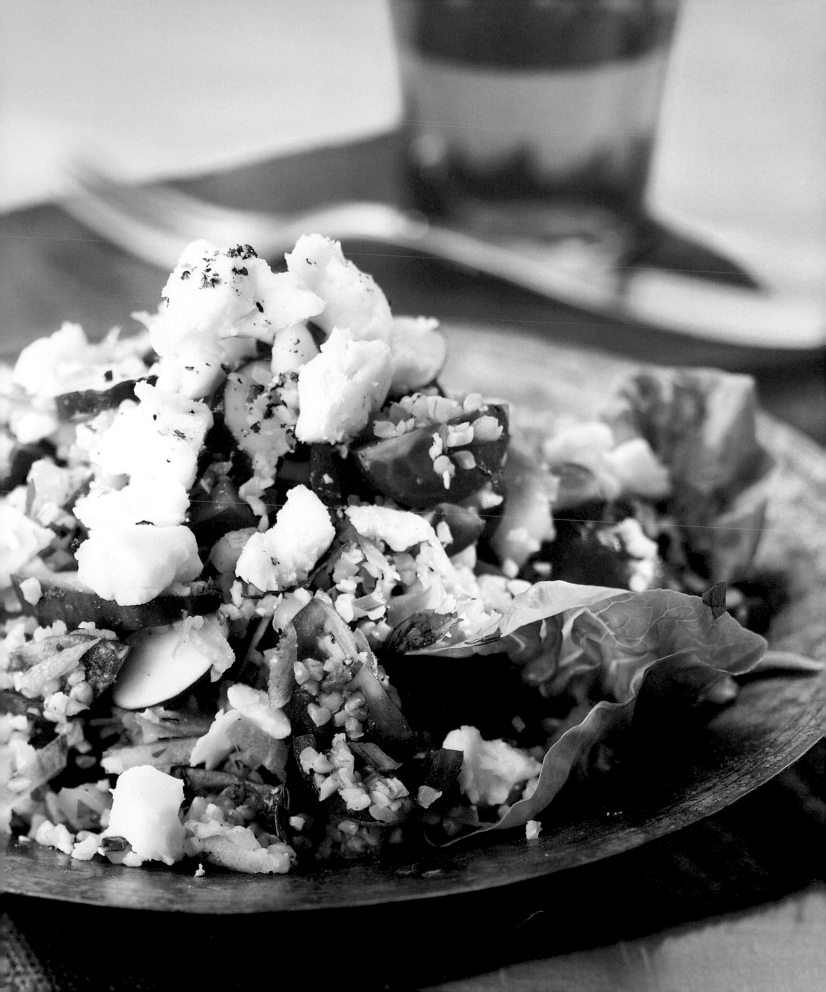

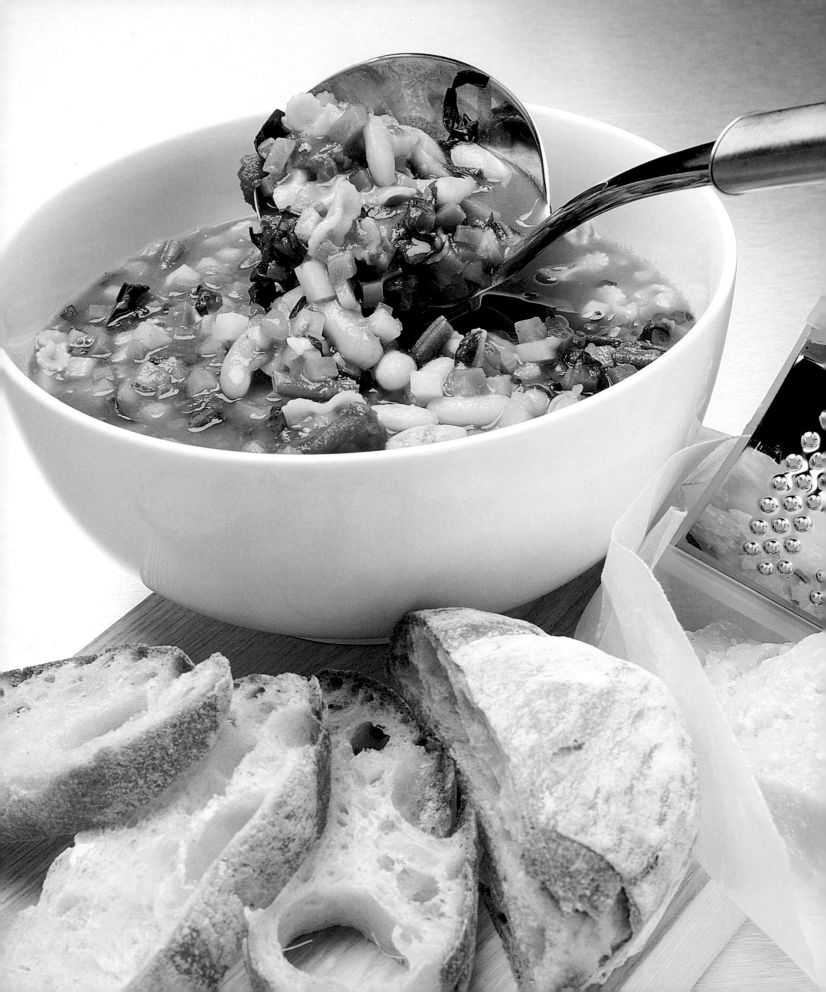

Minestrone

This minestrone makes the most of winter vegetables, and is full of vitamin goodness. Beans and pasta make it even more nourishing. Serve with chunks of fresh country-style bread for a satisfying meal.

Serves 6

1 tbsp extra virgin olive oil

1 large onion, finely chopped

3–4 garlic cloves, finely chopped

200 g (7 oz) dried cannellini or borlotti beans, soaked overnight and drained

1 can plum tomatoes in juice, about 400 g

2 tbsp tomato purée

200 g (7 oz) carrots, finely diced

150 g (5½ oz) swede, finely diced

150 g (5½ oz) celeriac, finely diced

250 g (8½ oz) peeled pumpkin flesh, finely diced

1 tsp fresh thyme leaves

1 bay leaf

3 allspice berries, finely crushed

200 g (7 oz) potatoes, peeled and finely diced

150 g (5½ oz) green beans, cut into short lengths

100 g (3½ oz) small pasta shapes, such as farfallini (bows) or conchigliette (shells), or broken-up spaghetti

125 g (4½ oz) spinach, chopped

4 tbsp shredded fresh basil

salt and pepper

55 g (2 oz) Parmesan cheese, freshly grated, to serve

Preparation time: 30 minutes, plus overnight soaking

Cooking time: about 1½ hours

1 Heat the oil in a large saucepan. Add the onion and garlic, cover and cook for 4–5 minutes, stirring occasionally, until the onion is translucent. Add the cannellini or borlotti beans and pour in 2 litres (3½ pints) water. Bring to the boil and boil for 10 minutes, then reduce the heat, cover the pan and simmer for 30 minutes.

2 Add the tomatoes with their juice, breaking them up with a fork, then add the tomato purée, carrots, swede, celeriac and pumpkin. Stir in the thyme, bay leaf and crushed allspice. Bring back to simmering point, then cover the pan again and simmer for 20 minutes.

3 Stir in the potatoes and green beans. Continue simmering, covered, for 15 minutes. Stir in the pasta and cook, still covered, for a further 10 minutes or until the cannellini or borlotti beans are tender and the pasta is cooked.

4 Add the spinach and basil, and season to taste with salt and pepper. Simmer uncovered for 2–3 minutes until the spinach has wilted. Ladle the soup into warm bowls and serve at once, with the Parmesan cheese to sprinkle on top.

Some more ideas

• Butternut squash or any other type of squash can be used instead of the pumpkin.

• Add 100 g (3½ oz) rinded and chopped lean smoked back bacon with the onion and garlic in step 1. Alternatively, crisp-fried Parma ham can be sprinkled over the soup when serving.

Plus points

• Beans and pulses are an excellent source of soluble fibre. Unfortunately they can produce unpleasant side effects such as wind and bloating. To prevent this, be sure to cook them thoroughly – undercooked beans are difficult to digest and thus more likely to cause wind.

• Pasta scores healthily low on the Glycaemic Index, which means that it breaks down slowly into glucose and glycogen in the body and provides long-lasting energy.

Each serving provides

kcal 290, protein 16 g, fat 6 g (of which saturated fat 2 g), carbohydrate 45 g (of which sugars 9 g), fibre 9 g

✓✓	A, C, folate
✓	B$_1$, B$_6$, B$_{12}$, E, niacin

Moroccan-style pumpkin and butter beans

Middle Eastern spices flavour this low-fat vegetarian casserole, which is full of vegetables and other fibre-rich ingredients. It is a great recipe for a cook-ahead meal as the flavours mature and improve if the casserole is chilled overnight, then thoroughly reheated for serving. Try it with couscous.

Serves 4

600 ml (1 pint) boiling water

1 vegetable stock cube, crumbled, or
   2 tsp vegetable bouillon powder or paste

½ tsp turmeric

½ tsp ground coriander

pinch of ground cumin

200 g (7 oz) leeks, halved lengthways
   and sliced

225 g (8 oz) parsnips, cut into 1 cm (½ in)
   cubes

600 g (1 lb 5 oz) piece of pumpkin, peeled,
   seeded and cut into 1 cm (½ in) cubes

400 g (14 oz) yellow or green courgettes,
   sliced

1 red pepper, seeded and chopped

100 g (3½ oz) ready-to-eat dried apricots,
   chopped

1 can butter beans, about 400 g, drained

pinch of crushed dried chillies,
   or to taste (optional)

salt and pepper

To garnish

30 g (1 oz) pine nuts

chopped parsley or fresh coriander

Preparation time: about 10 minutes
Cooking time: about 20 minutes

1 Pour the boiling water into a flameproof casserole. Stir in the stock cube, powder or paste, the turmeric, ground coriander and cumin. Add the leeks and parsnips and bring to the boil. Reduce the heat to moderate, cover the pan and simmer the vegetables for 5 minutes.

2 Add the pumpkin, courgettes and red pepper to the pan, then bring the stock back to the boil. Stir in the apricots, butter beans and chilli flakes, if using, adding more to taste for a spicier result. Season with salt and pepper. Reduce the heat, cover the pan and simmer for 10 minutes or until all the vegetables are tender.

3 Meanwhile, toast the pine nuts in a non-stick frying pan over a moderate heat, stirring constantly, until just beginning to brown and giving off their nutty aroma. Tip the pine nuts onto a board and chop them coarsely.

4 Taste the casserole and adjust the seasoning, if necessary, then ladle it into deep bowls. Sprinkle with the chopped pine nuts and parsley or fresh coriander and serve.

Plus points

- Pumpkin is a rich source of beta-carotene and other carotenoid compounds. Save and roast or toast the seeds as a snack as they provide good amounts of protein and zinc.
- Dried apricots are an excellent source of beta-carotene and a good source of calcium.
- Parsnips provide useful amounts of potassium, folate and vitamin B$_1$.

Each serving provides

kcal 250, protein 12 g, fat 7 g (of which saturated fat 1 g), carbohydrate 35 g (of which sugars 21 g), fibre 11 g

✓✓✓	A, C, iron
✓✓	B$_1$, B$_6$, folate
✓	calcium

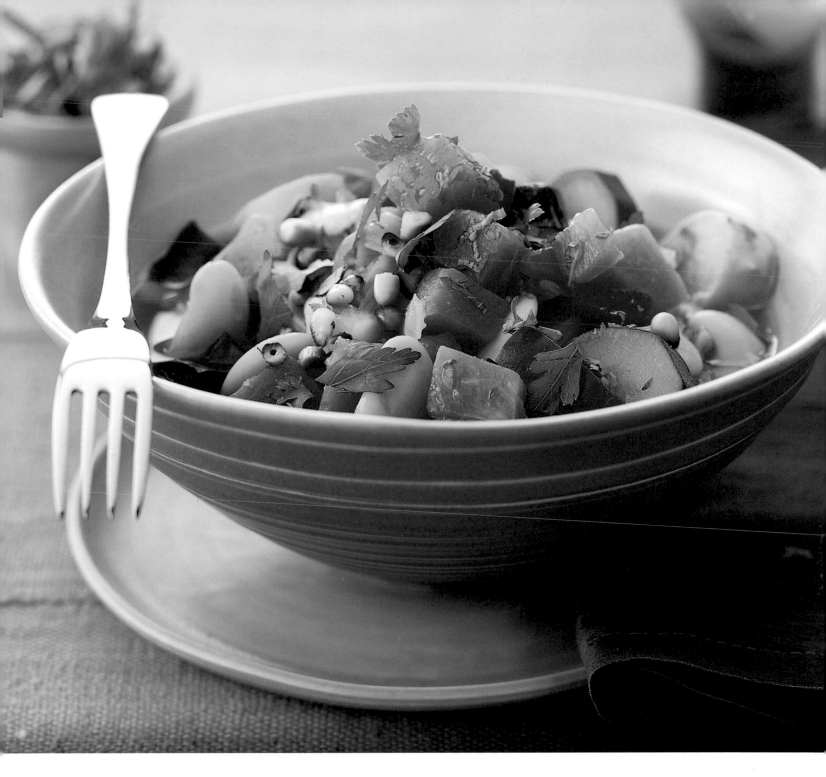

Some more ideas

• This casserole is delicious ladled over couscous. Place 340 g (12 oz) couscous in a heatproof bowl. Add salt to taste and pour in 600 ml (1 pint) boiling water to cover. Cover the bowl and leave to stand for about 5 minutes or until all the water has been absorbed and the couscous is plumped up and tender. Add 15 g (½ oz) butter and fluff up the couscous with a fork to separate the grains.

• Try other vegetables with the pumpkin – for example, broccoli florets can be added with the pumpkin instead of the courgettes. The distinctive flavour of turnips is also good with the other vegetables.

• For a fresh, peppery flavour, garnish the casserole with 55 g (2 oz) grated red radishes or large white radish (mooli).

Lentil risotto

Lentils add extra flavour and texture to this Italian-style mushroom risotto and also make it more nutritious. Serve with roasted or griddled Italian vegetables, such as peppers and courgettes, or a mixed salad, for a satisfying lunch, and one that is particularly tempting on a cold winter's day.

Serves 4

170 g (6 oz) green lentils
500 ml (17 fl oz) vegetable stock
  (see page 28)
1 tbsp extra virgin olive oil
1 onion, finely chopped
1 garlic clove, crushed
3 celery sticks, chopped
1 red pepper, seeded and diced
1 tsp ground coriander
1 tsp ground cumin
225 g (8 oz) mushrooms, sliced
170 g (6 oz) risotto rice
200 ml (7 fl oz) dry white wine
3 tbsp coarsely chopped fresh coriander,
  plus extra to garnish
50 g (1¾ oz) Parmesan cheese,
  cut into shavings
salt and pepper

Preparation time: 30 minutes
Cooking time: 45 minutes

Each serving provides Ⓥ

kcal 429, protein 21 g, fat 9 g (of which saturated fat 3 g), carbohydrate 59 g (of which sugars 6 g), fibre 6 g

✓✓✓	A, B$_6$, C, copper, selenium, zinc
✓✓	B$_6$, niacin, calcium, iron, potassium
✓	B$_1$, B$_2$, folate

1 Cook the lentils in a saucepan of boiling water for 20 minutes, then drain and set aside. Place the stock in the saucepan and bring to simmering point over a moderate heat. Lower the heat so the stock is simmering gently.

2 Heat the oil in another large saucepan, add the onion, garlic and celery, and cook for 5 minutes or until softened, stirring occasionally. Add the red pepper and the ground coriander and cumin, and cook for 1 minute, stirring.

3 Add the mushrooms, rice and cooked lentils and stir to mix. Pour in the wine and add a ladleful of the hot stock. Bring to a gentle boil and bubble until most of the liquid has been absorbed, stirring frequently.

4 Add another ladleful of stock and cook until it is absorbed, stirring frequently. Repeat this gradual addition of the hot stock until it has all been added. The rice should be creamy and tender but still with some bite, and the lentils cooked.

5 Stir in the chopped coriander and season with salt and pepper to taste. Serve hot, sprinkled with the Parmesan shavings and extra chopped coriander.

Some more ideas

• Instead of green lentils, you can use brown or Puy lentils.

• Replace the Parmesan shavings with 2 chopped hard-boiled eggs.

• Make a pearl barley 'risotto'. Soften 2 sliced leeks and 1 crushed garlic clove in 1 tbsp extra virgin olive oil. Add 1 seeded and diced red or yellow pepper, 250 g (8½ oz) pearl barley, 2 tsp dried herbes de Provence, 200 ml (7 fl oz) dry white wine and 100 ml (3½ fl oz) hot vegetable stock. Simmer for 45 minutes, gradually adding a further 400–500 ml (14–17 fl oz) hot stock and stirring frequently, until the pearl barley is cooked and tender. Meanwhile, steam 225 g (8 oz) broccoli florets and cook 170 g (6 oz) frozen peas. Stir these into the barley risotto and heat gently until piping hot. Season with salt and pepper to taste and serve, topped with the Parmesan shavings.

Plus points

• Lentils are the small seeds of a variety of leguminous plants. They are a good source of protein, starchy carbohydrate, dietary fibre and B vitamins.

• Parmesan cheese, which is made from unpasteurised skimmed cow's milk, contributes protein to this dish, as well as calcium and vitamin B$_{12}$.

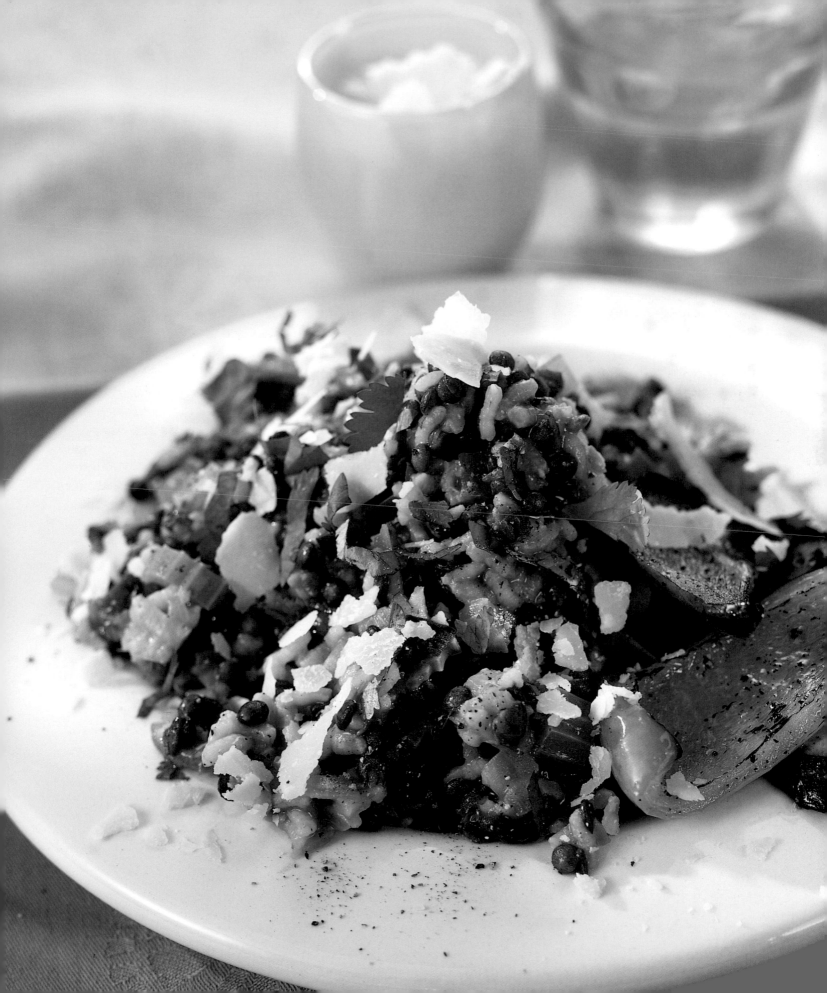

Spiced lentil dhal

Potato and cauliflower are a favourite combination for curry and they are delicious cooked with lentils in a mildly spiced sauce. Served with a fresh carrot chutney and fruit and nut raita, this healthy meal will be relished by meat-eaters as well as vegetarians. Serve with basmati rice or naan bread.

Serves 4

2 tbsp sunflower oil

1 large onion, coarsely chopped

1–2 garlic cloves, crushed

2 tbsp finely chopped fresh root ginger

2 tbsp mild curry paste

170 g (6 oz) red lentils

1 tsp ground cumin

1 tsp turmeric

1 tsp salt

400 g (14 oz) small new potatoes, halved

1 small cauliflower, broken into florets

1 red pepper, seeded and coarsely chopped

4 tomatoes, skinned and quartered

225 g (8 oz) baby spinach leaves

generous handful of fresh coriander leaves, coarsely chopped

Carrot and coriander chutney

3 carrots, coarsely grated

1 green chilli, seeded and finely chopped

juice of 1 lime

2 tbsp chopped fresh coriander

Banana and almond raita

2 firm bananas

280 g (10 oz) plain low-fat yogurt

55 g (2 oz) flaked almonds, toasted

Preparation time: 25 minutes

Cooking time: about 55 minutes

1 Heat the oil in a large saucepan. Add the onion, garlic and ginger, and cook for 5 minutes. Stir in the curry paste and stir for a further 2 minutes over a gentle heat.

2 Stir in the lentils, cumin, turmeric, salt and 1 litre (1¾ pints) water. Bring to the boil, then cover the pan and simmer gently for 10 minutes. Stir in the potatoes and cook for 10 minutes, then add the cauliflower and cook for another 10 minutes. Add the pepper and tomatoes, and simmer for 5 minutes.

3 Meanwhile, prepare the side dishes. Mix together the carrots, chilli, lime juice and coriander for the chutney. Transfer to a serving dish. For the raita, slice the bananas into a serving bowl. Stir in the yogurt and sprinkle with the almonds.

4 Stir the spinach into the curry and cook for 2 minutes or until just wilted. Stir in the coriander and serve, with the chutney and raita.

Each serving provides

kcal 550, protein 26 g, fat 17 g (of which saturated fat 3 g), carbohydrate 77 g (of which sugars 35 g), fibre 11 g

✓✓✓	A, B$_6$, C, E, folate, iron, phosphorus
✓✓	B$_1$, calcium, copper, potassium, zinc
✓	B$_2$

Some more ideas

• The vegetables can be varied according to whatever is available or preferred. For example, try chunks of courgette and aubergine with, or instead of, the cauliflower, or small whole okra or cut green beans with the tomatoes.

• Additional pulses can be added. Black-eyed beans and chickpeas are particularly good. If using dried pulses, soak them overnight, then drain and cook them in boiling water for 45–60 minutes or until almost tender before adding them to the curry. Canned pulses, well drained, should be added towards the end of the cooking time.

Plus points

• This curry is full of vegetables. Together with the lentils they provide valuable dietary fibre, vitamins and minerals.

• Vegetables play a protective role in fighting degenerative diseases and this recipe shows that eating 5 portions of fruit and vegetables daily can be easy, tasty and exciting.

• Uncooked accompaniments and salads boost the vitamin content of a meal as well as providing a variety of complementary textures and flavours.

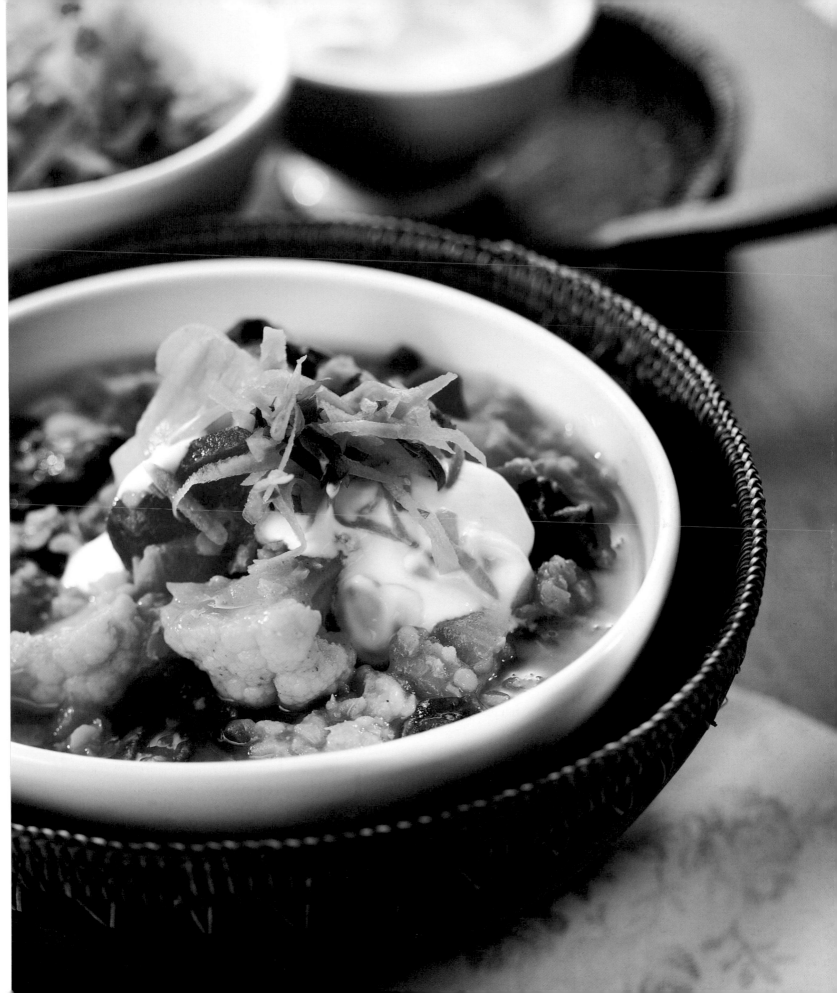

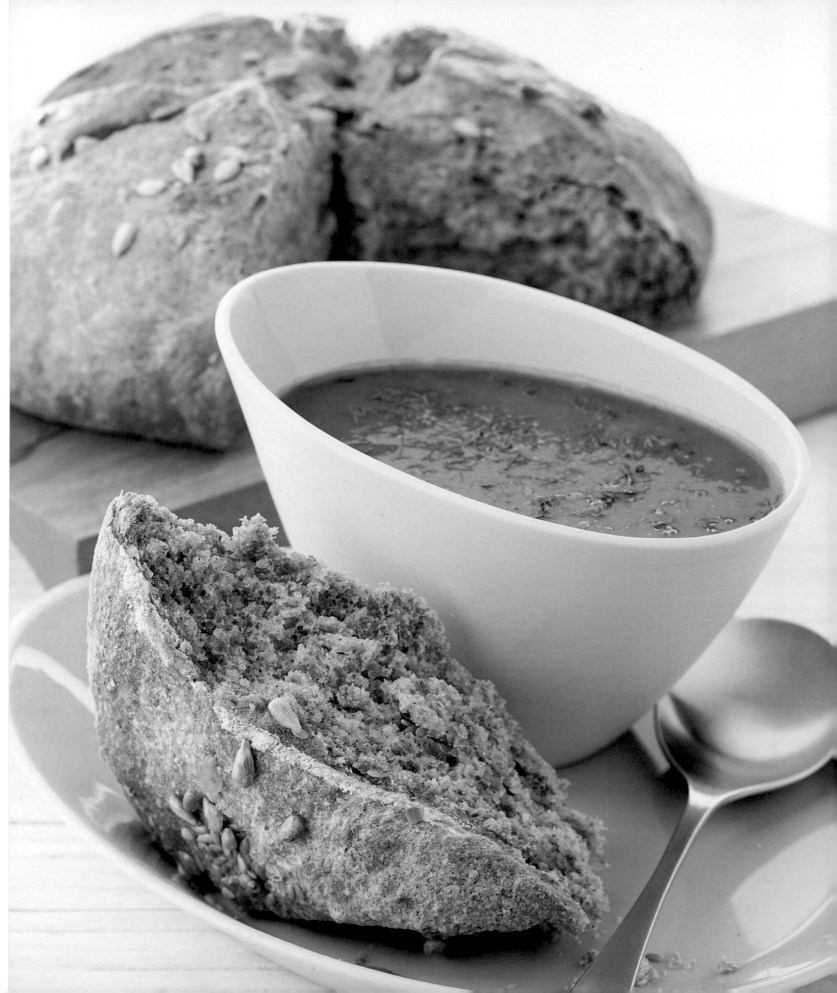

Multigrain seeded loaf

Serve this nutty-textured loaf very fresh, cut into wedges. It's good with a hearty bowl of soup or cheese and pickles. The mix of seeds can be varied to your own taste, or you can use just one kind.

Makes 1 round loaf (cuts into 8 wedges)

300 g (10½ oz) strong white (bread) flour

200 g (7 oz) strong wholemeal (bread) flour

100 g (3½ oz) buckwheat flour

75 g (2½ oz) polenta

2 tsp salt

1 sachet easy-blend dried yeast, about 7 g

1 tsp light muscovado sugar

3 tbsp sunflower seeds

2 tbsp pumpkin seeds

2 tbsp linseeds

2 tbsp sunflower oil

450 ml (15 fl oz) tepid water

a little semi-skimmed milk to glaze

Preparation time: 30 minutes, plus about 2 hours rising

Cooking time: 30–35 minutes

Each wedge provides Ⓥ

kcal 390, protein 11 g, fat 11 g (of which saturated fat 1 g), carbohydrate 65 g (of which sugars 2 g), fibre 5 g

✓✓✓	E
✓✓	B₁, B₆, folate, niacin, copper, selenium, zinc
✓	calcium, iron

1 Sift the white, wholemeal and buckwheat flours into a large bowl, tipping in any bran left in the sieve. Stir in the polenta, salt, yeast and sugar.

2 Mix together all the seeds, then set aside 1 tbsp for the topping. Stir the rest into the flour mixture.

3 Make a well in the centre of the dry ingredients and pour in the oil and most of the water. Gradually work the dry ingredients into the liquid to make a soft dough, adding the rest of the water as needed. Turn the dough out onto a work surface and knead for 10 minutes or until smooth and elastic.

4 Place the dough in a large, lightly greased bowl and cover with a damp tea-towel. Leave in a warm place for 1½ hours or until doubled in size.

5 Turn the risen dough out onto a lightly floured surface and knock it back with your knuckles, then knead firmly for a few minutes. Shape into a 20 cm (8 in) round and place on a lightly greased baking sheet. Cover with oiled cling film and leave to rise for 20–30 minutes or until well risen and springy to the touch.

6 Towards the end of the rising time, preheat the oven to 230°C (450°F, gas mark 8). Uncover the loaf and, using a sharp knife, cut deeply to mark it into 8 wedges. Brush with milk and sprinkle with the reserved seeds.

7 Bake for 15 minutes, then reduce the oven temperature to 200°C (400°F, gas mark 6). Bake for a further 15–20 minutes or until the loaf is golden brown and sounds hollow when tapped on the base. Cool on a wire rack. This is best eaten on the day it is made.

Some more ideas

• Shape the dough into a 'bubble loaf'. Roll it into about 8 balls and pack them together in a round shape, just touching, on the baking sheet. After baking they can be pulled apart and served as rolls.

• Instead of polenta, use medium oatmeal, and replace the seeds with 3 tbsp rolled oats, 2 tbsp poppy seeds and 2 tbsp sesame seeds.

Plus points

• Seeds are packed with essential fatty acids. Linseed, for instance, is one of the best sources of omega-3 fats, while sunflower seeds are an excellent source of omega-6.

• Pumpkin seeds are one of the richest vegetarian sources of zinc, a mineral that is essential for the functioning of the immune system. They are a good source of protein and unsaturated fat and a useful source of iron, magnesium and fibre.

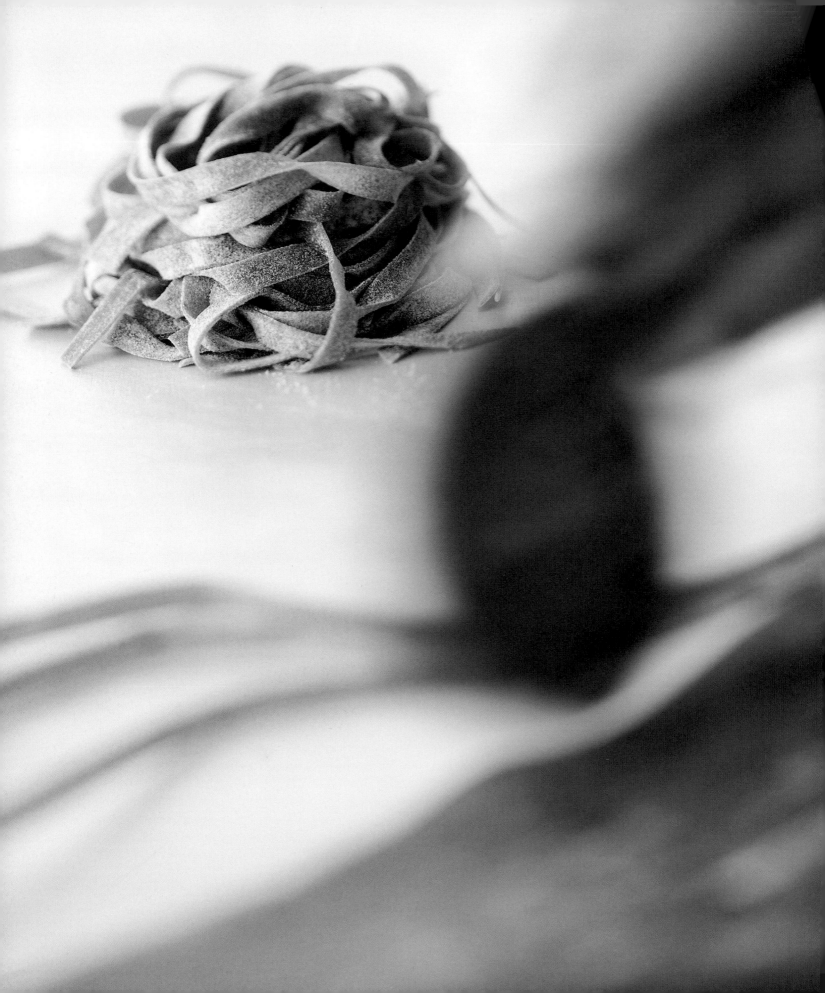

Pasta Power

Pasta is the perfect food for a modern healthy diet, being

low in fat and calories and high in starchy carbohydrates

and vitamins. And it is so versatile – ideal for everyday

eating as well as easily transformed into dishes to suit

any occasion. No wonder pasta is loved all over the world.

You can buy it dried or fresh, in hundreds of different

shapes, sizes and even flavours. Even better, make

and shape pasta dough yourself, flavouring it to surprise

and delight your family and friends. Cooking pasta is

as simple as boiling water, and

there is a vast choice of delicious

sauces to dress it, from the

simplest tomato or pesto to wild

mushrooms, seafood and truffles.

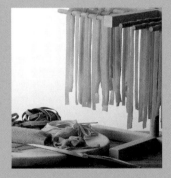

Pasta in a healthy diet

One of the world's most popular foods, pasta is a perfect staple for healthy eating. With a variety of shapes and colours, pasta is loved by families and gourmets alike.

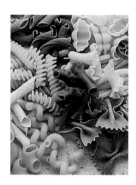

Why eat pasta?

Pasta has an ideal 'healthy eating' profile in that it is a low-fat, starchy (complex carbohydrate) food. Starchy carbohydrates should make up at least half of the daily calories in a well-balanced diet. Adding more pasta to meals is one of the easiest, most varied and nutritious ways to increase your starchy food intake.

There is a popular myth that pasta is fattening, but with the right sauces and accompaniments, the opposite is true – pasta is relatively low in calories and it helps to control hunger by making us feel full, leaving less room for fatty foods which are more likely to cause weight problems. Regular physical exercise in combination with a diet based around starchy carbohydrates is the best way to maintain a healthy waistline.

Great shape from simple grain

Pasta is traditionally made from durum wheat semolina. Durum wheat, grown in Italy, the Middle East and North America, is a 'hard' wheat with a high gluten content. Gluten is a protein that gives flour its strength and elasticity, which is what enables pasta dough to be rolled and shaped.

Pasta dough may be made from just flour, water and salt, or eggs or oil may be added to enrich the dough. Vegetable purées are used to colour pasta, but they are not present in sufficient quantity to make a major nutritional contribution.

Pasta can be made from a mixture of flour and durum semolina or standard wheat flour. Flours from other grains, such as buckwheat, rice or beans, are also used to make pasta – useful for people who cannot eat wheat or gluten.

Semolina is used to make gnocchi (small dumplings) and rolled into couscous. Couscous is a traditional North African staple, served in much the same way as pasta, to partner poultry, meat or vegetable stews and sauces.

Essential fibre

In addition to helping to control hunger pangs and reducing the likelihood of weight problems, diets rich in starchy foods have other plus points. Undigested fibre in starchy food passes to the colon, where it ferments and stimulates the production of healthy gut bacteria. These 'friendly bacteria' aid digestion and outnumber potentially harmful bacteria. This 'biomass' of good gut bacteria also helps to bulk faeces, preventing constipation and associated problems, such as piles.

The fermentation of the fibre produces fatty acids, which offer health benefits such as helping to regulate cell growth in the intestine, giving protection against colon cancer.

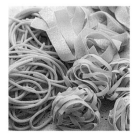

Brilliant for B vitamins

Pasta contains valuable vitamins, most notably B vitamins. B vitamins are water-soluble, and not stored for long in the body, so we need to eat them regularly. They are essential for healthy digestion and for the steady

Does it all add up?

While the human body is less likely to turn starchy carbohydrates into body fat than it is fatty foods, eating too much carbohydrate can cause a weight gain. Each gram of carbohydrate – starch or sugar – provides 4 kcal. So if you want to increase the starchy food in your diet, be sure that the quantity of calories eaten still matches the calories used up.

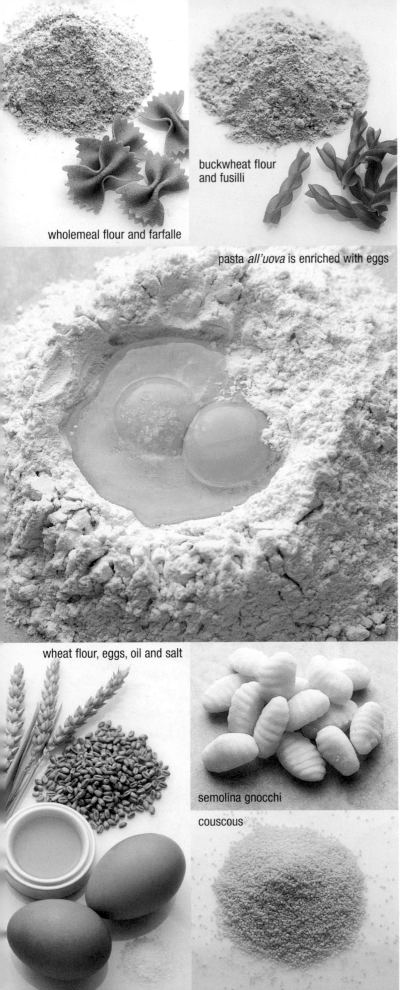

buckwheat flour and fusilli

wholemeal flour and farfalle

pasta *all'uova* is enriched with eggs

wheat flour, eggs, oil and salt

semolina gnocchi

couscous

and continuous release of energy from starchy foods. They are also important for healthy nerves, mental activity and memory. In particular, B_1 (thiamin) is needed to help to convert protein into muscle; B_2 (riboflavin), niacin and B_6 to convert food into energy; and B_6 for the creation of red blood cells and to prevent anaemia. All pasta provides B vitamins, although wholemeal varieties have more than white pasta, and in addition contain vitamin E from the germ of the wheat grain.

A source of minerals

Wholemeal pasta offers zinc and iron, essential to prevent anaemia. Selenium (mainly found in wholemeal pasta) is, like zinc, an antioxidant needed to make enzymes that destroy harmful free radicals, a by-product of normal cell function. Antioxidant nutrients prevent free radicals initiating cancer, heart disease and other health problems.

Pasta power

Athletes appreciate the value of pasta: most elite athletes eat a high-carbohydrate diet for a few days before an event, plus a starchy pre-event meal to boost energy and endurance. This is called carbohydrate loading. The body turns starch into glucose and glycogen, which is stored in muscles and liver, producing a better source of energy than sugar.

For most of us carbohydrate loading is unnecessary, but we can eat starchy food after exercise (as opposed to sugary or fatty food) to replenish depleted energy effectively.

Pasta and energy – the GI factor

GI stands for Glycaemic Index, which is a ranking of foods based on their effect on blood sugar levels. Low-GI foods break down slowly, releasing energy gradually into the bloodstream, which results in a smaller rise of blood sugar. High-GI foods cause a larger rise of blood sugar. Low-GI foods are more desirable because they can help to control hunger, appetite and weight, and lower raised blood fats. Pasta is a low-GI food, and the less processing during manufacture the lower the score: wholemeal pasta has a lower GI than white pasta, and thicker shapes score lower than thin varieties.

Know your pasta – Italian style

When planning your menu, choose the pasta first and add lots of vegetables and smaller quantities of fish, poultry or meat.

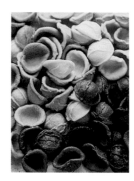

A pasta primer

Buying pasta can be quite an adventure – plain or filled, white, wholemeal or multi-coloured, big or small? Pasta comes in an almost bewildering variety of shapes and sizes, and many have several names that may be simply regional or peculiar to a particular manufacturer. Here are some Italian terms to make it easier to choose.

• Pasta di semola grano duro indicates that it is made from durum wheat flour, and all'uova that it is enriched with eggs.

• The word endings to pasta names can indicate the size of the shape: oni is large, for example conchiglioni (large shells); ette or etti are small, as in spaghetti, cappelletti (small hats) or orecchiette (small ears); and ini are smaller still.

• Spinach makes pasta verde (green); beetroot makes pasta alla bietola or rossi (red); and squid ink is added to make pasta seppia or neroli (black).

Although the description 'fresh' implies greater nutritional status, both fresh and dried pasta offer the same benefits.

Shaping up

Campanelle are bells with frilly edges, as are ballerine.

Capelli d'angelo, which literally means 'angel hair', are long and extremely thin strands.

Cannelloni are large tubes that are filled and baked.

Casarecce are rolled lengths forming an s-shape at each end.

Conchiglie are shells; conchigliette are a smaller version, while conchiglie grande are jumbo ones for stuffing.

Ditali are thimbles or tubes; ditalini are very small ones.

Farfalle are in the shape of bows, also described as bow ties or butterflies. Small bows are farfallette or farfallini.

Fettuccine are long, flat ribbons, about 5 mm (¼ in) wide.

Fusilli are spirals or corkscrews, also called coils or springs. They may be long or short. Another name for these is rotini.

Gemelli are narrow spirals or twists with hollow ends.

Gnocchi are fluted shells. Another name for these is cavatelli.

Lasagne are flat rectangular or square sheets. Lasagnette are wide, flat noodles with ruffled edges; reginette are similar.

Linguine are long, flat ribbon noodles, thinner than fettuccine.

Lumache are described as snail-shaped.

Macaroni are smooth, thick tubes. They may be as long as spaghetti, or 'short-cut' and straight or curved (elbow macaroni). Cavatappi are ridged spiral macaroni.

Orecchiette are small ear shapes.

Pappardelle are flat noodles about 2 cm (¾ in) wide.

Penne are short, straight tubes, cut diagonally to give them quill-like ends. They may be ridged (penne rigati) or smooth.

Radiatori look like little grills.

Rigatoni are short, ridged tubes, fatter than penne.

Spaghetti, the most familiar form of pasta outside Italy, are long, string-like strands. Spaghettini are thinner.

Tagliatelle are long, flat ribbon noodles, like fettuccine.

Vermicelli are a finer version of spaghetti.

Well filled

Filled pasta can be bought dried, but fresh is superior – the flavour and quality of dried stuffed pasta, particularly the filling, can be disappointing. These are the classic shapes.

Agnolotti are rectangular or crescent-shaped envelopes, traditionally filled with meat.

Capelletti are small stuffed hat-shaped pasta.

Ravioli are small or large square, round or oval parcels.

Tortelloni are large stuffed squares.

Tortellini are little stuffed rings, made by folding circles or squares in half, then pinching the corners together.

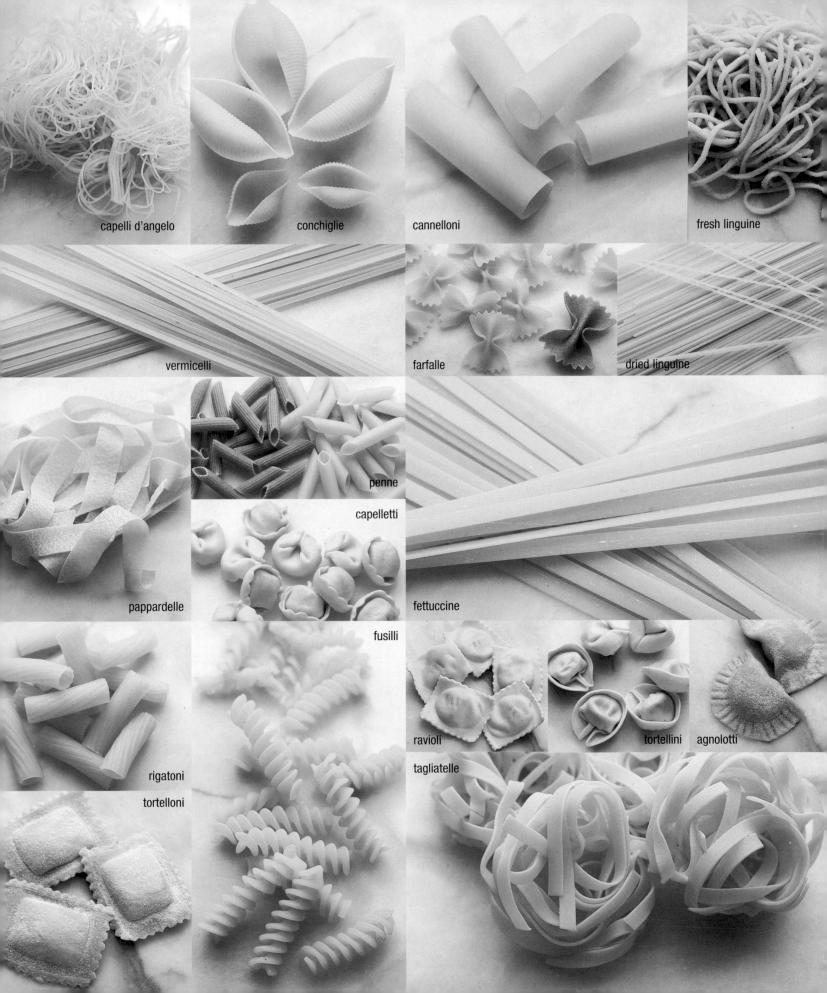

capelli d'angelo

conchiglie

cannelloni

fresh linguine

vermicelli

farfalle

dried linguine

pappardelle

penne

capelletti

fettuccine

rigatoni

fusilli

ravioli

tortellini

agnolotti

tagliatelle

tortelloni

Oriental and non-wheat pasta

Chinese cooks may not have invented pasta, but they certainly spread the healthy habit of eating noodles throughout the Far East.

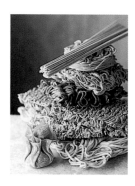

Noodles for breakfast

Noodle is the name given to flat ribbons of pasta (Italian and other types) and it is also applied to some round varieties. In the Orient, noodles are made from the staple grain of the region; for example, there are rice or buckwheat noodles, and even noodles made from mung or soya beans and vegetables. Dumpling wrappers are also a type of pasta dough.

Noodles are not confined to main meals. In Japan, for example, small local noodle restaurants, bars and stalls in towns and villages serve a wide variety of nutritious hot and cold vegetarian and non-vegetarian noodle dishes from breakfast through lunch and well into the evening. Similar enthusiasm for noodles exists in Malaysia, Thailand, Indonesia, Vietnam, Korea and the Philippines, where traditional meals incorporate noodles as a basic starchy food in a diet rich in vegetables and fruit.

Oriental noodle know-how

Cellophane noodles, also called transparent or bean thread noodles, are made from ground mung beans. These fine, white noodles are sold dried, in bundles. Before being added to soups or other dishes, they are soaked in water or stock, which makes them slippery and translucent.

Rice noodles, in China, are made from a mixture of rice flour, wheat starch and water. There are very fine, string-like noodles, sometimes called rice vermicelli, which are often broken up for use in soups, or deep-fried which causes them to puff up dramatically. Rice sticks are flat noodles, sometimes only about the length of a chopstick. They are most often served in a broth or sauce. Somen are fine rice noodles from Japan, used mainly in soup.

Soba, brown in colour, are the best-known Japanese noodles. Made from buckwheat flour, they are quite substantial – like wholemeal pasta – and are often served with a dipping sauce.

Spring rolls and egg rolls are made using slightly opaque, paper-thin wrappers. Chinese spring roll wrappers are made from wheat flour; the Vietnamese version is based on rice flour. Spring roll and rice paper wrappers may be bought frozen (thaw before use) or you can buy the prepared spring rolls. Try baking them on non-stick baking trays instead of deep-frying, for a low-fat result.

Wheat noodles, made from wheat flour and often enriched with egg, can be bought fresh or dried, in a wide variety of widths, flat or round. They need very little cooking – often just soaking. The Japanese have their own version of Chinese-style wheat noodles, called ramen.

Wonton wrappers, pale yellow in colour, are made from a wheat flour and egg dough. The small square or round wrappers are available fresh or frozen, and can be used to make wontons as well as other dumplings such as dim sum or

---

Health bites

Oriental noodles are every bit as nutritious as other types of pasta, with specific benefits depending on the grain from which they are made. Many non-wheat noodles are gluten-free, which makes them a suitable starchy food for people intolerant of wheat or gluten, also found in barley and rye.

Remember that crispy noodles, popular in fast-food and take-away restaurants, absorb a lot of oil or animal fat during deep-frying, so enjoy them now and again rather than every day.

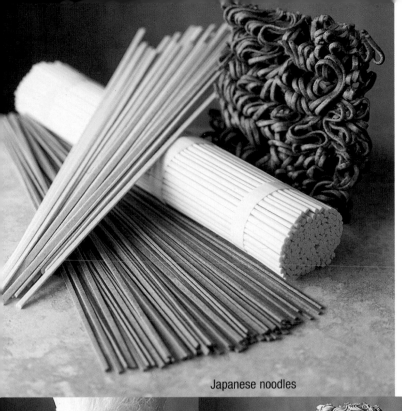

Japanese noodles

Preparing and cooking

Most Oriental noodles are either soaked or cooked in boiling water before being added to soups, vegetable dishes or stir-fries. They can also be served with a sauce, as for Italian-style pasta, or as a side dish. Noodle stir-fries, with lots of fresh vegetables and a moderate amount of lean meat, fish, shellfish, tofu or beans, make extremely well-balanced meals.

Alternative grains for making pasta

There is a wide range of Italian-style pasta made from grains other than wheat, including corn, barley, rice, soya-bean flour and vegetables. Combinations such as rice and soya-bean flours provide a good source of vegetarian protein and fibre. Many of these products are found in large supermarkets and healthfood shops as well as from mail-order suppliers.

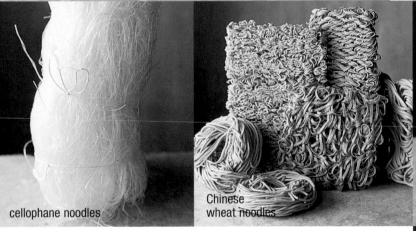

cellophane noodles

Chinese wheat noodles

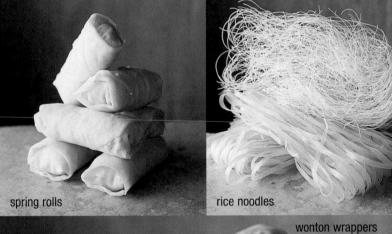

spring rolls

rice noodles

wonton wrappers

pot-stickers. Once filled, the dumplings can be fried, boiled or steamed (a good low-fat choice), or used in soup. Traditional wonton stuffings include pork, prawns and mushrooms.

Buying and storing Oriental noodles

Fresh noodles can be stored in their unopened packet in the fridge for up to 3 days. They can also be frozen: open freeze them on a tray and pack in freezer boxes or bags when hard, so that small quantities can be cooked from frozen as required. Check 'use by' dates on the packets before buying.

Dried noodles should be stored as for other types of dried pasta. Once opened, store in an airtight container. Check 'best before' dates before buying.

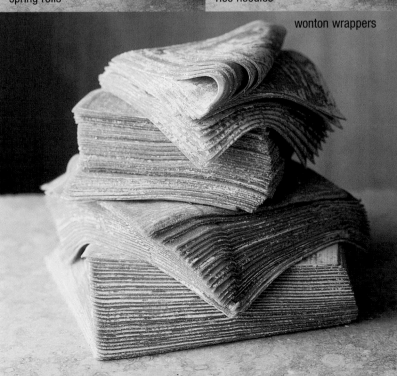

Buying and cooking pasta

Dried pasta has a long shelf-life, and fresh pasta is the perfect stand-by in the freezer. For hassle-free healthy eating, put pasta on your shopping list.

Buying tips
- Often the tastiest fresh pasta and the largest range of unusual dried shapes are available from Italian food shops, so if you have one near you, check it out.
- Check the 'best before' dates on packs of dried pasta. Unlike 'use by' dates on highly perishable food, it is not illegal to sell goods that are older than the 'best before' dates. However, the quality will probably have deteriorated. Try to buy from a store with a good turnover of stock.
- For everyday or frequent eating, look for stuffed pasta shapes that are lowest in fat. The best-quality fillings are those containing mainly the key ingredient; for example, on a packet of ricotta and spinach ravioli, the ricotta and spinach should be the first two ingredients listed. A long list of other ingredients, such as modified starches, water or other 'fillers' and additives, tends to indicate that the filling contains less of the main ingredient(s).
- Examine the pasta in the pack closely and choose shapes that look as though they have a generous amount of filling.
- As a general guide, bought fresh pasta with a low-fat filling, such as mushroom and garlic, will contain not more than 5 g fat per 100 g (3½ oz). This information is given on the nutritional labelling panel on the packet.
- Long-life products, such as vacuum-packed stuffed pasta shapes, tend to have a less pleasing flavour than fresh pasta.

Storing pasta
After opening, store any unused dried pasta in an airtight container. Cut the 'best before' date off the packet and put it in the container for future reference. Keep pasta in a cool, dry place.

Store fresh pasta in the fridge. Once a packet is opened, use it within 2 days, or freeze any unused pasta in freezer bags or an airtight container; it will keep for up to 8 months. If the

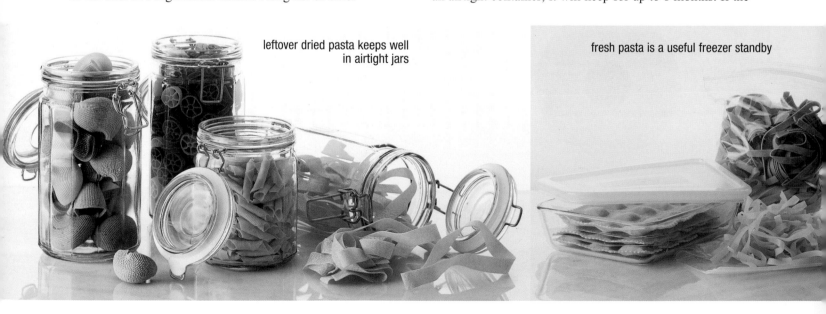

leftover dried pasta keeps well in airtight jars

fresh pasta is a useful freezer standby

pasta pieces are large, open freeze them on a tray covered with cling film, then transfer them to a freezer bag or container once they are hard. This keeps pieces separate, so that the required number can be removed very easily. Cook pasta from frozen for about 3 minutes.

Cooking pasta

- Use a large pan so that the pasta can move freely in the boiling water.
- Bring the pan of water to the boil, allowing 1 litre (1¾ pints) water to every 100 g (3½ oz) pasta.
- If using salt, add it to the water before adding the pasta. It is not necessary to add oil to the water, except for lasagne sheets which are more likely to stick together.
- Add the pasta to the boiling water. Cover the pan until the water comes back to the boil, then remove the lid. Stir once to prevent the pasta from sticking together.
- Once the pasta is cooked, drain in a large colander. If serving the pasta hot, do not rinse as this washes off the starch that gives taste and texture. Occasionally, pasta is rinsed before use in salads or baked dishes, such as lasagne.
- Save some cooking water either to dress pasta or to thin sauces.

The question of salt

Many cooks recommend adding 1 tsp coarse sea salt to every 1 litre (1¾ pints) water when cooking pasta. However, as pasta already contains salt, and reducing salt intake is often a step towards improving the diet, you may wish to use less. If you gradually reduce the amount of salt used in your cooking and eating, you will give your palate time to adjust to less salty food.

Cooking times

Check and follow packet instructions as cooking times vary, particularly for Oriental noodles and specialist non-wheat pasta. Typically, Italian-style dried white and coloured pasta takes 8–12 minutes to cook and wholemeal pasta 12–15 minutes, depending on size and thickness. The pasta is ready when it is al dente – tender but still firm, offering some resistance when bitten. At this stage, some cooks add a cup of cold water before draining to halt the cooking.

Fresh pasta, bought or home-made, cooks very quickly – usually in 3–5 minutes, although some types are cooked in just 1 minute.

Pasta portions

As a general guide, for a pasta dish with a light dressing or sauce, allow 50 g (1¾ oz) dried pasta and 100 g (3½ oz) fresh pasta per person for a light meal or starter, and 85 g (3 oz) dried or 115–150 g (4–5 oz) fresh pasta for a main course. Portions can vary considerably according to the quantities of other ingredients used, especially when lots of satisfying vegetables are served, and according to appetite.

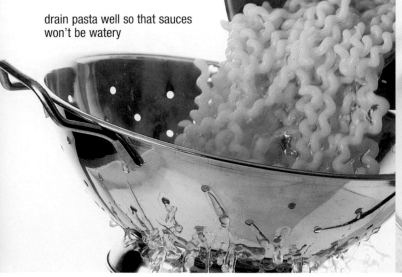

drain pasta well so that sauces won't be watery

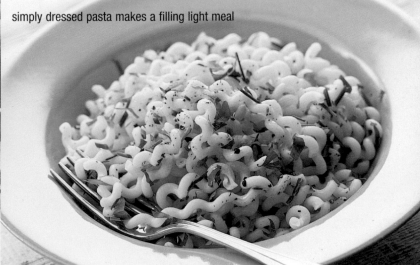

simply dressed pasta makes a filling light meal

Making pasta and its sauces

Making your own pasta allows you to vary the ingredients and flavours. And with freshly made sauce you can create a meal to suit any special occasion.

Home-made pasta

Pasta is surprisingly simple to make, and once you get the hang of handling the dough, you will be able to experiment with an enormous number of fillings and accompaniments. Making filled pasta also means that you can benefit from the freshest ingredients to boost nutrients and enjoyment.

All you need are a few standard kitchen items – rolling pin, sharp knife and metal pastry cutters. A pastry wheel is useful. If you decide to make pasta regularly, and in quantity, it is worth investing in a pasta machine. Hand-operated machines are very successful, but there are also electric pasta makers and attachments for food processors. Follow the manufacturer's instructions for using a machine.

Ingredients

Flour Some supermarkets and many Italian specialist shops sell special flour for making pasta. The flour may be 100% durum wheat semolina, such as an authentic Italian flour called doppio zero (double zero), which appears on the bag as 00 grade. Other flour sold for making pasta may be a combination of durum wheat semolina and ordinary flour.

Alternatively, use unbleached strong plain flour or plain wholemeal flour. A mixture of unbleached strong plain flour and buckwheat or rice flour can also be used. A small portion of soya flour will boost the protein content of the pasta.

Eggs Although much commercial pasta is made with just flour and water, most home-made pasta includes eggs. Standard medium eggs are ideal.

Oil Olive oil is authentic. Since the amount used is small, it will not have a great impact on the fat content of a dish.

Salt Fine sea salt offers the best flavour.

Tips for success

● Flour can vary in absorbency and egg sizes may differ, so results may vary on different occasions even with the same recipe. Weather and humidity also affect the dough.
● Sprinkle strands of freshly cut pasta liberally with semolina or flour to prevent them from sticking together.
● If you do not want to cook the dough immediately, you can freeze it, then cook it from frozen.

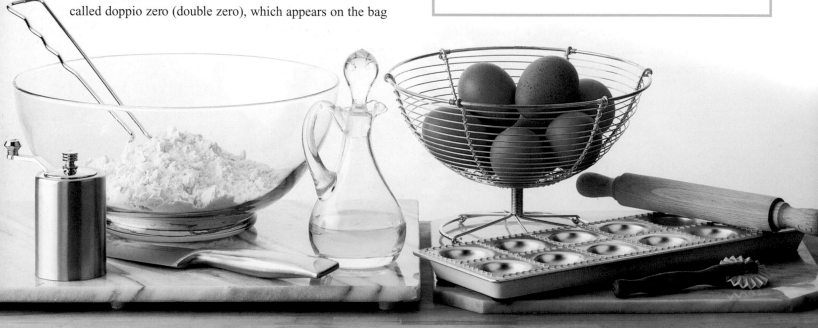

Fresh pasta

Makes about 675 g (1½ lb)
450 g (1 lb) strong plain flour
pinch of salt
4 eggs, beaten
1 tbsp extra virgin olive oil

Preparation time: 45 minutes, plus 30 minutes resting

1 Sift the flour onto a clean work surface or into a large mixing bowl. Make a well in the centre and add the salt, eggs and oil.

2 Using your hands, gradually mix the flour into the eggs and oil, until the mixture begins to form a firm dough. If necessary, add a few drops of water.

3 Knead the dough for about 10 minutes or until it is smooth and elastic. The dough should still be firm. Add a little extra flour if the dough becomes sticky.

4 Wrap the dough tightly in a polythene bag or with cling film and set it aside to rest for 30 minutes before rolling and cutting. Do not place in the fridge.

5 Cut the dough into quarters, as smaller portions are easier to manage. Roll out the dough very thinly on an unfloured surface, turning it over and around occasionally to prevent it from sticking, then cut it into the chosen shapes such as lasagne, cannelloni or noodles.

6 Noodles and unfilled pasta may be cooked immediately or allowed to dry for up to 30 minutes before cooking. It is a good idea to leave pasta to dry on clean tea-towels if it is slightly sticky. Hang noodles over a pasta drying rack, or lightly flour them and coil into nests.

Using a food processor

Check the manufacturer's instructions for kneading firm doughs. It is best to use the dough blade attachment. Knead it in the machine for 5–10 minutes.

Cutting simple shapes

Lasagne Cut neat rectangles or squares 7.5–10 cm (3–4 in) wide, or to fit the baking dish.

Cannelloni Instead of buying tubes, cut rectangles or squares and roll them around the filling – make your cannelloni small or chunky and long, as you wish.

Noodles Flour the rolled-out dough, fold it over several times or roll it loosely, and then cut it across into slices. Thin slices give fine noodles; thick slices make wide noodles. Experiment with all widths, from skewer-fine to noodles as wide as a ruler. Carefully unravel the noodles with your fingers.

Squares and diamonds Cut strips, then, without moving them, cut across to make squares or diamond shapes (cut at an angle to make the slanting sides).

Storing freshly made pasta

Leave the pasta to dry for 30 minutes to prevent the pieces from sticking together, then put in a polythene bag or covered container in the fridge. Use within 24 hours. To freeze the pasta for longer storage, spread the pasta out on a tray covered with cling film and open freeze until firm, then pack in polythene bags.

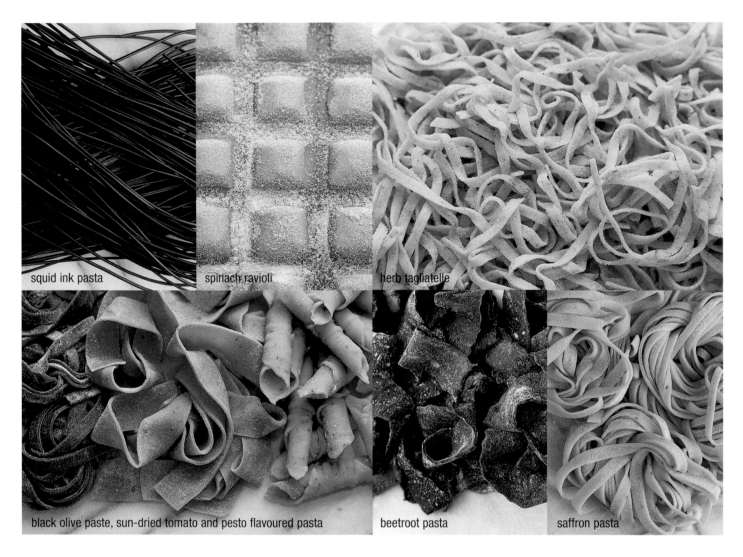

squid ink pasta

spinach ravioli

herb tagliatelle

black olive paste, sun-dried tomato and pesto flavoured pasta

beetroot pasta

saffron pasta

Flavouring pasta dough

Pasta can be coloured and flavoured with a wide variety of vegetable purées and pastes, such as tomato (and sun-dried versions), spinach, beetroot and carrot. Squid ink (available in packets from specialist outlets) can turn pasta dramatically black. Fresh and dried herbs, saffron, ground peppercorns, black olive paste, garlic, wholegrain mustard and spices such as cumin and curry powder can also be added to make interesting pasta.

Spinach Wash 225 g (8 oz) fresh spinach and place in a large saucepan. Cover and cook over a high heat, shaking the pan, for about 3 minutes. (The water clinging to the leaves is sufficient moisture in which to cook the spinach.) Drain well in a sieve, then chop finely or purée in a blender or food processor. Press out all excess water in a sieve, to give a thick paste. Use only 2 eggs for the dough. Add the spinach with the eggs and oil, then mix in the flour as in the basic recipe.

Beetroot Purée 1–2 small cooked beetroot. Use only 3 eggs for the pasta dough, and add the beetroot purée with the eggs.

Herbs Add a handful of finely chopped fresh herbs when mixing in the flour. Flat-leaf parsley, coriander, basil, oregano, marjoram and thyme are all delicious.

Saffron Add 1 tsp powdered saffron or a pinch of saffron threads infused in 1 tbsp boiling water.

Pesto sauce, sun-dried tomato paste or black olive paste Omit the oil and add 2 tbsp of the chosen sauce or paste.

Pasta saucery

The secret of pasta's versatility is its compatability with almost any other ingredient. From extravagant seafood to humble herbs and vegetables, sauces served with pasta can reflect all cooking styles. With only a few basic ingredients, a dressing can be conjured up to turn pasta into a delicious meal for every occasion.

In Italy, sauces for pasta were traditionally a celebration of regional produce, both the luxurious and common-or-garden. From truffles and fabulous wild fungi in the north, and aromatic pesto in Genoa, to fish and seafood in the south, and glowing tomatoes in Naples, there are plenty of authentic options. Today, pasta sauces are a vibrant reflection of the wide variety of fresh ingredients available from all over the world. With Mediterranean vegetables matched by spices and flavourings from the Orient, modern pasta sauces are a fashionable fusion food.

A little sauce with a positive zing
The pasta should definitely be the main attraction. The ideal amount of sauce (to Italians and healthy eaters) is enough to coat the pasta lightly without leaving a covering or pool on the plate when the pasta has been eaten.

Sauces based mainly on vegetables, with moderate amounts of lean meat, fish or shellfish, and fresh herbs, positively zing with flavour, colour and good nutrition. The vegetables pack a powerful antioxidant punch from their vitamins and minerals to boost and complement the energy-giving pasta.

Which sauce for which pasta?
There are no hard and fast rules – pasta is so good because it is so versatile – but some shapes have an affinity for certain types of sauce.
• Long thin strands of pasta go well with simple sauces, such as pesto, or can be dressed simply with a little butter or oil to keep the strands separate.
• Thicker strands of pasta and ribbon noodles go well with a meat, cheese or creamy sauce or a smooth tomato sauce.
• Tubular pasta, twists, shells and similar shapes go well with chunkier vegetable sauces.

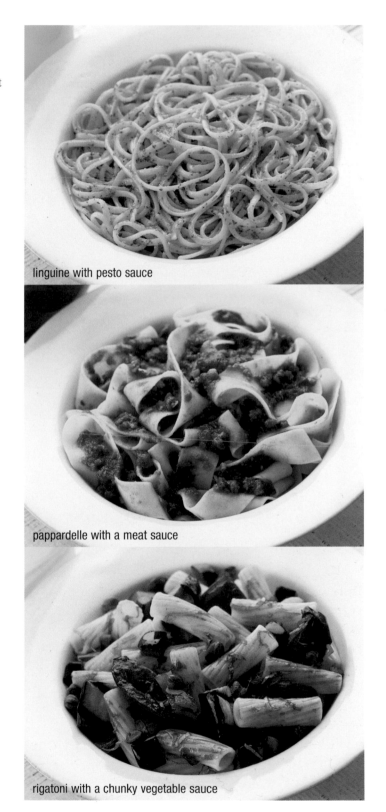

linguine with pesto sauce

pappardelle with a meat sauce

rigatoni with a chunky vegetable sauce

Fresh tomato sauce

There are many versions of this delicious, indispensable sauce. This one is a basic recipe for fresh tomatoes. Vine-ripened or full-flavoured summer tomatoes are best, but when they are not available, the sauce can be made with canned tomatoes.

Makes about 600 ml (1 pint), to serve 4

2 tbsp extra virgin olive oil

1 large onion, finely chopped

1 garlic clove, chopped

1 kg (2¼ lb) tomatoes, skinned, seeded and chopped

150 ml (5 fl oz) red wine or vegetable stock

2 tbsp chopped fresh basil or 1 tsp dried basil

pinch of sugar

salt and pepper

To serve (optional)

8–10 sprigs of fresh basil, shredded

4 tbsp freshly grated Parmesan cheese or 4 heaped tbsp
    Parmesan cheese shavings

Preparation time: 10 minutes
Cooking time: 25–35 minutes

1 Heat the oil in a large saucepan. Add the onion and garlic, and cook gently, stirring occasionally, for 5 minutes or until softened but not browned.

2 Add the tomatoes, wine or stock and basil. Cook over a moderate heat for 20–30 minutes or until the sauce is thick.

3 Purée the sauce in a blender or food processor until smooth, then rub it through a fine sieve if a particularly smooth result is required.

4 Add the sugar to balance the acidity of the tomatoes. Stir in salt and pepper to taste and reheat the sauce.

5 Use the sauce as required. Or pour it over freshly cooked pasta, toss well and top with shredded basil and freshly grated or shaved Parmesan cheese.

Some more ideas

• At the beginning of the tomato season, you can boost the flavour of the sauce by adding 1 tbsp tomato purée or sun-dried tomato paste.

• Use 2 cans chopped tomatoes, about 400 g each, with the juice, instead of fresh tomatoes.

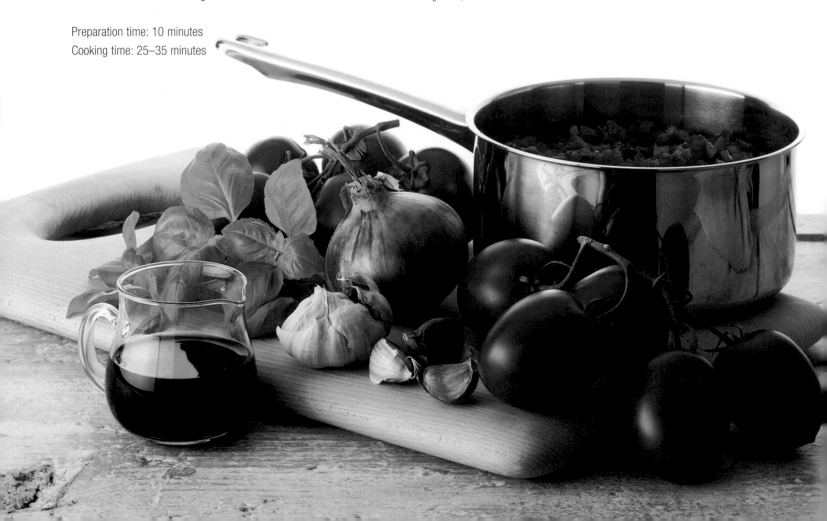

Pesto sauce

A little home-made pesto sauce goes a long way as it is packed with flavour. Toss this sauce into piping-hot pasta just before eating. Store any leftover pesto in a screwtop jar in the fridge (cover the surface of the pesto with a little extra oil).

Makes 150 ml (5 fl oz), to serve 4

2 garlic cloves
30 g (1 oz) pine nuts
30 g (1 oz) Parmesan cheese, freshly grated
20 g (¾ oz) fresh basil sprigs
5 tbsp extra virgin olive oil

Preparation time: 10 minutes

1 Place the peeled garlic in a food processor or herb chopper. Add the pine nuts and Parmesan, and process until the ingredients are finely chopped and thoroughly combined.

2 Add the basil, including all the soft stalks. (If the basil is picked from a mature plant with tough stalks, discard these before weighing the sprigs.) Process until the basil is chopped and the mixture begins to clump together.

3 Add the olive oil and process until combined. The sauce should have a fine, slightly grainy texture.

Garlic and herb dressing

Pasta is superb with a simple dressing of garlic, herbs and good olive oil. The secret is to warm the garlic with bay leaves in the oil, to mellow the garlic flavour slightly. Then the dressing should be left to stand for 30 minutes, or longer if possible, so that the flavour of the garlic can infuse the oil.

Serves 4

2 fresh bay leaves
4 garlic cloves, thinly sliced
5 tbsp extra virgin olive oil
grated zest of 1 lemon
4 tbsp snipped fresh chives
4 tbsp chopped fresh parsley
4 tbsp chopped fresh tarragon, sage, marjoram or dill,
    or a mixture of fresh herbs

Preparation time: 10 minutes, plus at least 30 minutes infusing

1 Crease the bay leaves in half and place them in a small saucepan with the garlic. Add about 1 tbsp olive oil and heat gently for 2 minutes or until the oil just begins to sizzle around the garlic. Remove from the heat.

2 Stir in the lemon zest, then pour in the remaining oil. Set aside to infuse for at least 30 minutes.

3 Remove the bay leaves and add the chopped herbs. Toss the dressing into hot pasta and serve.

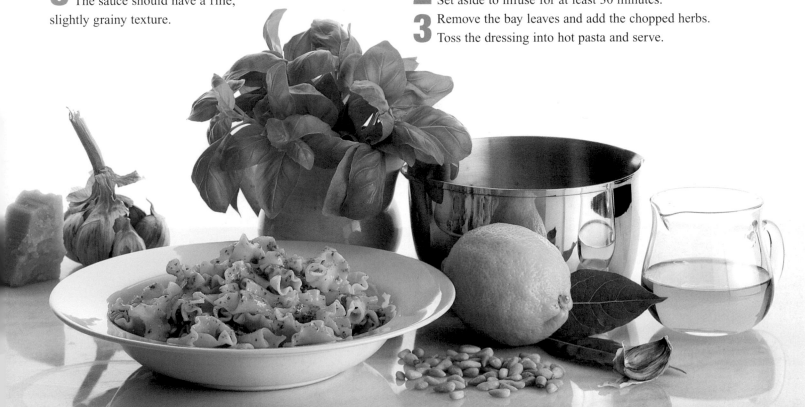

Béchamel sauce

This classic white sauce is used in a wide variety of dishes. Many flavouring ingredients can be added to make a number of different sauces.

Makes about 600 ml (1 pint), to serve 4

600 ml (1 pint) semi-skimmed milk
1 onion or 2 shallots, halved
1 bay leaf
6 black peppercorns
pinch of grated nutmeg or 1 blade of mace
55 g (2 oz) butter
55 g (2 oz) plain flour
salt and pepper

Preparation time: 5 minutes, plus 10 minutes infusing
Cooking time: 5 minutes

1 Pour the milk into a heavy-based saucepan and add the onion or shallots, bay leaf, peppercorns and nutmeg or mace. Bring just to the boil over a moderate heat, then remove from the heat, cover and set aside to infuse for 10 minutes. Strain the flavoured milk into a jug.

2 Melt the butter in the rinsed-out pan. Stir in the flour and cook gently, stirring occasionally, for 1 minute. Do not allow the flour to brown.

3 Remove the pan from the heat and gradually pour in the milk, stirring or whisking constantly. Return the pan to the heat and bring to the boil, still stirring or whisking.

4 Reduce the heat and simmer the sauce gently for 2 minutes, stirring occasionally, until it is smooth and thick.

5 Taste and add salt and pepper. Serve or use immediately.

Some more ideas

● For a cheese sauce, stir in 55 g (2 oz) grated mature Cheddar, Gruyère or Parmesan cheese and 1 tsp Dijon mustard just before serving.

● For an onion sauce, do not add the onion or shallots when infusing the milk. Finely chop 2 onions and cook in the butter over a low heat for 10 minutes or until softened but not browned, then stir in the flour. Purée the finished sauce in a blender or food processor if a smooth result is required.

● For a mushroom sauce, slice 300 g (10½ oz) button mushrooms and cook in the butter for 5 minutes before stirring in the flour.

● A one-stage béchamel sauce is quick, and it can be a good way of making a lower-fat sauce as the butter can be reduced or omitted. Pour the milk into a heavy-based saucepan and gradually whisk in the flour, sprinkling it lightly over the milk as you whisk. Slice the onion or shallots and add with all the remaining ingredients, including the butter, if using. Whisk the sauce over a moderate heat until it comes to the boil and thickens, then reduce the heat and simmer for 2 minutes. Strain the sauce, or use a draining spoon to remove the flavouring ingredients, and add seasoning to taste.

● For a cornflour-thickened béchamel, omit the butter and flour, and mix 4 tbsp cornflour to a smooth paste with a little of the milk. Infuse the remaining milk as above. Strain and heat to boiling point, then pour a little into the cornflour mixture, stirring. Return this to the milk in the saucepan. Bring to the boil, stirring until the sauce thickens, and simmer for 2 minutes.

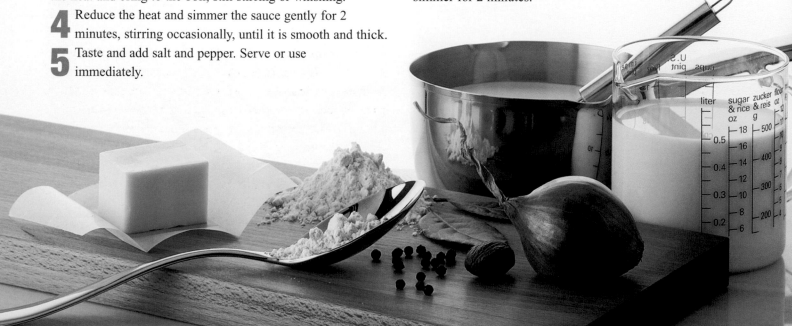

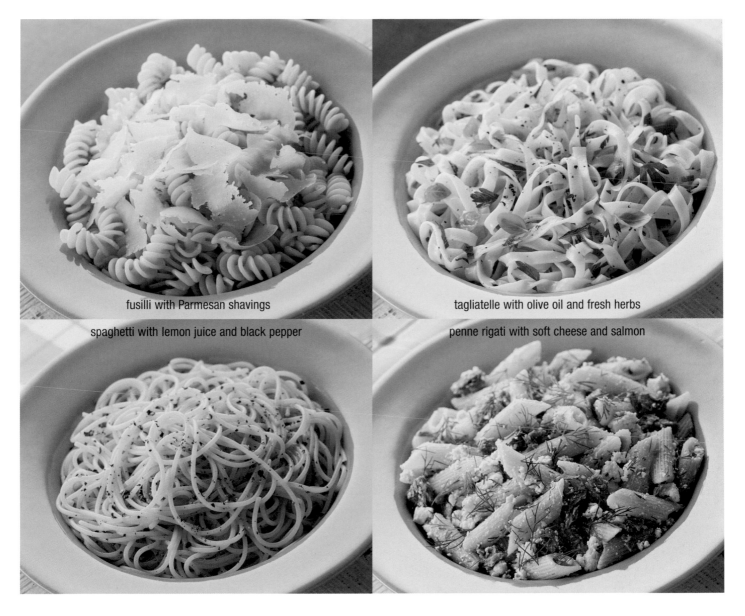

fusilli with Parmesan shavings

tagliatelle with olive oil and fresh herbs

spaghetti with lemon juice and black pepper

penne rigati with soft cheese and salmon

Simple and healthy partners for pasta

• Freshly grated or shaved good-quality Parmesan cheese (Parmigiano-Reggiano) is the traditional accompaniment for pasta served with vegetable or meat sauces (cheese does not always go well with fish or shellfish). Parmesan has a lot of flavour, so a little goes a long way, which means it does not over-burden the dish with fat. Pecorino is another sharp and salty cheese that is grated for sprinkling over pasta. Ewe's milk versions of pecorino are particularly useful for people who cannot tolerate cow's milk products.

• Finely chopped or torn fresh herbs, such as basil, parsley, flat-leaf parsley, coriander, chervil, sorrel, oregano, marjoram or thyme, are delicious tossed into pasta dressed with a little olive oil, melted butter or lemon juice and black pepper.
• Lemon juice and black pepper alone make a refreshing and very low-fat dressing for pasta. Add a little freshly grated lemon zest for extra zing.
• Reduced-fat soft white cheese or fromage frais, mixed with flaked poached or canned salmon or chopped fresh herbs, provides a lot of flavour without too much fat.

Penne primavera

This classic Italian dish is intended to make the very most of young spring produce, freshly picked from the vegetable plot. With today's choice of vegetables in supermarkets, the selection can be varied for year-round meals, and the recipe can also be made as a 'storecupboard supper' with good-quality frozen vegetables.

Serves 4

340 g (12 oz) penne or other pasta shapes

170 g (6 oz) young asparagus

170 g (6 oz) green beans, trimmed and
    cut into 3 cm (1¼ in) lengths

170 g (6 oz) shelled fresh peas

1 tbsp extra virgin olive oil

1 onion, chopped

1 garlic clove, chopped

85 g (3 oz) pancetta, chopped

115 g (4 oz) button mushrooms, chopped

1 tbsp plain flour

240 ml (8 fl oz) dry white wine

4 tbsp single cream

2 tbsp chopped mixed fresh herbs,
    such as parsley and thyme

salt and pepper

Preparation time: 15 minutes
Cooking time: 15 minutes

Each serving provides

kcal 560, protein 20 g, fat 17 g (of which saturated fat 6 g), carbohydrate 77 g (of which sugars 5.5 g), fibre 7 g

✓✓✓	C
✓✓	B₁, folate, niacin, copper, iron
✓	A, potassium, selenium

1 Cook the pasta in boiling water for 10–12 minutes, or according to the packet instructions, until al dente. Drain well.

2 While the pasta is cooking, cut the asparagus into 3.5 cm (1½ in) lengths, keeping the tips separate. Drop the pieces of asparagus stalk, the green beans and peas into a saucepan of boiling water. Bring back to the boil and cook for 5 minutes. Add the asparagus tips and cook for a further 2 minutes. Drain thoroughly.

3 Heat the oil in a saucepan. Add the onion and cook for 3–4 minutes or until softened. Add the garlic, pancetta and mushrooms, and continue to cook, stirring occasionally, for a further 2 minutes.

4 Stir in the flour, then gradually pour in the wine and bring to the boil, stirring. Simmer until the sauce is thickened. Stir in the cream and herbs with seasoning to taste. Add the vegetables to the sauce and heat gently for 1–2 minutes, without boiling.

5 Divide the pasta among 4 serving bowls and spoon the sauce over the top. Serve immediately.

Some more ideas

• For a vegetarian version, omit the pancetta and add 170 g (6 oz) shelled young broad beans, cooking them with the asparagus stalks and the green beans. Once drained, the skins may be slipped off the broad beans, if preferred. Add 4 shredded fresh sage leaves with the parsley and thyme, or try tarragon for a slightly aniseed flavour.

• Omit the pancetta and instead serve sprinkled with freshly grated Parmesan cheese – about 45 g (1½ oz) in total for the 4 portions.

• Use frozen peas instead of fresh, adding them with the asparagus tips.

Plus points

• Asparagus is a good source of many of the B vitamins, especially folate, which is important during the early stages of pregnancy to help to prevent birth defects such as spina bifida.

• Peas provide good amounts of the B vitamins B₁, niacin and B₆. They also provide dietary fibre, particularly the soluble variety, some folate and vitamin C.

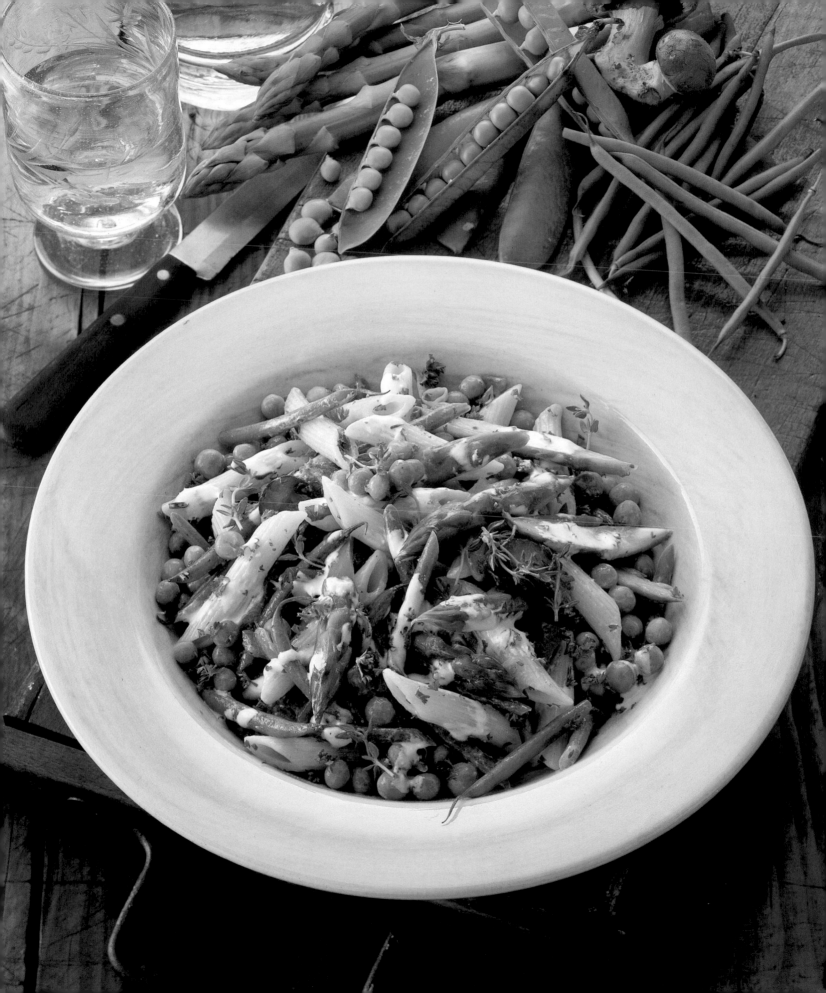

Rustic grilled vegetable and rigatoni salad

Grilled vegetables are delicious with chunky pasta in a tangy dressing. Serve this salad as a light lunch or offer it as an accompaniment for grilled poultry or meat, when it will serve 6 or 8.

Serves 4

200 g (7 oz) rigatoni
1 large red pepper, seeded and halved
125 g (4½ oz) tomatoes, cut into wedges
1 aubergine, trimmed and sliced lengthways
2 tbsp balsamic vinegar or lemon juice
3 tbsp extra virgin olive oil
2 tbsp shredded fresh basil
1 tbsp chopped capers
1 large garlic clove, crushed (optional)
30 g (1 oz) Parmesan cheese, freshly grated
　　salt and pepper

Preparation time: 35 minutes, plus cooling
　　and 30 minutes marinating

Each serving provides

kcal 310, protein 10 g, fat 12 g (of which
saturated fat 3 g), carbohydrate 42 g (of
which sugars 5.5 g), fibre 3 g

✓✓	A, C
✓	niacin, calcium, copper, potassium

1 Cook the rigatoni in boiling water for 10–12 minutes, or according to the packet instructions, until al dente. Drain and rinse under cold running water, then drain thoroughly and set aside to cool.

2 Preheat the grill to high. Grill the pepper halves, skin side up, for 5–10 minutes or until blistered and blackened. Place in a polythene bag, then leave until cool enough to handle.

3 Grill the tomatoes and aubergine for about 5 minutes or until slightly charred. Turn the vegetables so that they cook evenly, and remove the pieces as they are ready. Place the tomato wedges in a large salad bowl. Set the aubergine slices aside on a plate to cool slightly.

4 Cut the aubergine slices into 2.5 cm (1 in) strips and add to the tomatoes. Peel the peppers and cut them into 2.5 cm (1 in) strips, then add to the salad bowl. Mix in the pasta.

5 In a small bowl, mix the balsamic vinegar or lemon juice with the olive oil, basil, capers, garlic, if using, and Parmesan cheese. Lightly toss this dressing into the salad. Season to taste. Set the salad aside to marinate for about 30 minutes so that the flavours can mingle before serving.

Some more ideas

• For a hearty vegetarian main course salad, stir in 1 can cannellini or red kidney beans, about 400 g, well drained.

• Grilled courgettes and asparagus can be added to the salad. Slice the courgettes lengthways. Grill alongside the aubergine and tomatoes.

• Replace the aubergine with well-drained, bottled char-grilled artichokes.

Plus points

• Aubergines are a useful vegetable for making satisfying meals without a high calorie content. They contain just 15 kcal per 100 g (3½ oz).

• Grilling or baking is a healthy cooking method for vegetables like aubergines, which can absorb large amounts of fat when they are fried.

• Adding a little Parmesan cheese to pasta dishes contributes useful calcium as well as a wonderful flavour.

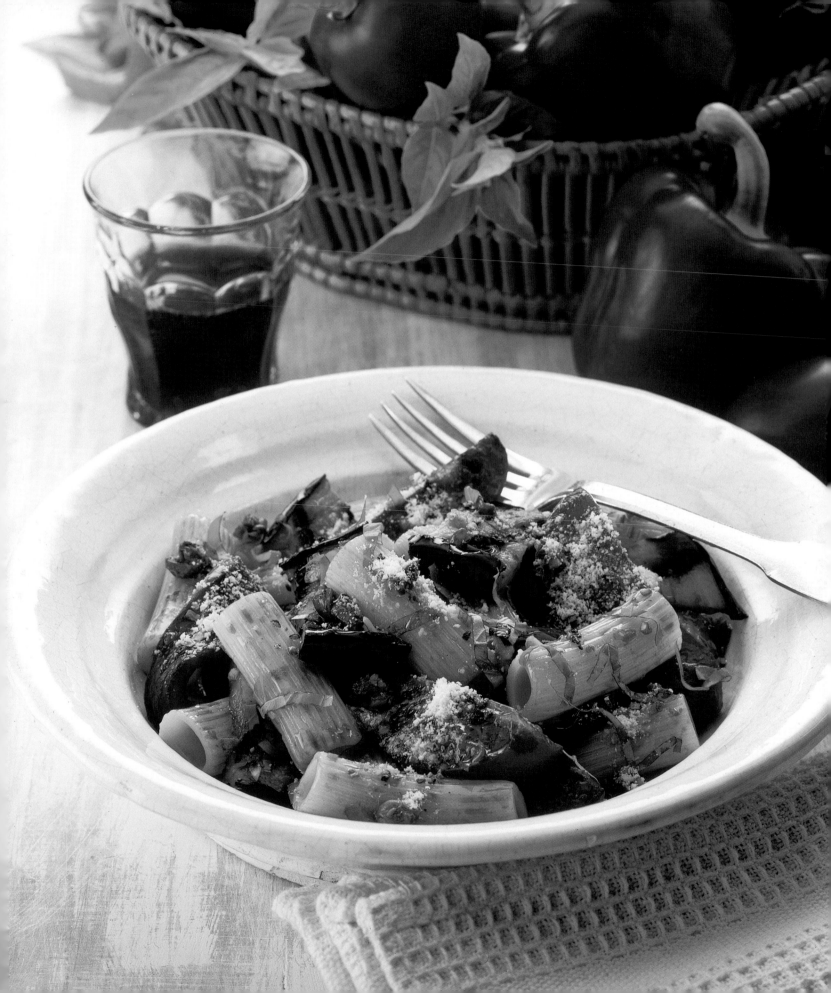

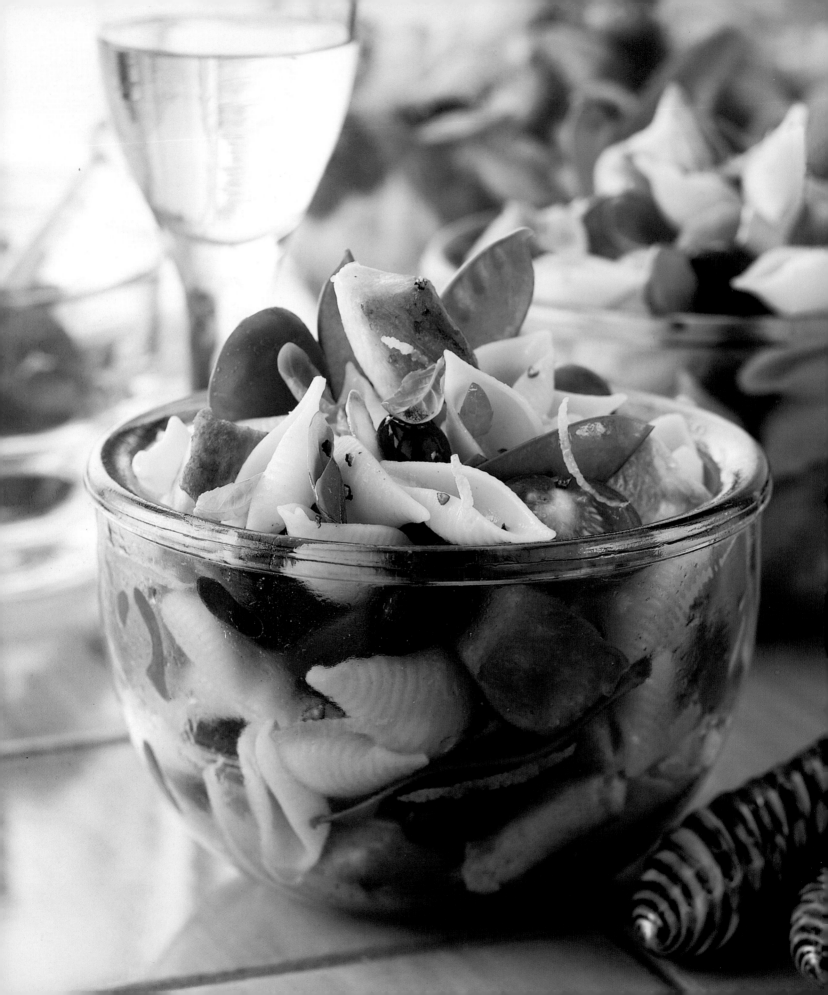

Pasta and chicken salad with basil

Tempt your family with this healthy and filling pasta salad. Quick to prepare, it makes an ideal midweek supper and won't spoil if someone is late home. Tossing the pasta with lemon juice and white wine not only adds flavour but also means that the quantity of oil can be reduced, so saving on fat.

Serves 4

300 g (10½ oz) pasta quills or shells

100 g (3½ oz) mange-tout

3 tbsp extra virgin olive oil

finely shredded zest and juice of 1 lemon

4 tbsp dry white wine

400 g (14 oz) skinless boneless chicken breasts (fillets), cut into bite-sized chunks

2 garlic cloves, thinly sliced

200 g (7 oz) baby plum tomatoes, halved, or 3 plum tomatoes, each cut into 6 wedges

50 g (1¾ oz) stoned black olives

1 small bunch of fresh basil, about 20 g (¾ oz)

salt and pepper

Preparation time: 15 minutes
Cooking time: 15 minutes

Each serving provides

kcal 470, protein 34 g, fat 12 g (of which saturated fat 2 g), carbohydrate 60 g (of which sugars 4 g), fibre 4 g

✓✓   B₁, B₆, C, niacin, copper, iron, selenium

✓   A, B₂, E, folate, potassium, zinc

1 Drop the pasta into a large saucepan of boiling water. When the water returns to the boil, cook for 10–12 minutes, or according to the packet instructions, until al dente. Add the mange-tout for the final minute of cooking. Drain, rinse with cold water and drain again well.

2 Mix 2 tbsp of the oil with the lemon zest and juice and the wine in a large salad bowl. Season to taste. Add the pasta and mange-tout, and toss to coat with the dressing. Set aside to cool slightly.

3 Meanwhile, heat the remaining 1 tbsp of oil in a large frying pan. Add the chicken and garlic, and stir-fry over a high heat for 5–6 minutes or until the chicken is lightly browned and thoroughly cooked. Add to the pasta.

4 Scatter the tomatoes and olives over the top. Sprinkle with the basil leaves, tearing larger ones into pieces. Toss the salad together and serve while the chicken is still warm.

Some more ideas

• For a chicken and couscous salad, use 200 g (7 oz) couscous instead of the pasta. Pour 600 ml (1 pint) boiling water over the couscous and leave to soak for 5 minutes. Drain, then toss with the lemon zest and juice, oil and some seasoning (omit the wine). Stir-fry the strips of chicken, adding 250 g (9 oz) sliced courgettes for the last 2 minutes of cooking. Add to the couscous, together with the tomatoes and olives, and flat-leaf parsley instead of basil. Toss well and serve.

• Use leftover cooked chicken. Mix the cooked chicken with the pasta and mange-tout, and omit step 3. Either leave out the garlic or add 1 crushed garlic clove to the dressing in step 2.

Plus points

• The vitamin C provided by the freshly squeezed lemon juice and the tomatoes will aid the absorption of iron from the chicken.

• Pasta is an excellent source of starchy carbohydrate and it is low in fat. It also contains valuable vitamins, in particular the water-soluble B vitamins that we need to take in regularly.

Spaghetti with Brie and cherry tomatoes

Here is a colourful pasta dish full of fresh summery flavours. The asparagus and tomatoes are very lightly cooked before tossing with the hot pasta and cubes of Brie – the tomatoes gently burst and release their sweet juices, and the heat makes the cheese just start to melt.

Serves 4

400 g (14 oz) spaghetti

2 tbsp extra virgin olive oil

2 plump garlic cloves, finely chopped

170 g (6 oz) thin asparagus, cut into 5 cm (2 in) pieces

300 g (10½ oz) cherry tomatoes, halved

large handful of fresh basil leaves, roughly torn

170 g (6 oz) Brie cheese, cut into cubes

salt and pepper

Preparation and cooking time: 30 minutes

Each serving provides Ⓥ

kcal 553, protein 22 g, fat 19 g (of which saturated fat 8 g), carbohydrate 77 g (of which sugars 6 g), fibre 4 g

✓✓	A, C, folate, niacin, calcium, copper, zinc
✓	B₁, B₂, B₆, B₁₂, E, iron, potassium

1 Cook the pasta in a large pan of boiling water for 10–12 minutes, or according to the packet instructions, until al dente.

2 Meanwhile, heat the oil in a large frying pan, add the garlic and cook for about 30 seconds. Don't let it brown. Tip in the asparagus and add 4 tbsp of water. Cook over a moderate heat for 3–5 minutes, stirring frequently, until the asparagus is just tender and most of the water has evaporated.

3 Add the cherry tomatoes and basil, and cook for a further 2 minutes or until the tomatoes start to soften but still hold their shape. Season with salt and pepper to taste.

4 Drain the pasta in a colander, then pour it into a large serving bowl. Add the vegetable mixture and the Brie, and toss gently to mix. Serve hot, sprinkled with a grinding of pepper.

Some more ideas

• Replace the Brie with Camembert.

• For spaghetti with Brie, asparagus and fresh tomato salsa, cook the pasta as in the main recipe, adding the asparagus to the pan for the last 3 minutes of the cooking time. Meanwhile, finely chop 300 g (10½ oz) ripe tomatoes and mix with 1 finely chopped small red onion, 4 tbsp chopped parsley, 1 crushed garlic clove, 2 tbsp extra virgin olive oil, and salt and pepper to taste. Drain the pasta and asparagus, and tip them into a large serving bowl. Add the salsa and the cheese, and toss gently to mix.

• Make rigatoni with mozzarella and rocket. Replace the spaghetti with rigatoni (or penne), and the Brie with 150 g (5½ oz) mozzarella. Omit the asparagus and water, and increase the quantity of tomatoes to 500 g (1 lb 2 oz). In step 4, add 100 g (3½ oz) rocket with the mozzarella, tossing with the pasta just until the leaves wilt and the cheese begins to melt.

Plus points

• Cheese and tomatoes are a traditional combination, and together they provide protein and many essential vitamins and minerals.

• Brie is made from full-fat cow's milk, but because it has a high water content it contains less fat than hard, dense cheeses such as Cheddar.

• Basil, a member of the mint family, is believed to aid digestion and relieve the headaches that often occur with a cold.

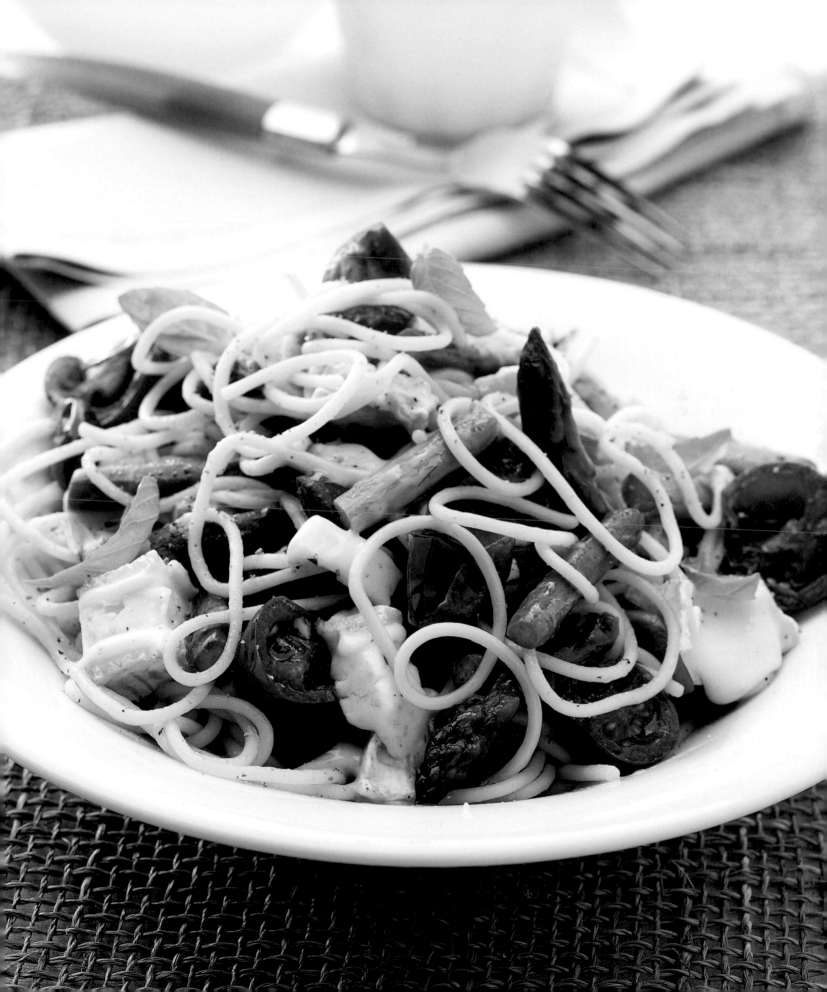

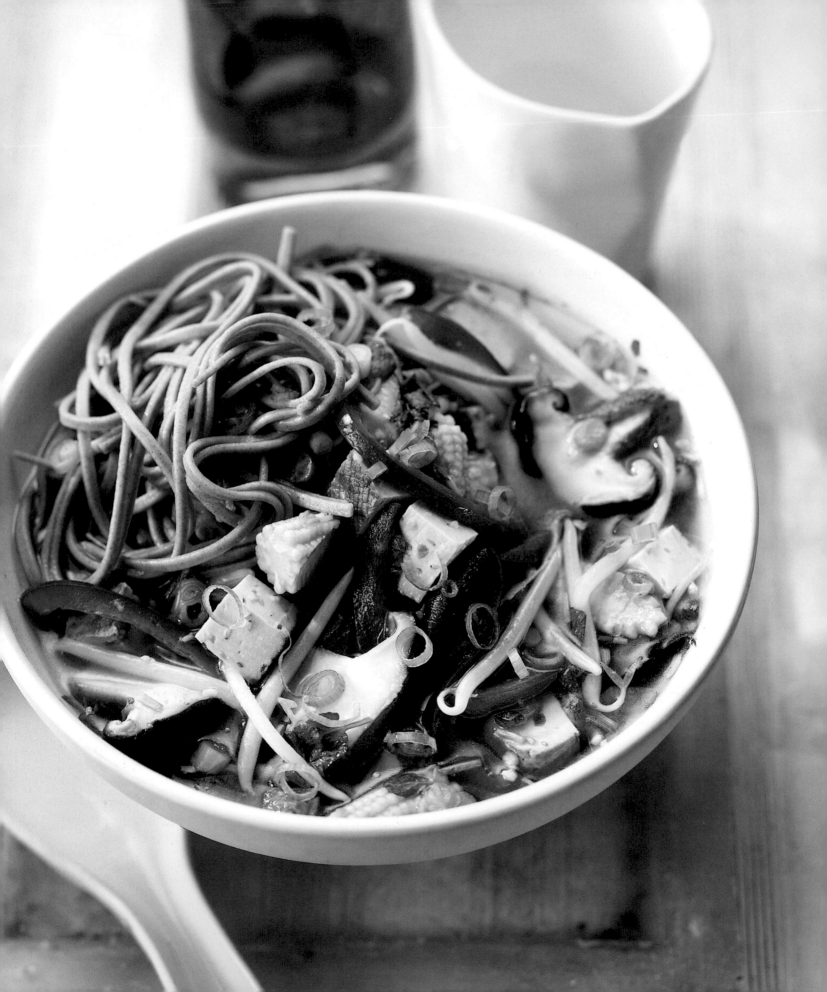

Japanese soup noodles with smoked tofu and bean sprouts

As interest in Oriental cuisines increases, supermarkets are stocking a wider variety of noodles. To make this tempting lunch dish, Japanese soba – hearty noodles made from buckwheat – are simmered in a soy and ginger stock with smoked tofu and an appetising mixture of vegetables.

Serves 4

150 g (5½ oz) soba (Japanese buckwheat noodles)

1 tbsp sunflower oil

1 tbsp finely grated fresh root ginger

2 garlic cloves, crushed

1 red pepper, seeded and thinly sliced

100 g (3½ oz) baby corn, sliced diagonally

100 g (3½ oz) shiitake mushrooms, sliced

1.7 litres (3 pints) vegetable stock

3 tbsp light soy sauce

3 tbsp medium dry sherry

2 spring onions, very thinly sliced

55 g (2 oz) watercress, roughly chopped

85 g (3 oz) bean sprouts

250 g (8½ oz) smoked tofu with almonds and sesame seeds, cubed

Preparation time: 15 minutes

Cooking time: 10 minutes

Each serving provides

kcal 346, protein 13 g, fat 13 g (of which saturated fat 2 g), carbohydrate 41 g (of which sugars 5 g), fibre 3 g

✓✓✓	A, C, E, calcium
✓✓	copper, iron
✓	B₁, B₆, folate, niacin, zinc

1 Bring a large pan of water to the boil, add the noodles and boil for 5 minutes or until softened. When they are ready, drain them well.

2 While the noodles are cooking, heat the oil in another large saucepan. Add the ginger and garlic, and cook, stirring frequently, for about 1 minute. Add the red pepper, baby corn and shiitake mushrooms, and cook for a further 3 minutes, stirring frequently, until the vegetables are softened.

3 Pour in the vegetable stock and add the soy sauce and sherry. Bring to the boil and simmer for 3 minutes. Stir in the spring onions, watercress, bean sprouts and tofu, and cook for about 1 minute more or until the bean sprouts soften slightly.

4 Divide the noodles among 4 large serving bowls. Ladle the vegetables and soup on top and serve immediately.

Another idea

● To make scented Thai noodles with prawns and lemongrass, cook 150 g (5½ oz) cellophane noodles in boiling water for about 3 minutes or until softened. Meanwhile, stir-fry 1 tbsp grated fresh root ginger, 1 tbsp finely chopped lemongrass and 2 crushed garlic cloves in 1 tbsp sunflower oil for 1 minute. Add 1 seeded and sliced red pepper and 100 g (3½ oz) sugarsnap peas, and cook for a further 3 minutes. Pour in 1.7 litres (3 pints) vegetable stock together with 3 tbsp each light soy sauce and dry sherry. Bring to the boil and simmer for 3 minutes. Add 300 g (10½ oz) raw tiger prawns, peeled, 115 g (4 oz) baby spinach leaves, 150 g (5½ oz) bean sprouts, 4 thinly sliced spring onions and 2 tbsp chopped fresh coriander. Simmer until the prawns change from grey-blue to pink, then remove from the heat and stir in the grated zest and juice of 2 limes and 2 tbsp fish sauce. Put the drained noodles in serving bowls, ladle over the soup and serve.

Plus points

● Soba are Japan's most popular noodles. They are made from buckwheat, which though eaten as a cereal is actually the fruit of a plant related to rhubarb. Buckwheat is a good source of B vitamins and contains some calcium.

● Tofu is a good source of non-animal protein and offers good amounts of iron and B vitamins as well as useful amounts of calcium. It is low in saturated fat.

Hong Kong-style chow mein with pork and green vegetables

A mixture of green vegetables adds colour, crispness and food value to this simple noodle stir-fry with pork and dried mushrooms. Chinese egg noodles are prepared more quickly than Western pasta – they only need brief soaking – so this dish can be made from start to finish in less than 30 minutes.

Serves 4

25 g (scant 1 oz) dried Chinese mushrooms
   or shiitake
chicken or vegetable stock
340 g (12 oz) Chinese egg noodles
2 tbsp sunflower oil
1 large garlic clove, crushed
1 tbsp finely chopped fresh root ginger
1 fresh red or green chilli, seeded and
   finely chopped, or to taste
2 tsp five-spice powder
200 g (7 oz) pork fillet, trimmed and
   cut into strips
2 green peppers, seeded and thinly sliced
100 g (3½ oz) small broccoli florets
2 celery sticks, thinly sliced
2 tbsp soy sauce
1 tbsp rice wine (sake or mirin) or dry sherry
100 g (3½ oz) bean sprouts
2 tbsp finely chopped fresh coriander
2 tsp toasted sesame oil
fresh coriander leaves to garnish

Preparation time: about 20 minutes
Cooking time: about 6 minutes

1 Place the mushrooms in a small bowl and pour in enough boiling water to cover them. Leave to soak for 10 minutes. Line a sieve with muslin or kitchen paper and place it over a bowl, then pour the mushrooms and their soaking liquid into it. Measure the strained liquid and make it up to 100 ml (3½ fl oz) with chicken or vegetable stock if necessary, then set aside. Discard any tough stalks from the mushrooms, slice them and set aside.

2 While the mushrooms are soaking, place the noodles in a large mixing bowl and pour in enough boiling water to cover them generously. Leave to soak for 4 minutes, or according to the packet instructions, until tender. Drain well and set aside.

3 Heat a wok or large frying pan over a high heat. Add 1 tbsp of the sunflower oil and, when it is hot, stir in the garlic, ginger, chilli and five-spice powder. Stir-fry for 30 seconds, taking care not to let the flavourings burn.

4 Add the strips of pork and continue stir-frying for about 2 minutes or until they are cooked through. Use a draining spoon to remove the pork from the wok and set it aside.

5 Add the remaining oil to the wok and heat until it is almost smoking. Stir in the peppers, broccoli, celery and mushrooms, and stir-fry for 2 minutes. Stir in the mushroom liquid, soy sauce and rice wine or sherry, then return the pork to the wok. Continue cooking, stirring constantly, for about 1 minute or until the pork is reheated.

6 Stir in the noodles, then the bean sprouts and toss together briefly, just long enough to heat the ingredients without softening the bean sprouts, as they should retain their crunch.

7 Stir in the chopped coriander and sprinkle with the sesame oil. Serve the chow mein immediately, garnished with coriander leaves.

Plus points

• The average fat content of lean pork is just 3.5% (3.5 g per 100 g), much the same as that contained in chicken breast, which (without skin) contains 3.2 g per 100 g. Pork is also a good source of zinc, and it provides useful amounts of iron and the B vitamins, particularly B_1, B_6, B_{12} and niacin.

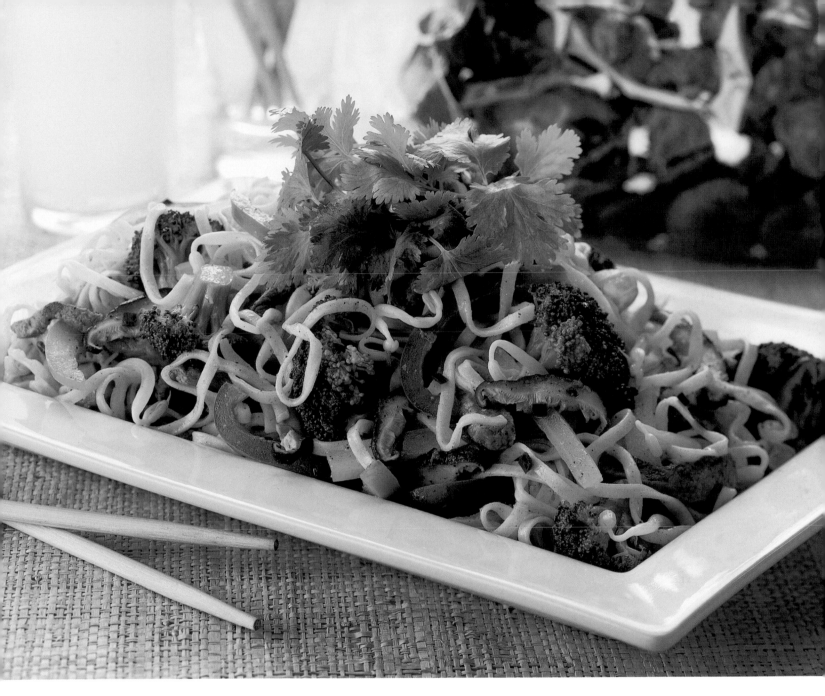

Some more ideas

• Replace the pork with skinless boneless chicken breasts (fillets), cut into thin slices, or peeled raw tiger prawns.

• Use wheat-free Chinese rice noodles for anyone on a gluten-free diet.

• For a delicious vegetarian version, omit the pork fillet and add 300 g (10½ oz) mange-tout or sugarsnap peas. Baby sweetcorn, halved lengthways, sliced carrots, chopped French beans, cauliflower florets and sliced fresh mushrooms are also all suitable.

Each serving provides

kcal 488, protein 17 g, fat 13 g (of which saturated fat 3 g), carbohydrate 73 g (of which sugars 3 g), fibre 2.5 g

✓✓✓	C
✓✓	B_1, B_{12}, niacin
✓	B_6, folate, iron, potassium, zinc

Macaroni and mushroom cheese

Introduce vegetables to old favourites for up-to-the-minute healthy family meals.
This well-loved pasta dish is delicious with mushrooms, peas and peppers added.
Using a small amount of powerful Roquefort cheese ensures that the sauce is creamy
and full flavoured, but not too high in fat.

Serves 4

225 g (8 oz) macaroni or rigatoni

170 g (6 oz) frozen peas

2 tbsp sunflower oil

1 red pepper, seeded and chopped

225 g (8 oz) mushrooms, quartered if large

30 g (1 oz) plain flour

600 ml (1 pint) semi-skimmed milk

1 tbsp Dijon mustard

55 g (2 oz) Roquefort cheese, chopped

salt and pepper

Topping

30 g (1 oz) mature Cheddar cheese, grated

55 g (2 oz) fresh wholemeal breadcrumbs

Preparation time: 30 minutes

Cooking time: 10–15 minutes

Each serving provides

kcal 515, protein 22 g, fat 17 g (of which
saturated fat 7 g), carbohydrate 73 g (of
which sugars 13 g), fibre 6 g

✓✓✓	A, C, calcium, copper
✓✓	B_1, B_2, E, folate, niacin, potassium, selenium
✓	B_6, B_{12}, iron

1 Preheat the oven to 220°C (425°F, gas mark 7). Cook the pasta in boiling water for 10–12 minutes, or according to the packet instructions, until almost al dente. Add the peas for the final 2 minutes of cooking. Drain the pasta and peas well.

2 Heat the oil in a heavy-based saucepan and cook the red pepper for 1–2 minutes. Add the mushrooms and cook for 2–3 minutes or until softened, stirring occasionally.

3 Stir in the flour, then gradually stir in the milk and bring to the boil, stirring. Simmer until thickened.

4 Add the mustard and Roquefort cheese with seasoning to taste (remember, though, that Roquefort is quite salty) and stir until the cheese has melted. Add the pasta and peas and mix in thoroughly. Pour the mixture into an ovenproof dish.

5 Mix the Cheddar cheese with the breadcrumbs and sprinkle this over the pasta mixture. Bake for 10–15 minutes or until lightly browned and bubbling hot. Serve immediately.

Some more ideas

- Instead of baking the macaroni cheese, place it under a moderately hot grill until bubbling and the topping is golden.
- Button Brussels sprouts are delicious with pasta in a blue cheese sauce. Cook 225 g (8 oz) sprouts in boiling water until just tender, then drain well and cut in half. Take care not to over-cook the sprouts – they are at their best while still slightly crunchy. Use instead of the mushrooms, adding the sprouts with the pasta.

Plus points

- Frozen vegetables often contain more vitamin C than fresh vegetables. For example, frozen peas retain 60–70% of their vitamin C content after freezing and maintain this level throughout storage.
- Roquefort cheese is high in fat and salt, but it has such a strong flavour that a little goes a long way. It is a good source of protein, calcium and phosphorus, and it provides useful amounts of the B vitamins B_1, B_2, B_6 and niacin.

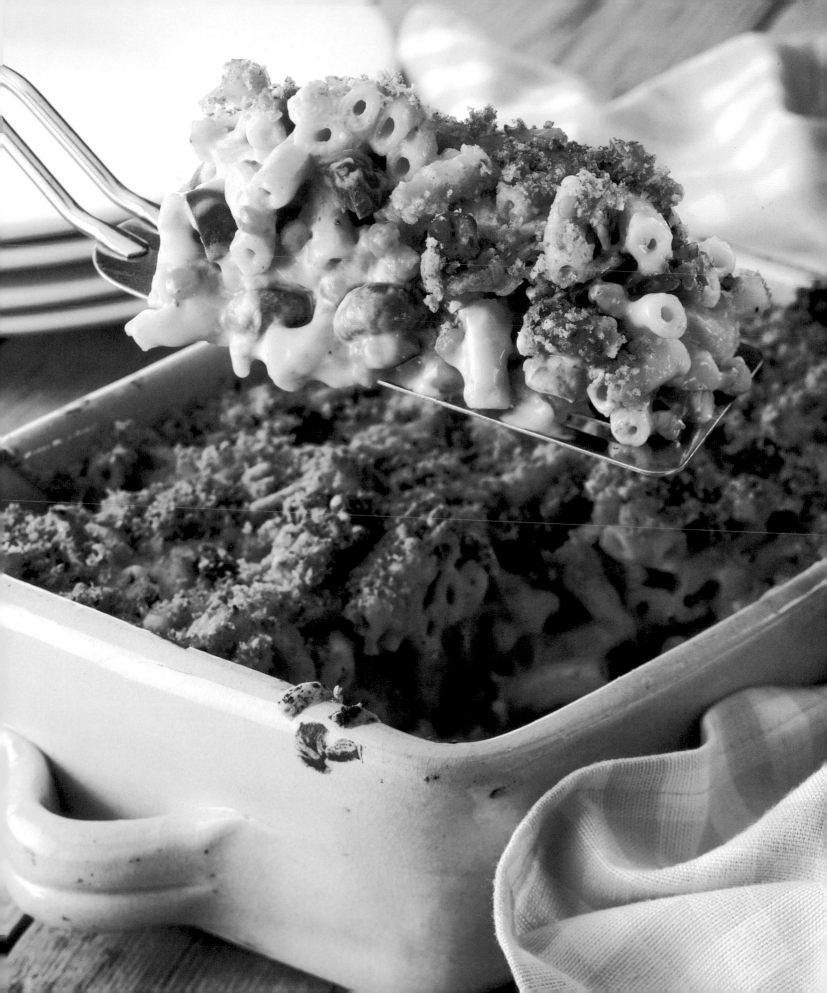

Seafood lasagne

Packed with seafood and lots of vegetables, this lasagne is a superb vitamin-rich, nutritious meal. Choose vegetables that are fresh and in season – when fresh peas, asparagus and runner beans are past, try broccoli, kale and sautéed mushrooms. Serve with bread and a salad of interesting mixed leaves.

Serves 6

3 tbsp extra virgin olive oil

1 small bulb of fennel, diced

1 onion, chopped

4 garlic cloves, coarsely chopped, or to taste

2 tbsp coarsely chopped fresh parsley

$\frac{1}{4}$–$\frac{1}{2}$ tsp fennel seeds

$\frac{1}{4}$–$\frac{1}{2}$ tsp dried mixed Italian herbs

pinch of crushed dried chillies

125 g (4$\frac{1}{2}$ oz) prepared squid

125 g (4$\frac{1}{2}$ oz) salmon fillet, skinned and
  cut into chunks

125 g (4$\frac{1}{2}$ oz) raw tiger prawns, peeled

125 g (4$\frac{1}{2}$ oz) shellfish cocktail mix

150 ml (5 fl oz) dry white wine

150 ml (5 fl oz) fish or vegetable stock

grated zest of $\frac{1}{2}$ lemon

2 bay leaves

1 carrot, roughly chopped

1 kg (2$\frac{1}{4}$ lb) tomatoes, diced

5 runner beans, cut into bite-sized pieces

1 courgette, sliced or diced

250 g (9 oz) asparagus tips

170 g (6 oz) shelled fresh or frozen peas

400 g (14 oz) no-precook lasagne

250 g (9 oz) ricotta cheese

2 eggs, lightly beaten

85 g (3 oz) Parmesan cheese, freshly grated

freshly grated nutmeg

salt, pepper and cayenne

Preparation time: about 1$\frac{1}{2}$ hours
Cooking time: 30 minutes

1 Preheat the oven to 180°C (350°F, gas mark 4). Heat 2 tbsp of the oil in a large saucepan. Add the fennel, onion and half of the garlic. Cook for about 5 minutes or until the onion has softened, then add the parsley, fennel seeds, Italian herbs and chilli flakes. Cook for 1–2 minutes.

2 Add the squid and salmon, and cook for about 1 minute, then stir in the prawns and cocktail mix. Cook for only a moment – about 30 seconds – then use a draining spoon to transfer the seafood to a bowl and set aside.

3 Add the wine, stock, lemon zest, bay leaves and carrot to the juices remaining in the pan. Boil for 5 minutes, or until the liquid is reduced to about 100 ml (3$\frac{1}{2}$ fl oz). Stir in the tomatoes and continue to cook over a high heat for 3–4 minutes or until reduced to a well-flavoured sauce.

4 Add the runner beans and remaining garlic. Cover and cook for 10 minutes. Stir in the courgette and season to taste. Cover and cook for 5 minutes, then add the asparagus and peas. Cook, covered, for 5 minutes.

5 Lightly grease a deep 28 cm (11 in) lasagne dish with a little of the remaining oil. Place about two-thirds of the vegetables in the dish, lifting them out of the sauce with a slotted spoon and discarding the bay leaves, then top with a layer of lasagne, overlapping the sheets slightly. Add the seafood and a second layer of overlapping lasagne. Pour on the remaining vegetables and sauce. Top with the remaining sheets of lasagne.

6 Mix the ricotta cheese with the eggs and Parmesan. Season with a little nutmeg, salt, pepper and cayenne. Pour this evenly over the top of the lasagne and drizzle with the remaining olive oil.

7 Bake for 30 minutes, or until the lasagne is heated through and the top is speckled golden brown. Serve immediately.

Plus points

• Oily fish, such as salmon, is rich in omega-3 fatty acids, which are a type of polyunsaturated fat believed to help protect against coronary heart disease and strokes.

• The Mediterranean diet is thought to be healthier than the average diet in the UK. One of the reasons for this is the use of olive oil, a monounsaturated fat, rather than butter and other saturated fats.

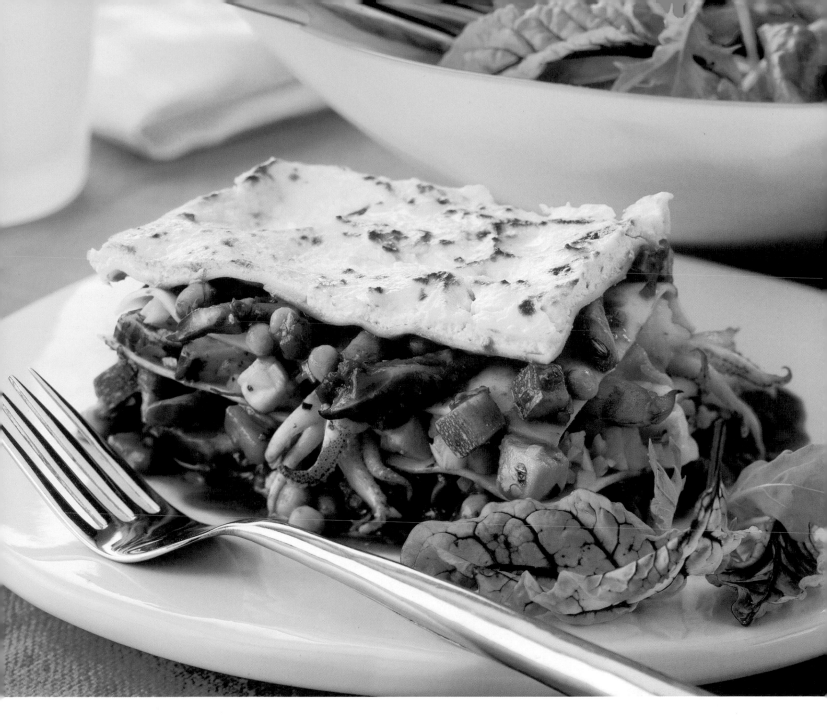

Some more ideas

● When fresh tomatoes are lacking in flavour, add 1 tbsp tomato purée and a pinch of sugar to the sauce.

● For a vegetarian lasagne, omit the seafood and step 2 of the recipe. Increase the vegetables – use 10–12 runner beans and 3 courgettes – and add 1 can flageolet beans, about 400 g, well drained.

● Vary the vegetables according to availability. For example, leave out the runner beans and increase the peas to 250 g (9 oz); use 2 celery sticks instead of the bulb of fennel; replace the fresh tomatoes with 2 cans chopped tomatoes, about 400 g each.

● If you don't like squid, or any other of the fish and seafood ingredients listed, simply leave them out and increase another seafood item.

Each serving provides

kcal 595, protein 38 g, fat 22 g (of which saturated fat 8 g), carbohydrate 60 g (of which sugars 11 g), fibre 6 g

✓✓✓	A, B_1, B_{12}, C, calcium, copper
✓✓	E, folate, niacin, iron, potassium, selenium
✓	B_2

Pumpkin, ricotta and sage gnocchi

There are numerous versions of gnocchi in Italy. For the one here, a flour-based dough of ricotta and mashed pumpkin, flavoured with sage and Parmesan cheese, is shaped into the little dumplings. A colourful roasted pepper and onion sauce completes the dish. Serve with a baby spinach and watercress salad.

Serves 4

2 red peppers, halved and seeded

1 onion, halved

500 g (1 lb 2 oz) pumpkin or acorn squash, cut into wedges and seeded

1 tbsp extra virgin olive oil

250 g (8½ oz) ricotta cheese

1 egg, beaten

3 tbsp chopped fresh sage

30 g (1 oz) Parmesan cheese, freshly grated

200 g (7 oz) plain flour, plus extra for rolling

salt and pepper

fresh sage leaves to garnish

Preparation and cooking time: 1½–2 hours, plus 1–2 hours drying

Each serving provides   Ⓥ

kcal 404, protein 18 g, fat 15 g (of which saturated fat 7 g), carbohydrate 52 g (of which sugars 11 g), fibre 5 g

✓✓✓	A, C, calcium
✓✓	B₁, E, zinc
✓	B₂, B₆, B₁₂, folate, niacin, copper, iron, potassium

1 Preheat the oven to 200°C (400°F, gas mark 6). Spread out the pepper and onion halves, cut side down, on a baking sheet. Place the pumpkin or squash wedges, skin side up, on another baking sheet. Bake the peppers and onion for 30–35 minutes, and the pumpkin or squash for 45–55 minutes, or until all the vegetables are tender.

2 Transfer the peppers and onions to a blender or food processor and add the oil. Blend until almost smooth. Season with salt and pepper to taste. Pour into a saucepan and set aside.

3 Leave the pumpkin or squash until cool enough to handle, then scrape the flesh from the skins into a bowl. Mash until smooth. Beat in the ricotta, egg, chopped sage and Parmesan, then gradually work in the flour to make a soft dough.

4 Flour a work surface. Divide the dough into quarters and, with floured hands, roll each piece into a long, 2 cm (¾ in) thick rope. Cut into 2 cm (¾ in) lengths. Press the back of a fork into each piece of dough to make a pattern. Leave the gnocchi at room temperature to dry for 1–2 hours.

5 Bring a large saucepan of water to the boil. Drop in the gnocchi, 10–12 at a time, and poach them for 2–3 minutes or until they bob up to the surface. Remove with a draining spoon and drain well on kitchen paper. Transfer to a warmed ovenproof serving dish and keep warm in a low oven until all the gnocchi are cooked.

6 Meanwhile, gently warm the roasted pepper sauce over a low heat. Spoon the sauce over the gnocchi, garnish with sage leaves and serve.

Plus points

• Like other cheeses, ricotta is a good source of calcium. In addition, it offers good quantities of phosphorus, another mineral involved in ensuring bones and teeth are healthy. Phosphorus is also important in the release of energy from food.

• Pumpkin has a high water content, which makes it particularly low in calories – just 15 kcal per 100 g (3½ oz).

• Puréed vegetable sauces such as this are delicious low-fat dressings for pasta.

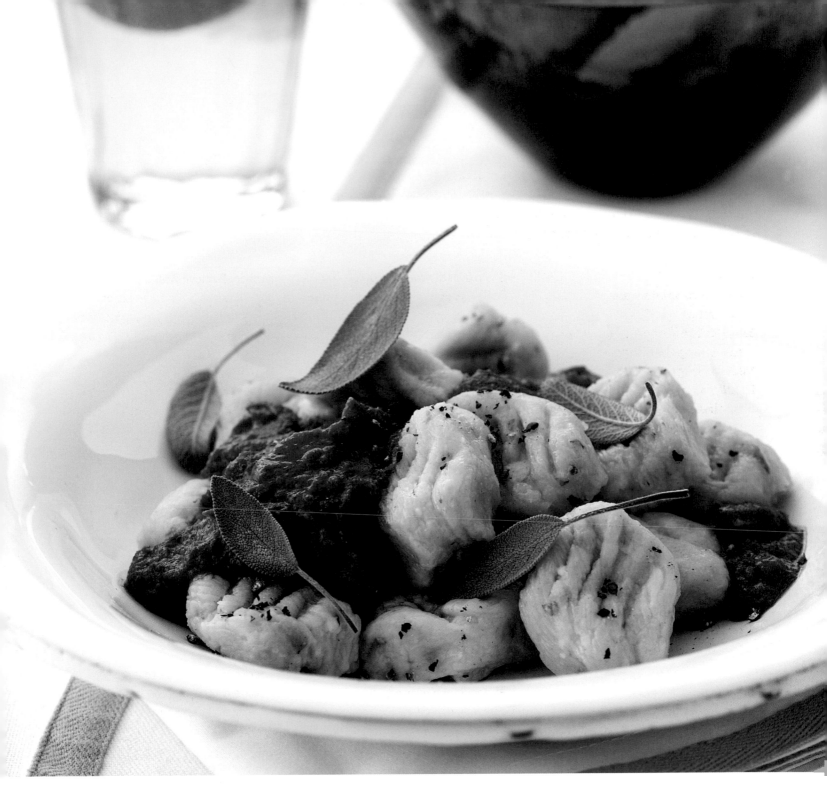

Another idea

● For ricotta and fresh herb gnocchi, combine 250 g (8½ oz) ricotta cheese, 85 g (3 oz) finely chopped rocket, 20 g (¾ oz) finely chopped parsley, 3 tbsp snipped fresh chives, 1 beaten egg and 30 g (1 oz) freshly grated pecorino cheese. Add 200 g (7 oz) plain flour, 1 tsp freshly grated nutmeg, and salt and pepper to taste, and mix to a soft dough. Shape and cook as in the main recipe. Serve with a roasted tomato sauce: toss 500 g (1 lb 2 oz) small plum tomatoes and 2 garlic cloves in 1 tbsp extra virgin olive oil, then roast in a preheated 200°C (400°F, gas mark 6) oven for 20–25 minutes. Purée until smooth, and season to taste.

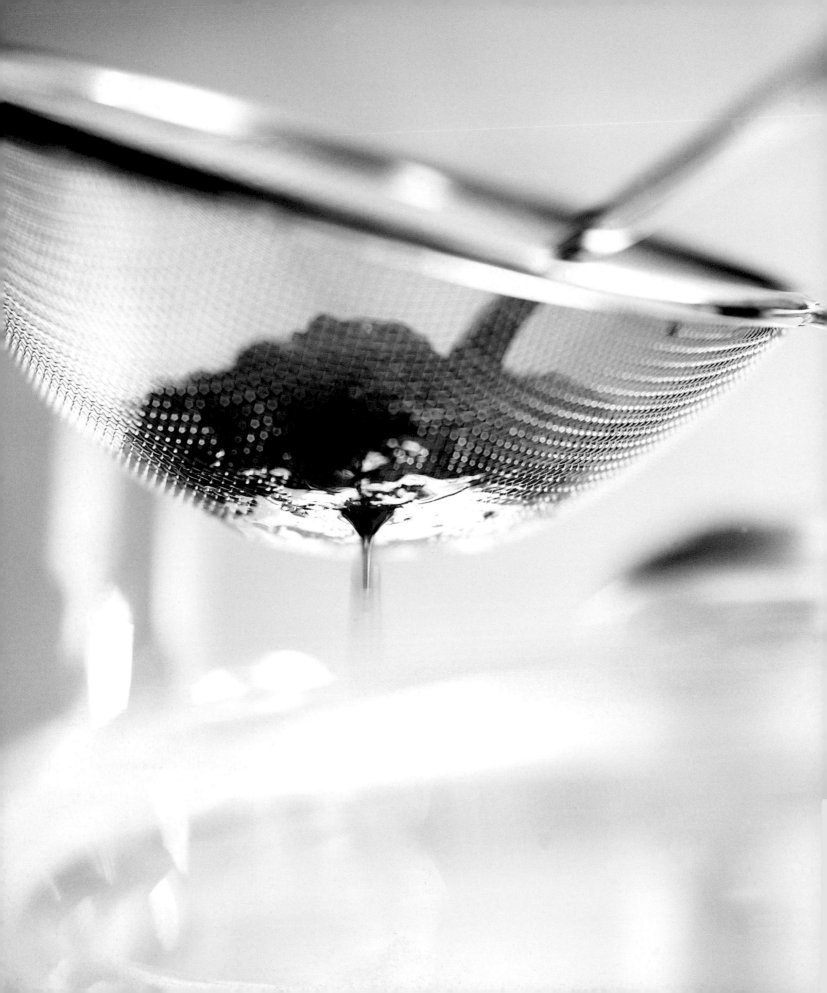

Super Fruit

Fruit is packed with vital vitamins, minerals and essential fibre, all of which help to protect you against ill health and keep you feeling at your best. The more fruit you eat, the greater the benefits, and with so many kinds to choose from, there will always be something to tempt you. Fruit is an ideal basis for healthy desserts, as well as being an attractive addition to salads and many savoury dishes. And it is the ultimate convenience food, easy to carry and eat anywhere. This chapter gives an overview of why fruit is so good for you, what to look for when buying fruit, and how to make sure you get the most from its great taste and health benefits.

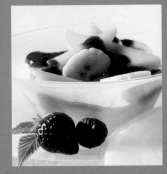

Fruit in a healthy diet

All fruit is good for us, be it fresh, frozen, dried or canned, so you can enjoy it whatever the season.

Why eat fruit?

In nutritional terms, fruit is full of vitamins and minerals, in particular vitamin C and beta-carotene and the minerals potassium, magnesium and selenium, plus different types of fibre. All of these are essential for general vitality and health.

Eating more fruit also improves the chances of avoiding cancer – an increasing number of studies show that people who eat a lot of fruit and vegetables are at less risk of heart disease, stroke and cancer, particularly colon and stomach cancer and probably breast cancer. The exact components in fruit and vegetables that offer protection have yet to be identified, but antioxidant vitamins and minerals play an important role, possibly in conjunction with different types of fibre and other natural plant chemicals.

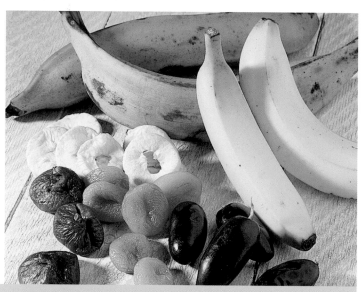

▲ Best fruit for energy – plantains, bananas, fresh dates, dried fruit such as apples, figs and apricots

▼ Best fruit for bioflavonoids – citrus (skin and pulp), apricots, cherries, grapes, papaya, cantaloupe melon

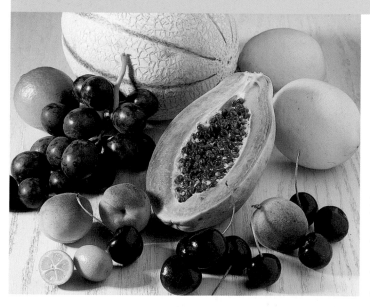

What fruit nutrients can do

• Antioxidants – vitamins C, E and beta-carotene and the minerals zinc, selenium, manganese and copper – have the ability to delay or prevent oxidation, the process that produces highly reactive and damaging free radicals. Free radical damage ages us and causes 'oxidative' changes that increase the risk of heart disease and cells that can initiate cancers. Vitamin E also protects against cancer and heart disease, premature ageing, cataracts and other diseases. It strengthens blood capillary walls and helps to generate new skin. Antioxidants also maintain normal cell function.

• Bioflavonoids are another type of antioxidant. They work with vitamin C to boost immunity and to strengthen blood capillaries, and act as anti-inflammatory agents.

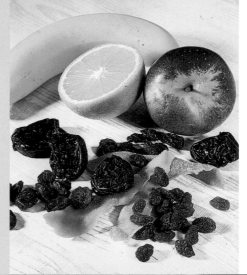

Best fruit for fibre – bananas, oranges, apples, dried fruit ▶
Best fruit for vitamin C – kiwi fruit, oranges, strawberries, blackcurrants ▼

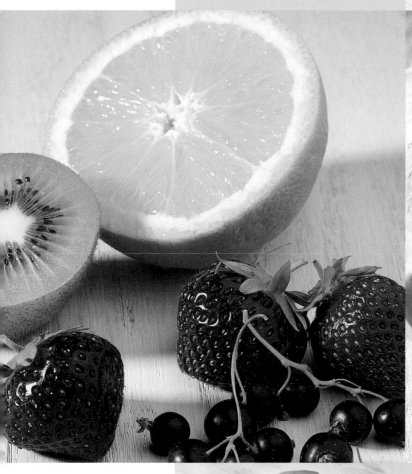

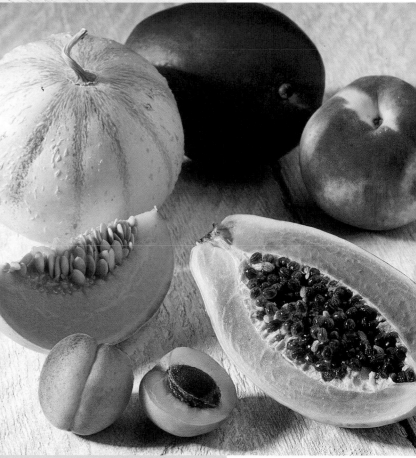

▲ Best fruit for beta-carotene – cantaloupe melon, mango, peaches, papaya, apricots
◀ Best fruit for minerals – bananas (potassium), apricots, particularly dried (iron), prunes (potassium and iron)

• B vitamins are vital for healthy nerves and releasing energy from food during digestion. Although in general fruit is not as good a source of B vitamins as, say, cereals, one of the B vitamins, folate (also referred to as folic acid), is found in oranges and other citrus fruit and in bananas.

• Fibre comes in several varieties, many of which are found in fruit. Soluble fibre (like the gummy pectin in fruit that makes jams gel) helps to lower levels of harmful blood cholesterol. Insoluble fibre, from the skin and fibrous structure of fruits, helps to prevent constipation and associated problems.

• Potassium works to balance sodium, thus helping to prevent high blood pressure. Most Western diets contain too little potassium and too much sodium, particularly in processed foods. Potassium-rich fruit like bananas and oranges are useful aids to getting the balance right.

Which are the best fruits to eat?

Eating a wide variety is more beneficial than focusing on any particular type of fruit because there is no proof that one single fruit is better than any other at protecting against specific diseases. To spread your intake across different types of fruit, regularly choose from yellow-orange fruit (mangoes, peaches, apricots, melon), citrus fruit, berry fruit (strawberries, raspberries, blackcurrants, blueberries), exotic fruit (guava, passion fruit, papaya, kiwi, dates) and others such as apples, pears, bananas, pineapple and plums.

Whenever possible choose fruit in season and eat it raw to maximise the vitamin and mineral intake – even quick cooking reduces nutrient content. Remember, though, that cooked, canned and frozen fruit are still quite high in nutrients – in fact, frozen fruit will contain more vitamins than tired 'fresh' fruit. Fruit canned in fruit juice has less sugar than that canned in syrup, and it has a more 'fruity' flavour.

Is organic fruit better?

Many people feel that fruit grown without artificial pesticides is the ideal option. However, not eating enough fruit and vegetables is more harmful to health than hazards from any possible pesticide residues. Government regulations are designed to minimise residues in fruit, which surveillance shows do not usually exceed Maximum Residue Levels.

The golden rule is that fruit should always be thoroughly washed, as this removes some of the surface pesticides, waxes and other treatments. If you plan to use the zest of citrus fruit, it is wisest to buy organic or unwaxed fruit because the waxes contain fungicide.

How can desserts be healthy?

Healthy desserts might sound a contradiction in terms. Yet puddings based on fruit can make a delicious nutritional contribution to a meal. Puddings need not be high in fat and sugar to be satisfyingly rich and sweet. A good example is bread pudding packed with dried fruit – this helps to meet the daily requirements for many nutrients.

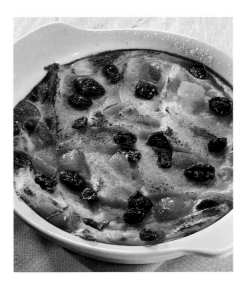

Fruity bread pudding
A bread pudding with lots of dried fruit added provides vitamins from the fruit, starchy carbohydrates (bread), protein (eggs) and dairy foods (milk).

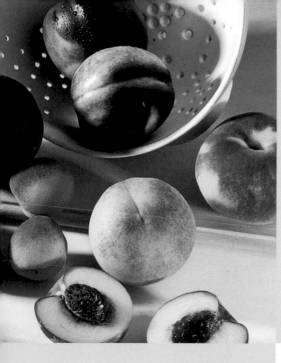

Eating lots of different fruit is the best way to take advantage of the vital nutrients each has to offer

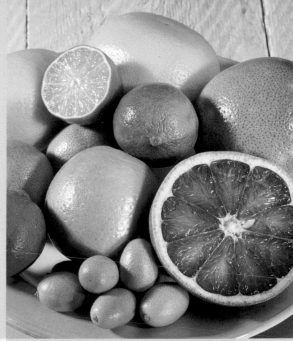

▲ Yellow-orange fruit, such as peaches, nectarines and apricots, provide beta-carotene, as well as B vitamins and vitamins A and C

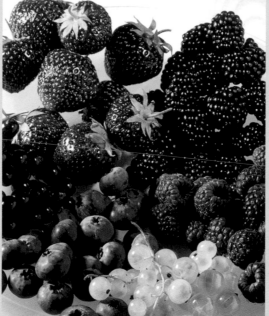

▲ Citrus fruits are packed with vitamin C and also provide fibre

Berries of all kinds give us vitamins C and E, plus fibre ▶

Other fruits contribute gummy fibre (apples), energy (pears), potassium (bananas), vitamin C (pineapple), and vitamin E and the antioxidant beta-carotene (plums) ▼

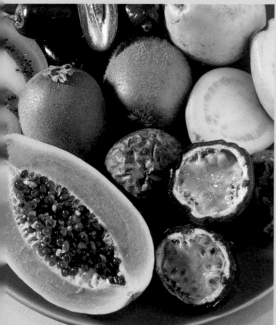

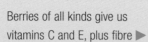

◀ Of the many and varied exotic fruits, fresh dates provide vitamin C, fibre and lots of energy, guava gives us vitamin C and fibre, passion fruit has vitamins A and C, papaya offers vitamins A and C and fibre, and kiwi fruit is loaded with vitamin C plus some potassium

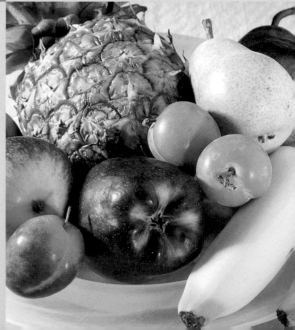

A new look at favourite fruits

The tremendous health potential of familiar fruits means that we should look at them in a new light and try to eat them more often.

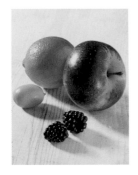

An ABC of common fruit

While we think of fruit as supplying mainly vitamin C, some fruit also contain small but useful amounts of beta-carotene, which the body can convert to vitamin A, plus the B vitamins, vitamin E, and minerals such as iron and zinc. All the fruits here are low in calories and fat free. A portion size is given to help you count your 5-a-day.

When buying and storing fruit, buy the freshest you can find, and buy it in fairly small quantities that you know you will use up quickly. The vitamin content, particularly vitamin C, will vary according to freshness.

Apple (1 medium-sized fruit)

It has long been said that 'an apple a day keeps the doctor away'. One study has shown that eating up to 3 apples a day for a month can help to lower blood cholesterol levels. This is probably because apples contain gummy fibre (pectin) and an antioxidant called quercetin. So now we might add to the adage '... and 2 apples a day keeps the specialist away!' In addition, eating apples can help to prevent gum disease.
• Choose firm, bright crisp apples. Store in the fridge for up to 2 weeks, and bring to room temperature before eating.

Apricot, peach and nectarine (3 apricots, 1 medium-sized peach or nectarine)

Apricots provide vitamins B_1 (thiamin), niacin and B_6, and are a useful source of the antioxidant beta-carotene. An average serving of 3 apricots also provides useful amounts of fibre and potassium as well as vitamin C. Peaches and nectarines share a similar health profile, with more vitamin C, less vitamin A and slightly less fibre than apricots. The darker the colour of the fruit, the higher the carotenoid content, so white-flesh peaches and nectarines will contain less beta-carotene.
• Choose firm plump fruit that yields slightly to the touch and has even-coloured skin. Do not buy fruit that is green near the stalk. It is unripe and will just go soft. Store in the fridge for up to a week, or ripen in a paper bag at room temperature.

Banana (1 medium-sized fruit)

Bananas contain high levels of natural sugars, and are a better source of energy than refined sugary foods because they have a lot more to offer. They are unusual amongst fruit because they are a useful source of vitamin B_6 and vitamin E, as well as providing folate. A medium-sized banana even contains a good amount of vitamin C, and the potassium content (10% RNI) helps to redress our typically high sodium intake, as well as replacing minerals lost through perspiration. Bananas really are a super fruit!
• If eating immediately, choose yellow fruit with a few brown specks; otherwise select fruit with green ends to ripen. Do not store in the fridge as this turns banana skins black. Instead, keep at room temperature, or in a cool place to slow ripening.

Berry fruit (1 cupful or approx 100 g/¾ oz)

The purple, dark red and blue colours that characterise many berries, such as blackcurrants, blackberries, loganberries, raspberries and strawberries (as well as dark cherries and black grapes), come from antioxidant anthocyanin flavonoids, which may help to strengthen walls of small blood vessels.
• Blackberries have similar nutrient levels to blackcurrants, but contain even more vitamin E – 2.4 mg per portion, making them the richest fruit source of vitamin E.
• Blackcurrants are outstandingly high in vitamin C, containing more than five times the RNI in a portion. In addition to vitamin C, blackcurrants also contain useful amounts of potassium, fibre and vitamin E.

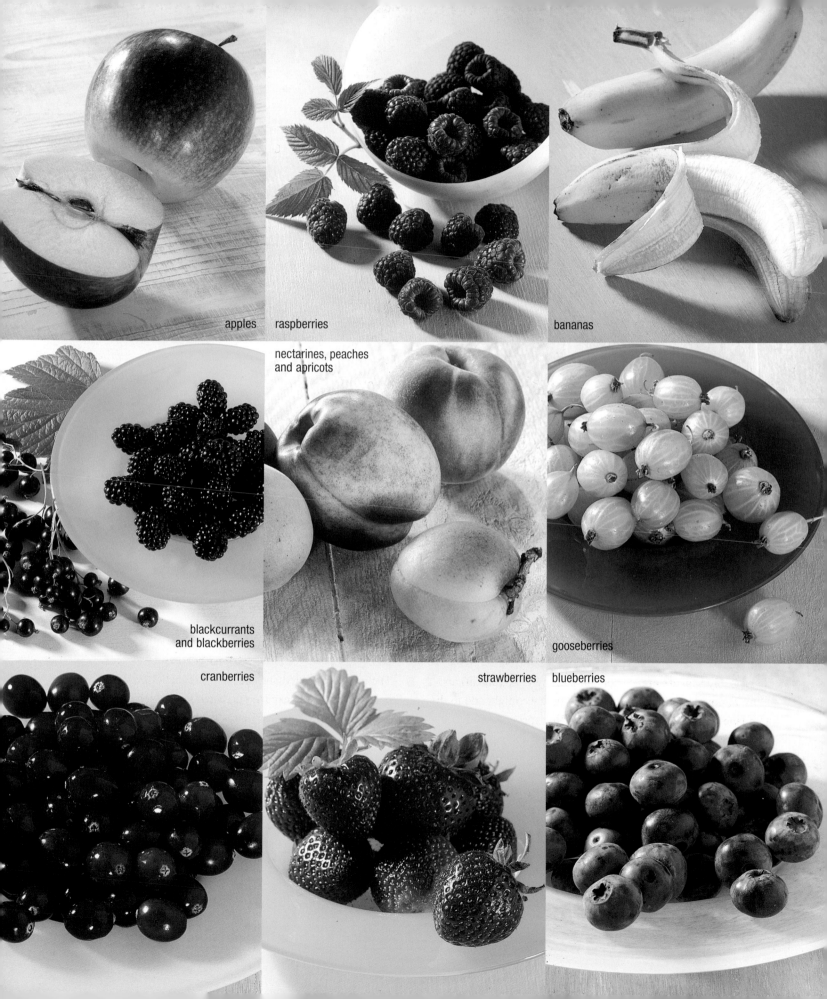

apples   raspberries   bananas

nectarines, peaches
and apricots

blackcurrants
and blackberries   gooseberries

cranberries   strawberries   blueberries

• Blueberries contain antioxidants and nutrients similar to those found in cranberries.

• Cranberries are a good source of vitamin C and provide useful amounts of fibre. A regular intake of cranberry juice can be used to help treat or prevent urinary tract infections such as cystitis, because they contain a compound that prevents the most common bacteria which cause cystitis from becoming attached to the bladder wall.

• Gooseberries can be enjoyed during their short summer season as a good source of vitamin C and a useful source of soluble fibre.

• Raspberries contain half the vitamin C of strawberries.

• Strawberries are an excellent source of vitamin C, with a portion containing nearly twice the RNI for that vitamin – gram for gram they contain more vitamin C than oranges. They are also a useful source of folate.

• Choose firm, plump berries with a 'bloom' (e.g. blueberries and blackberries) or that are shiny (blackcurrants). Do not buy berries if there are white patches or any mould on them, or if damage to the packaging has caused juice to run out of the fruit. Use as soon as possible, storing in the fridge for no more than 1–2 days, unwashed and uncovered as they go mouldy quickly. When ready to use, rinse berries briefly in cold water and pat dry gently on kitchen paper.

Cherries (20 cherries or 80 g/scant 3 oz)

These are a useful source of vitamin C. In addition, they have a mild laxative action.

• Buy and store as berries.

Citrus fruit (1 medium-sized orange, ½ grapefruit, 20 kumquats)

All citrus fruit – oranges, grapefruit, lemons, limes, mandarins, satsumas, kumquats and so on – are very nutritious. They are an excellent source of vitamin C – one medium-to-large orange provides twice the RNI of vitamin C – and the membrane that encases each juicy segment is a common source of flavonoids and fibre. Pink grapefruit contains beta-carotene.

• Choose firm, well-shaped fruit that feel heavy for their size. Do not buy fruit with bruises or soft patches or that are shrivelled. Store in the fridge, or at room temperature. The thick skin helps to prevent citrus fruit from drying out.

Grapes (1 cupful or approx 100 g/3½ oz)

Deliciously sweet, grapes are a useful source of potassium and copper. Those with red and black skins have antioxidant properties as they are high in bioflavonoids (which is passed on to the wine made from the grapes).

• Choose plump fruit, either shiny or with a bloom. Do not buy if they are shrivelled, going brown or split. Store in the fridge for up to 4–5 days.

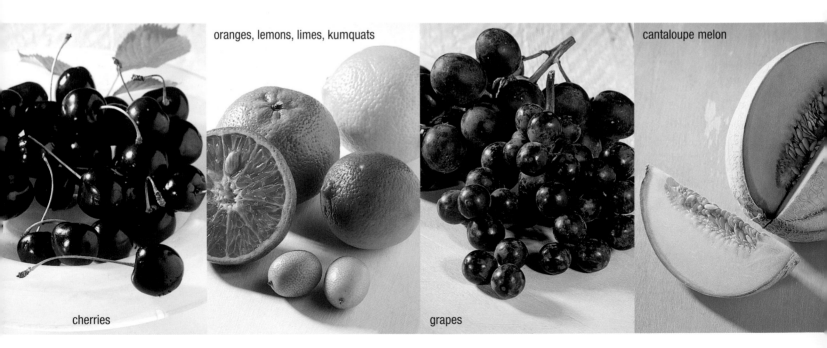

oranges, lemons, limes, kumquats

cantaloupe melon

cherries

grapes

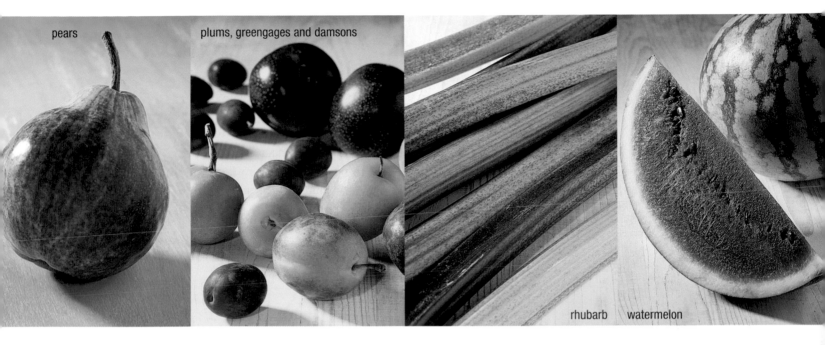

pears

plums, greengages and damsons

rhubarb   watermelon

Melon (1 medium-sized wedge)

All melons provide vitamins B and C, although those with orange flesh, such as cantaloupe, contain more of these vitamins. The orange-fleshed melons also offer beta-carotene.

• Only some varieties are scented, so aroma is not necessarily an indication of ripeness, and melons do not have to be soft at the stalk end to be ripe. Do not buy if damaged or bruised. Store either in the fridge for up to 2 weeks (melons do not continue to ripen after picking) or at room temperature. Once cut, wrap and store in the fridge.

Pear (1 medium-sized fruit)

Although not nutritionally outstanding, pears make a great energy-boosting snack because they are slightly higher in calories than apples and many other fruits. Pears are one of the most easily digested fruits. It is rare to have an allergic reaction against them, so they are often included in exclusion diets used for identifying foods that cause allergies.

• Choose firm fruit that feels slightly soft and has a bright and even-coloured skin. Do not buy fruit with brown marks or soft spots. Store at room temperature for up to 2 days or, if ripe, keep in the fridge.

Plum, greengage and damson (2 large or 3 medium-sized fruit)

These contain useful amounts of fibre and beta-carotene, as well as vitamins C and E.

• Choose well-coloured fruit with unblemished skins. Do not buy soft fruit with brown patches or fruit with any hint of fermentation. Also avoid hard or shrivelled fruit. Store in the fridge for up to 2 days; use as soon as possible because plums go over-ripe quickly.

Rhubarb (6 tbsp stewed)

Although treated as a fruit in cooking, rhubarb is actually a vegetable. It is a good source of potassium.

Watermelon (1 medium-sized wedge or 200 g/7 oz)

Use this fruit as a nutritious and refreshing thirst-quencher – it contains over 90% water, plus some carotenoids, making it a useful source of vitamin A. Watermelon is also a good source of vitamin C (40% RNI).

• Buy and store as for melon.

The vitamin C–iron connection

Fruits such as oranges, strawberries and kiwi that are very rich in vitamin C have been shown to improve the body's uptake of iron from vegetable sources. This is especially useful for vegetarians and for the increasing number of people cutting down on red meat, which is the traditional source of this important mineral in the diet.

Fruits from round the world

Tropical and exotic fruits are wonderful in fruit salads, but also add exciting flavours to savoury dishes. It's well worth getting to know them better.

An ABC of tropical fruit

Exotic and tropical fruits brighten our shops with their colours and shapes. Those featured here offer a potent combination of antioxidant minerals and vitamins A, C and E, which is often reflected in their vibrant colours.

Yellow and orange fruit, such as mango, papaya, persimmon, carambola or star fruit, and tamarillo, are particularly good sources of antioxidants such as beta-carotene and vitamin C. The fresh fruit contains more nutrients than canned and has firmer texture and bright colours.

For the fruit discussed here, an average portion is 1 cupful or 100 g (3½ oz) of the edible flesh.

Asian pear

Crunchy, juicy and slightly sweet, this type of pear is a useful source of vitamin C and provides some fibre. Also called nashi (the Japanese word for pear), Chinese pear and Oriental pear, it may be small and yellow-green in colour or large and brown, and the skin may be smooth or sprinkled with russeting, according to the particular variety. When cooked, Asian pears never become completely tender, but retain their shape and firm texture.

• Asian pears are hard when ripe, unlike common pears. Store them in the fridge, where they will keep well for a long period – longer than apples. They are delicious raw and chilled, as well as cooked.

Cactus pear or prickly pear

The fruit of several varieties of cactus, this has sweet, brightly coloured pulp that smells of watermelon, and a multitude of hard black seeds. The flesh is rich in fibre and also supplies vitamin C and potassium.

• Choose fruit that has a fresh colour and no mouldy spots. If it gives when gently pressed it is ripe (it should not feel soft and squishy). Fruit that is firm can be left to ripen at room temperature. Once it is ripe, store it in the fridge, where it will keep for up to a week.

Cape gooseberry

The juicy dense flesh of this fruit, also called physalis, provides vitamin C and fibre as well as beta-carotene. Sweet with a slightly sharp aftertaste, it adds an intriguing flavour to both sweet and savoury preparations, either raw or cooked.

• Choose yellow or orangy gooseberries, avoiding any that are greenish. If spread out, still in their papery husks, on an uncovered plate, cape gooseberries will keep in the fridge for up to a month.

Carambola or star fruit

This fruit is a useful source of vitamins A and C, plus potassium and fibre. Its juicy, crisp flesh and attractive shape make it a decorative addition to puddings as well as to savoury dishes, and it does not discolour once cut.

• Choose juicy-looking fruit with a good colour; avoid any with brown or shrivelled edges. If the fruit is at all green, leave it to ripen at room temperature until the skin is completely yellow; the fruit should have a lovely perfume when ripe. Once fully ripe, store the fruit in the fridge, where it will keep for up to 2 weeks.

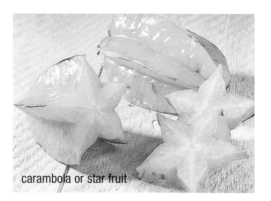
carambola or star fruit

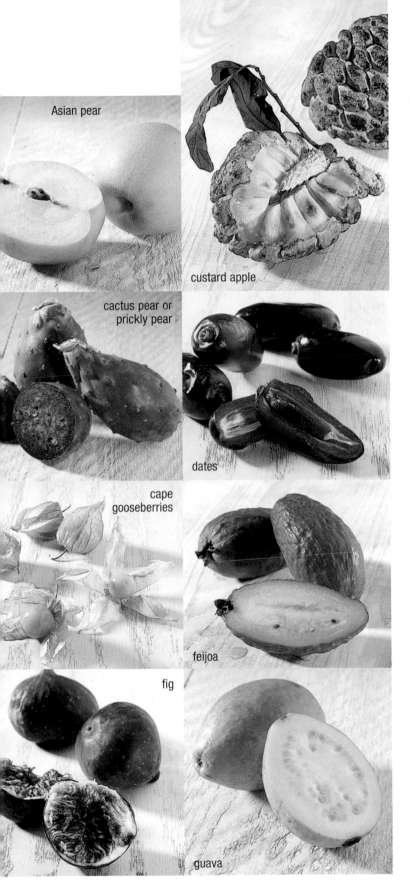

Asian pear

custard apple

cactus pear or prickly pear

dates

cape gooseberries

feijoa

fig

guava

Custard apple

Looking like a plump, yellowish-green pine cone, the custard apple, or cherimoya, has sweet, slightly granular flesh with large shiny seeds. It is a good source of fibre and also provides vitamin C and niacin.

● Choose fruit that is even in colour, with no dark or splotched areas. When ripe it will just give when gently pressed (like an avocado). To ripen, keep at room temperature; thereafter store in the fridge for up to 4 days.

Date

Fresh dates are energy dynamos – these little batteries contain 30 calories (kcal) per date. They also provide vitamin C (a 100 g/3½ oz portion, which is about 4 dates, supplies almost a third of the RNI) and useful amounts of fibre.

● Choose plump, glossy fruit and store it in the fridge, where it will keep for up to 2–3 days.

Feijoa

This elongated oval fruit has a thin green skin and slightly tart, softish granular flesh. An excellent source of vitamin C, it also provides small amounts of the B vitamins. Feijoa is delicious both raw and cooked.

● Choose fruit that is fragrant. If it is not tender, leave it at room temperature for a few days – eat only when ripe and creamy-soft, otherwise feijoa can be rather bitter.

Fig

Although not an outstanding source of any particular nutrient, figs have small, but not negligible, amounts of many vitamins and minerals and fibre.

● Figs bruise easily, so are best bought before fully ripe. When ready to eat, they will be soft and the skin will split.

Guava

A portion of fresh guava can contain over five times the RNI of vitamin C, and even canned guava contains four times the RNI. Guava is also a useful source of fibre. The hard, edible seeds are as high in vitamins as the sweet juicy flesh, so you may want to try eating them too.

● When tender-ripe, guava has an intense floral aroma. Fruit that is slightly green, but still tender with some aroma, will ripen at room temperature, so buy it if that is all that is available. Once fully ripe, it can be kept in the fridge for up to 2 days (do not refrigerate unripe guavas).

Kiwi fruit

Just one kiwi fruit contains nearly the total RNI for vitamin C, so put aside your prejudices – caused probably by this fruit's overuse in restaurants when it first appeared here. It is also a useful source of potassium, and is low in calories, at about 29 kcal per fruit.

● When buying kiwi, choose firm fruit that yields only slightly when pressed. Avoid fruit that is damaged or soft, as it will be mushy and lack flavour. Kiwi continues to ripen after picking (it is picked while still hard), so keep it at room temperature and then, once ripe, store it in the fridge for up to 2 weeks.

Lychee

Eating 3–4 raw lychees will provide two-thirds of your daily RNI of vitamin C. As these fruit are so luscious and beautifully perfumed, this is much more pleasurable than swallowing a vitamin pill.

● Choose lychees that feel heavy and full, with no cracks or shrivelling of the shell. The rosier they look, the fresher they will be. The fruit, still in shells, keeps well in the fridge – up to 2 weeks, although some of the perfume will be lost.

Mango

The luscious mango, with its richly coloured flesh, is one of the best fruit sources of vitamin A (from beta-carotene), providing over half the daily needs in one portion, which is about half a large mango. It is also an excellent source of vitamin C, and provides useful amounts of copper and fibre.

● Green mangoes are not necessarily unripe as skin colour depends on the variety. For those varieties that become yellow or red when ripe, choose fruit that feels full, with taut skin and no soft spots. The fruit should have a pleasant perfume (sniff the stalk end) – the stronger the scent, the more ripe it is. Keep the fruit at room temperature until ripe, then use it without delay, as mangoes do not benefit from prolonged storage in the fridge.

Papaya

Also called pawpaw, this is another nutritious 'all rounder' with good antioxidant value – an excellent source of vitamin C, useful source of vitamin A and providing useful amounts of fibre. The softish seeds in the centre of the yellow or sunset-pink papaya flesh are edible.

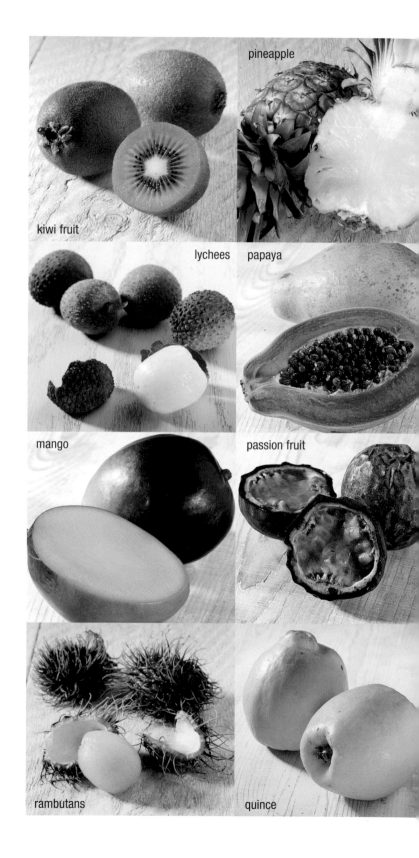

kiwi fruit

pineapple

lychees   papaya

mango

passion fruit

rambutans

quince

• Papaya is easily bruised, so it is usually harvested when very green and hard. It will continue to ripen after picking, although it will never have as rich a flavour as fruit ripened on the tree. Choose fruit whose skin has a good colour and no mouldy or bruised patches. Do not refrigerate unripe fruit; instead, let it ripen at room temperature.

Passion fruit

Although not nutritionally a champion, a passion fruit does contribute some vitamins A and C, and if you don't strain out the seeds it is a good source of fibre. Its major culinary contribution is its intense exotic fragrance. The granadilla is a close relative of passion fruit.

• Choose fruit that is large and heavy. Fruit with a dimpled skin is ready to use. If you can only find fruit with smooth skin, leave it at room temperature for a few days to wrinkle and ripen. Ripe fruit can be stored in the fridge for 1 week.

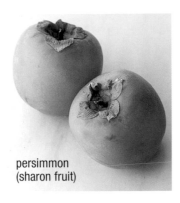
persimmon
(sharon fruit)

Persimmon

A good source of both vitamins C and A as well as fibre, the persimmon also provides some potassium. The variety most commonly available is the sharon fruit, which has flesh similar in texture to a firm plum.

• While some varieties of persimmon cannot be eaten until they are completely ripe and soft (otherwise they are mouth-puckeringly bitter), the sharon fruit can be enjoyed even when quite firm. Choose fruit with skin that is rich in colour. When ready to eat it will give to gentle pressure.

Pineapple

We are so used to pineapple that it hardly seems exotic, but it is certainly tropical in origin. Fresh pineapple is a good source of vitamin C.

• Choose pineapple with a fresh appearance, and avoid fruit with any soft bruised areas or leaves that are yellow or brown at the tips. A good indication of ripeness is a sweet aroma at the stalk end. Pineapple does not ripen after picking, although keeping it at room temperature for a few days will decrease the fruit's acidity and make it taste sweeter. A whole ripe pineapple can be stored in the fridge for up to 3 days.

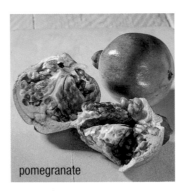
pomegranate

Pomegranate

This fruit offers good vitamin C and fibre content plus a lot of visual appeal, that adorns sweet and savoury dishes. The refreshingly acid-sweet pulp is a beautiful glistening deep pink with crunchy seeds inside.

• Choose fruit that is heavy for its size, with richly coloured, firm skin that has no blemishes. Pomegranate will keep well in the fridge for up to 3 months.

Quince

A portion of quince is a good source of vitamin C, although as this fruit requires cooking to be edible most of that vitamin is lost. Quince also provides a useful amount of fibre, and it is this fibre, or pectin, that makes quince so ideal for naturally jelled confections.

• Choose fruit that is aromatic. Once ripe (it will be yellow all over), it can be kept in the fridge, but wrap each fruit individually as quince bruises easily.

Rambutan

Called a 'hairy lychee' because its flesh is very like that of a lychee, the rambutan contains half the vitamin C of lychees.

• Choose fruit that feels heavy and full. If tender and ripe, store in the fridge.

Tamarillo

This egg-shaped fruit has a smooth, glossy, deep-red skin, and the dark apricot-coloured flesh inside resembles that of a tomato. In fact, its flavour is more like a pleasantly tart tomato than a sweet fruit – all of which explains why it is also called 'tree tomato'. A good source of vitamin C, this vitamin is retained if the fruit is used raw in a salad.

• Choose firm heavy fruit. When ripe it will give slightly when pressed and will be fragrant. Keep at room temperature until it ripens, then store in the fridge for up to a week.

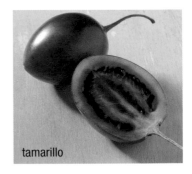
tamarillo

Concentrated fruity goodness

What dried fruits lack in size, they make up for in the concentration of their nutrients. And being small they make wonderful snacks, especially for children.

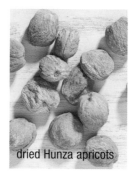
dried Hunza apricots

An ABC of dried fruit

Drying food is a traditional method of preservation. Reducing the moisture content and concentrating sugars means bacteria cannot thrive. The result of drying fruit, whether in the sun or by industrial processes, is higher levels of carbohydrates weight-for-weight than fresh fruit. This makes dried fruit a great source of energy and an excellent snack food, particularly popular with small children. However, the high calorie content can spoil small appetites for meals and is also something weight watchers should be aware of. The high sugar content also means that dried fruit is best not eaten frequently between meals as this could increase the risk of tooth decay.

Many dried fruits are a significant source of potassium, and they contain useful amounts of minerals such as iron, as well as fibre. Drying reduces the water-soluble vitamin C content, but some B vitamins (also water-soluble) remain.

- Apples contain lots of fibre (40% RNI in just 100 g/3½ oz), plus a small amount of iron.
- Apricots are a useful source of vitamin A (13% RNI in 100 g/3½ oz), plus fibre. They are one of the richest fruit sources of iron, a mineral lacking in many women's diets and essential to prevent anaemia.
- Bananas when dried have five times the calories of fresh.
- Blueberries provide a useful amount of fibre in 30 g (1 oz).
- Cherries are lower in sugars than many other dried fruit. They contain one-third the fibre of raisins.

- Cranberries contain only a little less fibre than raisins and sultanas, and have many other good things to offer (see page 302). They are sweetened when dried.
- Currants provide fibre and magnesium.
- Dates are a very palatable source of fibre – they provide 10% RNI in just 4 dates. They also contain an impressive combination of nutrients, with small but significant amounts of the minerals potassium and copper, and the B vitamins niacin, B_6 and folate.
- Figs are best known for their fibre – in 2 dried figs there is 12% RNI. But they also contain an interesting mixture of nutrients: a surprising 14% RNI of calcium, a good amount of magnesium, significant iron (19% RNI for men, 11% for women) and potassium (11% RNI).
- Mango retains some of its antioxidant attractions and a useful amount of fibre.
- Papaya retains a lot of its brilliant colour when dried. It is a useful source of fibre at 14% RNI in a 30 g (1 oz) portion, and contains calcium.
- Peaches when dried contain twice the iron of fresh peaches (23% RNI for men, 14% for women in 30 g/1 oz), and they offer vitamin A and the B vitamin niacin. Dried peaches are also a useful source of fibre.
- Pears offer 29% RNI of fibre per 85 g (3 oz) serving, plus 18% RNI potassium and some iron.
- Pineapple tends to contain more additives than other dried fruit (e.g. acidity regulators, citric acid, malic acid, preservatives, sulphur dioxide). This may be because dried pineapple snacks are often made from the woody core rather than the main body of the fruit, which is generally used for canning.

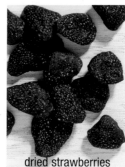
dried strawberries

- Prunes are very well known for their laxative role, with 3 prunes containing 10% RNI fibre. The same number of prunes also contains 10% RNI of iron for men and 6% for women, plus 7% RNI of potassium. In addition, prunes have an antioxidant role to play.
- Raisins and sultanas contain a useful amount of fibre. Their concentration of vitamins and minerals is lower than some dried fruit, but they are a useful source of potassium.

Sweet snacks

Most of the carbohydrate in dried fruit is in the form of sugars, but unlike refined sugar these foods are a valuable source of fibre and nutrients, making them a good snack food. They are also an excellent cooking ingredient – used with fresh fruit they can help reduce sugar or replace it.

Fruit and fibre – the GI factor

GI stands for Glycaemic Index, which is a ranking of foods based on their effect on blood sugar levels. Low-GI foods break down slowly, releasing energy gradually into the bloodstream, which results in a smaller rise of blood sugar. High-GI foods break down more quickly and cause a larger rise of blood sugar. Low-GI foods are more desirable because they can help to control hunger, appetite and weight, and lower raised blood fats. Fruit with a low GI include cherries, grapefruit, dried apricot, apple, banana, grapes, kiwi, mango, peach, pear and plum, and with intermediate GI cantaloupe, papaya, raisins and pineapple. Watermelon has a high GI.

Additives in dried fruit

Much dried fruit is treated with sulphur-based preservatives to prevent discoloration and to preserve and enhance the orange colour of fruits such as apricots and peaches. If dried fruits are unsulphured they are a less attractive brown colour and they do not have the sharp tang of sulphured fruit. Some people with asthma find sulphured foods trigger attacks. Potassium-based preservatives are used to prevent fungal and bacterial spoilage, particularly in ready-to-eat dried fruit that is partially hydrated for convenience. Fully dried fruit contains fewer additives. Dried fruit may also be coated with vegetable oil to make it glossy and prevent it from sticking and clumping.

Average calorie contents per 50 g (1¾ oz) of dried fruit

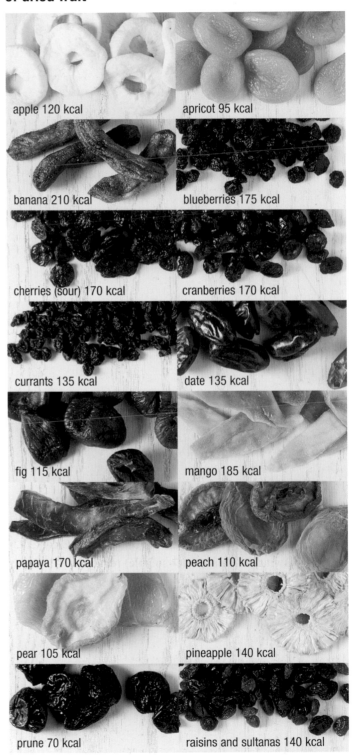

apple 120 kcal

apricot 95 kcal

banana 210 kcal

blueberries 175 kcal

cherries (sour) 170 kcal

cranberries 170 kcal

currants 135 kcal

date 135 kcal

fig 115 kcal

mango 185 kcal

papaya 170 kcal

peach 110 kcal

pear 105 kcal

pineapple 140 kcal

prune 70 kcal

raisins and sultanas 140 kcal

Preparing and cooking fruit

If you have bought good quality fruit, cook it as little as possible in order to retain the maximum vitamins and minerals.

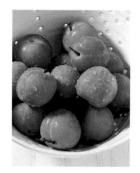

Golden rules for preparing fruit
- Wash fruit well to remove surface dirt and bacteria. Some surface pesticides will also be removed by washing. Rinse well in cold water, then drain or dry.
- Prepare fresh fruit as close to serving or cooking as possible.
- Avoid unnecessary peeling (vitamins and minerals are just below the skin, and the skin is a source of fibre).
- Do not chop too small.
- Dress cut surfaces with lemon juice to reduce nutrient loss.
- Cover and store prepared fruit in the fridge if not cooking or eating immediately.

- Never soak prepared fruit in water.
- Cook for the shortest time in the minimum amount of water, whether poaching fruit, boiling, stewing or microwaving. Steaming avoids contact with water, although some of the water-soluble vitamins will be lost.
- Avoid keeping fruit warm for long periods, or reheating it.

Saving vitamins and minerals
Vitamin A and its vegetable form beta-carotene are stable during mild heating, but losses occur at high temperatures. Vitamin E is destroyed gradually by heat, and the higher the temperature and the longer the cooking time, the greater the loss. Vitamin C leaches out during cooking because it is water-soluble. Minerals also leach into cooking water, but are not destroyed by normal cooking temperatures, so try to use the cooking water in the dish or include in syrups for fruit salad.

Good partners for fruit desserts

Cream on top – an occasional treat
Cream is a well-loved accompaniment for many fruit puddings as well as being used as an ingredient in both sweet and savoury dishes. You can enjoy cream as part of a healthy diet, eating a little occasionally and perhaps opting for creams that are lower in fat and calories. To help you choose, these are the fat contents and calories in different creams per level tablespoon: reduced-fat crème fraîche 2.25 g fat/28 kcal; single cream/soured cream 2.85 g fat/30 kcal; whipping cream 5.85 g fat/ 56 kcal; crème fraîche 6 g fat/58 kcal; double cream 7.2 g fat/67 kcal; clotted cream 9.45 g fat/88 kcal.

Yogurt – a better choice?
Yogurt is made by culturing milk with 'friendly' bacteria to thicken it (see page 184). Plain yogurt makes an excellent alternative to cream,

both as an accompaniment for fruit desserts and as an ingredient, but it's important to remember that yogurts contain differing amounts of fat and calories. To help you choose, these are the fat and calories for 1 level tablespoon of different yogurts: fat-free yogurt 0 g fat/7.5 kcal; low-fat plain yogurt 0.12 g fat/8 kcal; low-fat bio yogurt 0.12 g fat/10 kcal; whole milk plain yogurt 0.45 g fat/12 kcal; 'lite' Greek-style yogurt 0.75 g fat/12 kcal; Greek-style yogurt 1.35 g fat/17 kcal.

Frozen yogurt is a delicious lower-fat alternative to ice-cream. But it does contain a lot of sugar, and thus is high in calories.

The best of both
Whip a little whipping cream until stiff, then whip in the same amount of plain low-fat yogurt. Sweeten with a little honey or icing sugar and flavour with a few drops of pure vanilla extract, if liked.

Fruit coulis

Coulis are basically very simple fruit purées, made with raw or cooked fruit, sweetened if necessary. Coulis made with raw fruit will retain more of the vitamin C content, which is otherwise reduced through even the briefest cooking. Almost any soft fruit can be used for an uncooked coulis – kiwi, blackberries, peach, mango and papaya, to name just a few.

Berry coulis (uncooked)

Makes 200 ml (7 fl oz), to serve 4 with a dessert

125 g (4½ oz) raspberries
125 g (4½ oz) strawberries, sliced
1 tbsp fresh lemon juice or 1–2 tbsp kirsch
1 tbsp icing or caster sugar, or to taste

Preparation time: 10 minutes

1 In a bowl, mash the berries with a fork. Mix in the lemon juice and sugar. Alternatively, purée the fruit with the lemon juice and sugar in a food processor or blender.

2 Spoon the mixture into a fine nylon sieve placed over a bowl. Press the fruit through the sieve using a large spoon or spatula. Chill the coulis before serving.

Currant coulis (cooked)

Makes 200 ml (7 fl oz), to serve 4 with a dessert

125 g (4½ oz) redcurrants, stalks removed
125 g (4½ oz) blackcurrants, stalks removed
50 g (1¾ oz) sugar, or to taste
orange or lemon juice or crème de cassis (optional)

Preparation time: 15 minutes
Cooking time: 5 minutes

1 Place the fruit in a medium saucepan with the sugar. Cook over a low heat, stirring occasionally, until the sugar dissolves. The fruit should be soft with the juices running from it. Taste and add more sugar if necessary.

2 Press the fruit through a sieve as for the berry coulis. Taste and, if you like, sharpen the flavour with a little orange or lemon juice, or add crème de cassis for a sweeter flavour.

Some more ideas

• Gooseberries can be prepared in the same way. Use 250 g (9 oz) topped and tailed fruit and add 2 fresh elderberry flowerheads or 2 tbsp elderflower cordial and a little water to cook with the fruit. Serve with desserts or ice-cream. Or add less sugar and serve with cooked mackerel.

• For rhubarb coulis, use 250 g (9 oz) fruit, sweeten with sugar or honey and flavour with ground ginger.

• Make quick coulis with fruit canned in natural juice.

• Dried fruit (soaked to plump if needed), used alone or in combination with fresh fruit, make delicious coulis. Cook the dried fruit if necessary before puréeing.

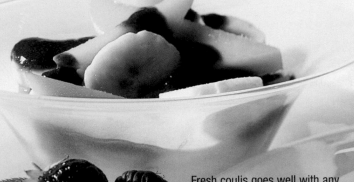

Fresh coulis goes well with any kind of fruit salad. You can liven up a milk pudding with currant coulis or serve fresh mango and banana with berry coulis.

Grilled fruit brochettes

Cooking fruit on skewers, just long enough to heat the fruit through and slightly caramelise its sugars, is an easy and fun way of enjoying fresh fruit. If you are having a barbecue, cook the fruit brochettes over the charcoal fire – but take care not to char the fruit or leave it too long in the smoke.

Serves 4

½ medium-sized ripe pineapple

2 just ripe, firm bananas

2 ripe but firm pears

4 ripe but firm fresh figs

2 ripe but firm peaches

juice of 1 lemon

4 tsp sugar

cape gooseberries to decorate

Raspberry-orange coulis

225 g (8 oz) raspberries

grated zest and juice of ½ orange

1½ tbsp sugar, or to taste

Preparation time: 20 minutes

Cooking time: 6–7 minutes

Each serving provides   Ⓥ

kcal 220, protein 3 g, fat 1 g (of which saturated fat 0.2 g), carbohydrate 54 g (of which sugars 53 g), fibre 7 g

✓✓✓ C
✓   B₁, niacin, copper, potassium

1 Soak 8 bamboo skewers in cold water for 20 minutes.

2 Meanwhile, make the coulis. Purée the raspberries with the orange zest and juice and the sugar in a blender or food processor. If you like, sieve the purée to remove the raspberry pips. Taste the coulis and add a little more sugar, if necessary. Set aside.

3 Preheat the grill. Prepare the pineapple, bananas, pears, figs and peaches, peeling as necessary and cutting into attractive bite-sized pieces. Thread the fruit onto the soaked skewers, alternating them to make a colourful arrangement.

4 Sprinkle the kebabs with half of the lemon juice and sugar. Grill them for 3–4 minutes or until lightly tinged with brown, then turn over, sprinkle with the remaining lemon juice and sugar and grill for a further 3 minutes or until the second side is lightly browned and caramelised a little.

5 While the kebabs are being grilled, pull back the papery skins on the cape gooseberries to form a star-like flower round the fruit.

6 Place 2 fruit kebabs on each plate, drizzle round the coulis, decorate with cape gooseberries and serve hot.

Some more ideas

- Use nectarines instead of peaches.
- Use apples when peaches are not in season.
- Serve the fruit kebabs raw, just the fresh fruit skewers resting in a pool of the coulis.

Plus points

- This delicious recipe provides useful amounts of important antioxidant vitamins – plenty of vitamin C from the raspberries and the orange and lemon juices, and vitamin A converted from the beta-carotene in the peaches. As the fruit is heated for only a very short time, most of the vitamin C is retained.
- There is plenty of dietary fibre – both soluble and insoluble – in this array of fruit, and this is essential to keep the digestive tract healthy. Insoluble fibre provides bulk and prevents constipation. The soluble fibre found in fruit can be fermented by bacteria in the gut, producing substances that help to protect against bowel cancer.

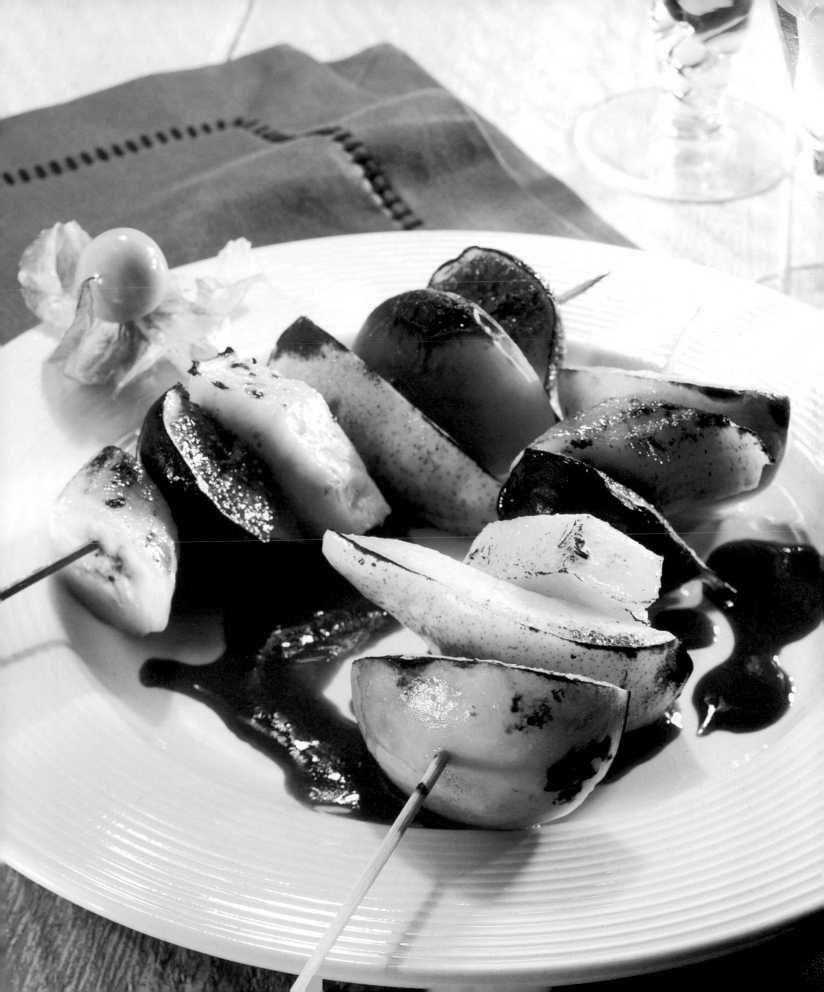

Exotic fruit salad

This simple but very special fruit salad is just bursting with the wonderful colours and fragrance of exotic fruits – papaya, mango, kiwi fruit and passion fruit. It's rich in vitamins too, making a delightfully refreshing and nutritious end to a meal. Arrange the fruit on a platter or mix together in a pretty bowl.

Serves 4

1 large papaya
1 large mango
2 kiwi fruit
6 tbsp orange juice
2 tbsp lime juice
2 passion fruit

Preparation time: 15 minutes

1 Peel and halve the papaya and scoop out the seeds. Slice the fruit crossways and arrange the slices in 2 rows on a serving platter, or cut into chunks and put into a large serving bowl.

2 Stone and peel the mango and cut lengthways into wedges. Arrange the wedges in a row between the papaya slices. Or cut into chunks and add to the serving bowl.

3 Peel the kiwi fruit and cut lengthways into wedges or chunks. Scatter them over the slices of mango and papaya.

4 Mix the orange juice with the lime juice. Halve the passion fruit and scoop out the seeds and pulp into the juice mixture. Spoon over the salad and serve immediately.

Some more ideas

- Instead of using orange juice, make a syrup. Put 2 tbsp sugar in a small saucepan with 6 tbsp water and dissolve it over a low heat, then bring to the boil and boil for 2 minutes. Remove from the heat and add the lime juice. Allow the syrup to cool while preparing the fruit.
- For an orange, kiwi and strawberry salad, peel 2 oranges and cut into segments, holding them over a bowl to catch the juice. Mix the segments with 2 kiwi fruit, cut into wedges, and 280 g (10 oz) strawberries, halved or sliced if large. Warm the juice from segmenting the oranges (about 4 tbsp) with 2 tbsp maple syrup or honey until just combined, then cool. Add a handful of freshly torn basil leaves, and drizzle over the fruit.
- Sprinkle the salad with 2 tbsp toasted coconut shreds.
- Instead of the papaya and mango, use a small melon, such as Ogen, and about 400 g (14 oz) peeled pineapple.

Each serving provides
kcal 120, protein 2 g, fat 0.5 g (of which saturated fat 0 g), carbohydrate 27 g (of which sugars 19 g), fibre 5 g

✓✓✓	C
✓✓	A, B_6, potassium

Plus points

- Mango, papaya, kiwi and passion fruit are all excellent sources of vitamin C. An average slice of papaya provides more than double the recommended daily requirement of vitamin C, and the mango provides 6 times the daily requirement of vitamin C.
- All the fruits in this salad provide a wealth of phytochemicals that help to protect against excessive free radical attack, which may spark off degenerative diseases.
- As well as being an excellent source of vitamin C and beta-carotene, mango provides useful amounts of vitamin B_6.

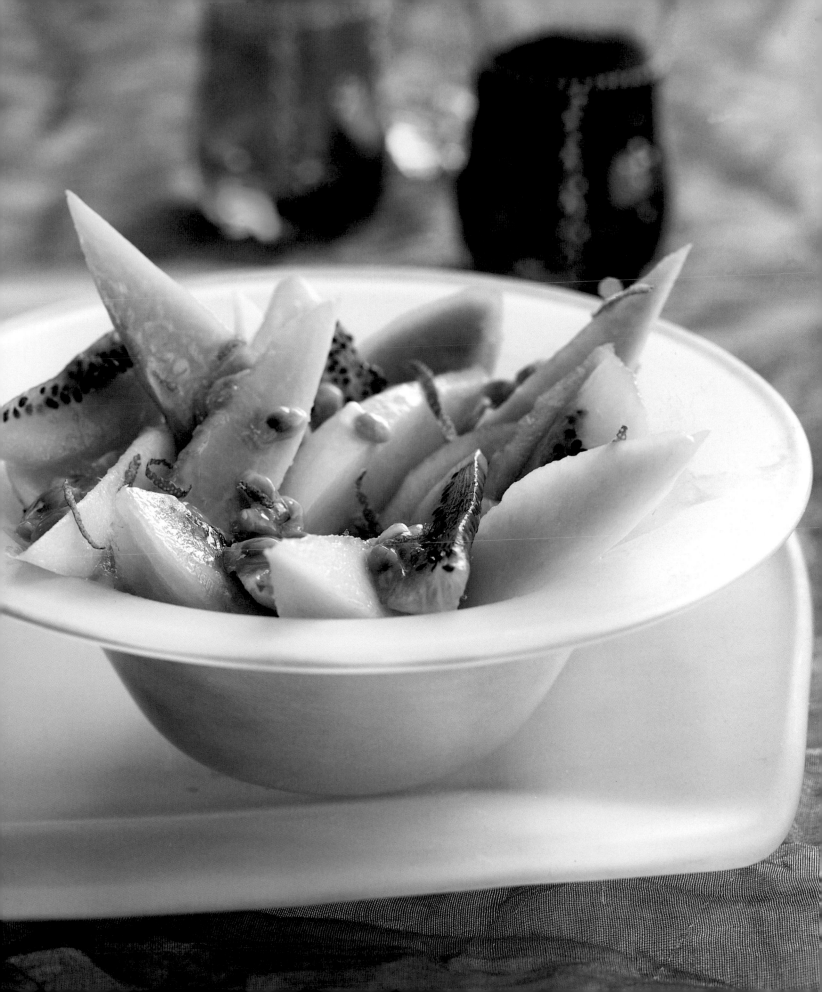

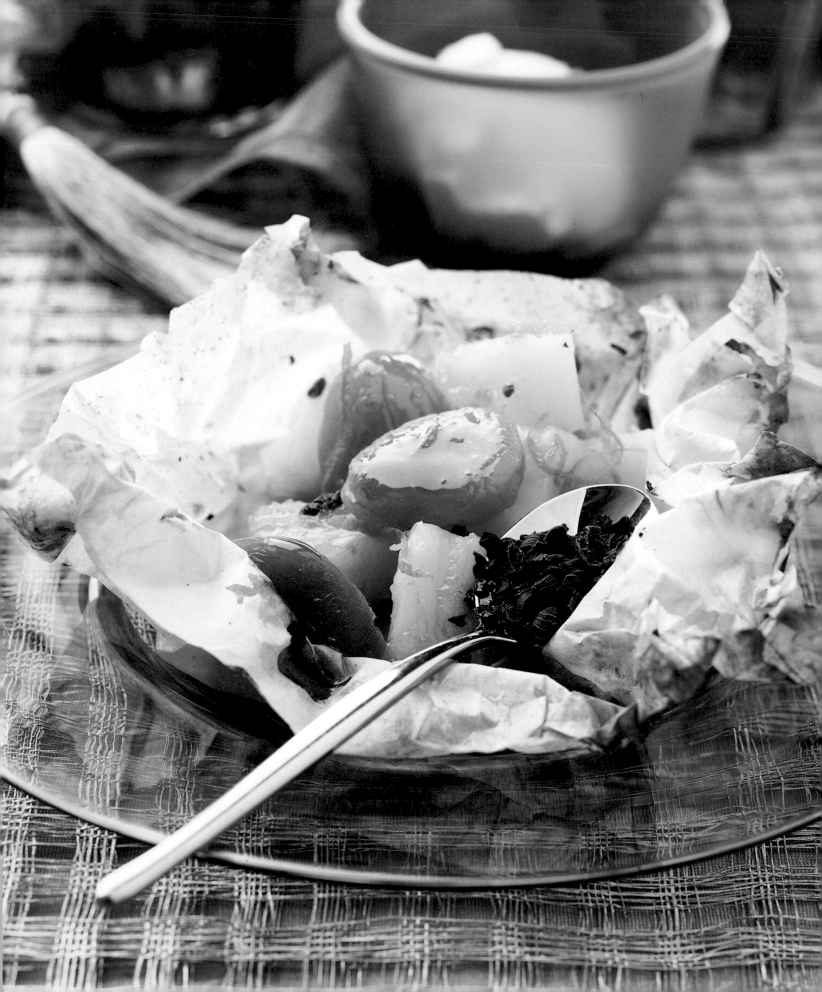

Hot fruity parcels

Baking fruit in paper parcels is a brilliant way of sealing in all the flavour and preserving the precious nutrients. It also makes a novel presentation method and saves on washing up! Serve this delicious fruity treat of fresh pineapple and dried apricots with a dollop of Greek-style yogurt or crème fraîche.

Serves 4

1 ripe pineapple

12 ready-to-eat dried apricots

2 tsp cardamom pods

grated zest of 1 orange

4 tbsp orange juice

4 tsp clear honey

55 g (2 oz) good plain chocolate (at least 70% cocoa solids), grated

Preparation time: 10 minutes

Cooking time: 20 minutes

1 Preheat the oven to 200°C (400°F, gas mark 6). Cut 4 sheets of baking parchment or greaseproof paper, each measuring about 30 cm (12 in) square.

2 Peel the pineapple and cut out the core. Cut the flesh into slices and then into cubes. Divide the cubes among the squares of paper and add 3 apricots to each one. Crush the cardamom pods and extract the seeds. Add to the parcels. Sprinkle over the orange zest and juice, and drizzle 1 tsp honey on top of each.

3 Wrap the paper loosely round the fruit, enclosing it completely, and seal tightly. Place the parcels on a baking tray and bake for 20 minutes.

4 Place the parcels on individual serving plates and unwrap them. Sprinkle grated chocolate into each parcel and serve.

85 g (3 oz) sweetened dried cranberries. Add a piece of cinnamon stick to each parcel in place of the cardamom seeds. Bake for about 15 minutes. After cooking, unwrap the parcels and sprinkle a few chopped walnuts over instead of the chocolate.

● For a special occasion, spoon 1 tsp brandy, Cointreau or Grand Marnier into each parcel in place of the orange juice and serve with good-quality vanilla ice cream.

● The parcels, made using foil instead of parchment or greaseproof paper, can be cooked on a barbecue for 5 minutes.

Each serving provides Ⓥ

kcal 230, protein 3 g, fat 4 g (of which saturated fat 2 g), carbohydrate 48 g (of which sugars 48 g), fibre 5 g

✓✓✓	C
✓✓	B₁, B₆, copper, potassium
✓	B₂, folate

Some more ideas

● Save time by using a tub of ready-sliced fresh pineapple in pineapple juice, about 350 g, drained.

● The fruit can be varied according to what is in season or what you have available. For example, instead of apricots use halved strawberries or thickly sliced firm bananas.

● For pear and cranberry parcels, use 4 peeled, cored and quartered ripe dessert pears and

Plus points

● Dried apricots are one of the richest fruit sources of iron. They also provide useful amounts of vitamin A (derived from beta-carotene) and fibre.

● Pineapple contains an enzyme called bromelin, which aids digestion. It is also a good source of vitamin C.

Baked almond-stuffed peaches

Baking fruit brings out its flavour wonderfully, and a stuffing is a simple way of making baked fruit special. Here peaches are filled with a mixture of dried apricots, almonds and amaretti biscuits. Many other fruits – nectarines, apples, pears or quinces – can be prepared in the same way, to ring the seasonal changes.

Serves 4

5 large ripe but firm peaches

10 ready-to-eat dried apricots, finely diced

6 amaretti biscuits, crumbled

2 tsp pure almond extract

1 tbsp brandy

1 egg white

55 g (2 oz) whole blanched almonds

Preparation time: 20 minutes

Cooking time: about 40 minutes

Each serving (fruit alone) provides ⓥ
kcal 200, protein 6 g, fat 9 g (of which saturated fat 1 g), carbohydrate 24 g (of which sugars 21 g), fibre 5 g

✓✓	C, E
✓	B$_2$, niacin, copper, potassium

1 Preheat the oven to 180°C (350°F, gas mark 4).

2 Cut the peaches in half and remove the stones. Arrange 8 of the halves, cut side up, in a shallow baking dish. Set aside. Finely dice the remaining 2 peach halves.

3 Combine the diced peach with the dried apricots, crumbled amaretti, almond extract, brandy and egg white. Stir to mix thoroughly.

4 Heat a small heavy ungreased frying pan and lightly toast the almonds, turning and tossing every so often, until they are lightly browned in spots. Remove and coarsely chop, in a food processor or by hand, to make a mixture of small chunks of nuts and ground nuts.

5 Add the chopped almonds to the fruit and amaretti mixture and mix well. Use to fill the hollows in the peach halves, heaping up the filling and pressing it gently together. Cover the baking dish with a tent of cooking foil.

6 Bake for 25–30 minutes, then remove the foil. Increase the oven temperature to 200°C (400°F, gas mark 6) and bake for a further 5–10 minutes or until the nutty topping is lightly browned. The peaches are best when warm, but they can be chilled before serving.

Some more ideas

• Nectarines can be used instead of peaches, with pistachios instead of almonds.

• Macaroons can be used instead of amaretti, but fewer according to size.

• For baked stuffed apples or pears, substitute sultanas for the diced dried apricots and add a few shakes of ground cinnamon to the filling. Allow 10 minutes longer baking time before removing the foil covering.

• Use quinces instead of peaches, allowing 15 minutes extra baking time.

• Use a mixture of peaches or nectarines, apples, pears and quinces, and make the filling from a mixture of these fruit. Allow 10–15 minutes extra baking time.

Plus points

• Peaches contain plenty of vitamin C (31 mg per 100 g/3½ oz) and this can help the body to absorb iron present in other foods – in this case from dried apricots. Iron deficiency anaemia is probably the most common deficiency disease in the UK, so every little bit helps. Dried apricots also provide vitamin A and plenty of potassium for regulating blood pressure.

• Almonds not only have a delicious and distinctive flavour, but also contain protein and plenty of vitamin E.

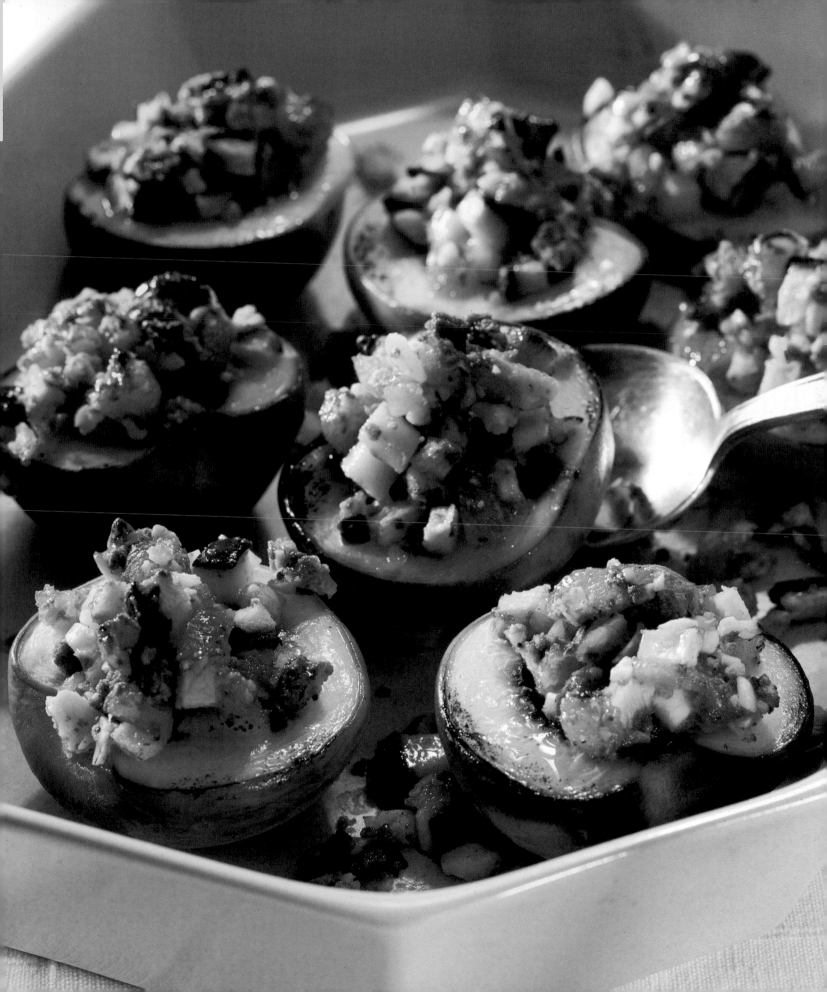

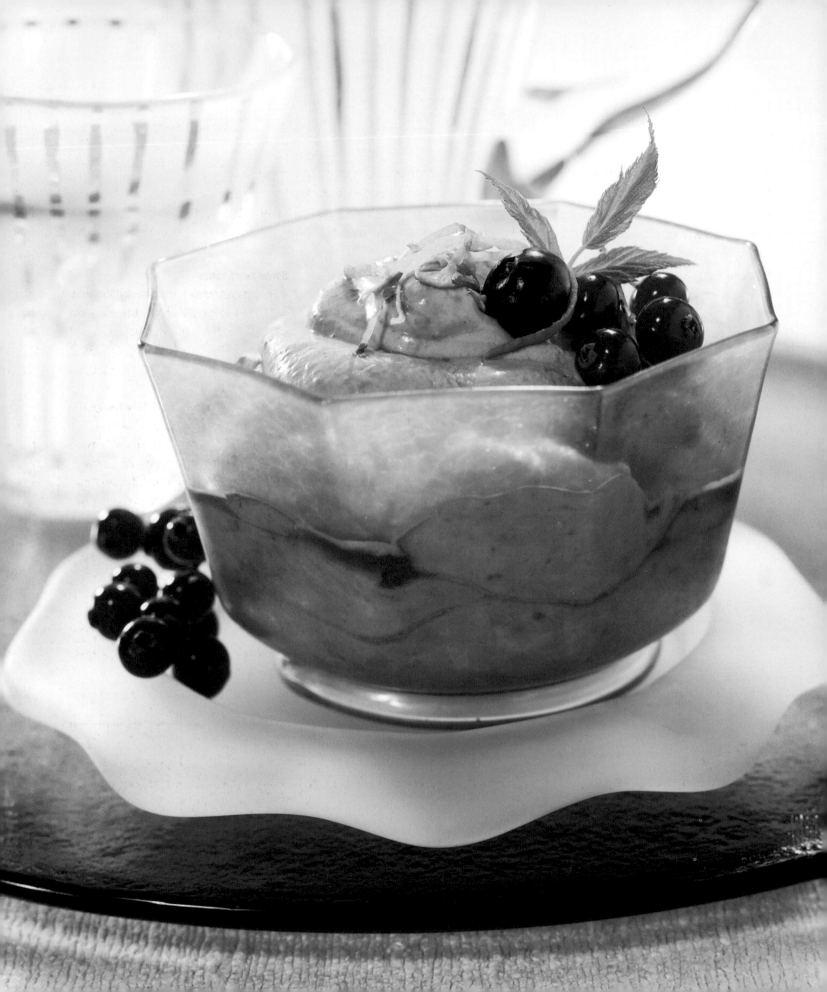

Summer fruit fool

A quick pudding to rustle up at a moment's notice, this can be made with almost any fruit in season. The usual whipped double cream in fruit fool is replaced here with a mixture of low-fat yogurt and whipping cream, yet despite the fat content being reduced, this is still a wonderfully rich and creamy dessert.

Serves 4

300 g (10½ oz) mixed soft fruit, such as raspberries, blackberries, blueberries or currants

55 g (2 oz) caster sugar

150 ml (5 fl oz) whipping cream

grated zest of ½ orange

150 g (5½ oz) plain low-fat bio yogurt

finely shredded orange zest to decorate (optional)

Preparation time: 20 minutes, plus cooling and chilling

1 Reserve about 55 g (2 oz) of the mixed fruit for decoration. Put the remaining mixed fruit in a saucepan with 2 tbsp water. Bring just to the boil, then reduce the heat and cook gently for 5 minutes or until soft and very juicy. Stir in the sugar.

2 Remove from the heat and leave to cool slightly. Pour into a food processor or blender and purée. Press the purée through a sieve to remove all the pips. Alternatively, just press the fruit through a sieve to purée it. Set aside to cool completely.

3 Whip the cream with the grated orange zest until thick. Add the yogurt and lightly whip into the cream, then mix in the cooled fruit purée.

4 Spoon into dessert dishes or goblets. Chill well before serving, decorated with the reserved berries and orange zest, if using.

Some more ideas

- For gooseberry fool, replace the soft fruit with 450 g (1 lb) gooseberries (don't reserve any for decoration) and increase the caster sugar to 115 g (4 oz). Cook the gooseberries for about 15 minutes or until softened. This gooseberry fool will serve 6.

- For a strawberry fool, slice 225 g (8 oz) ripe strawberries, reserving 4 whole ones for decoration, and sprinkle with the sugar. Leave for 30 minutes or until the juices are running from the fruit, then purée. Add to the cream and yogurt mixture. Serve decorated with the reserved strawberries, quartered or sliced.

- For a guava fool, roughly chop 225 g (8 oz) ripe guavas, with their skins, and purée in a food processor or blender with 45 g (1½ oz) sugar. Press through a sieve, then taste the purée and add a little more sugar if it isn't sweet enough. Fold into the cream and yogurt mixture with 1 tbsp orange liqueur. Guava is an excellent source of vitamin C.

Each serving provides

kcal 230, protein 3 g, fat 15 g (of which saturated fat 9 g), carbohydrate 22 g (of which sugars 22 g), fibre 2 g

✓✓✓	C
✓✓	A
✓	B₂, calcium

Plus points

- Yogurt is a good source of calcium. Throughout life, but particularly during adolescence and pregnancy, it is important for women to get enough calcium to keep bones healthy and prevent osteoporosis later.
- The mixed soft fruit are all rich in the antioxidant vitamin C, and their natural acidity helps to prevent the loss of this vitamin during the cooking. To retain as much vitamin C as possible, the sugar is added after the fruit is softened.

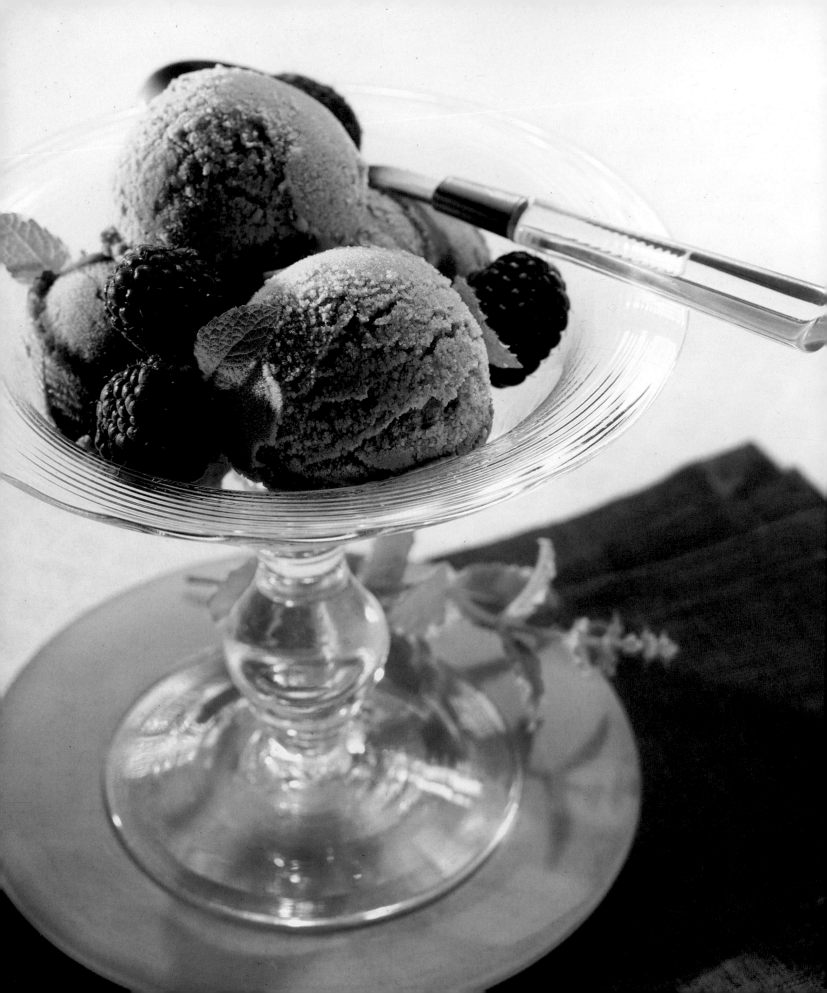

Raspberry frozen yogurt

This frozen yogurt, exotically flavoured with rosewater and crème de cassis, is much lower in sugar than bought frozen yogurt. Serve scoops on their own, or pile into sundae glasses with fresh fruit and sprigs of mint.

Serves 8

500 g (1 lb 2 oz) raspberries

4 tbsp seedless raspberry jam

2 tbsp rosewater

2 tbsp crème de cassis (optional)

500 g (1 lb 2 oz) Greek-style yogurt

3 tbsp icing sugar, or to taste

To decorate (optional)

raspberries

fresh mint leaves

Preparation time: 15–20 minutes, plus freezing (varies according to method used)

Each serving provides ⓥ

kcal 140, protein 5 g, fat 6 g (of which saturated fat 3 g), carbohydrate 19 g (of which sugars 19 g), fibre 2 g

✓✓	C
✓	folate, calcium

1 Put the raspberries into a saucepan and add the raspberry jam. Warm over a low heat for about 5 minutes or until the raspberries are pulpy, stirring occasionally.

2 Press the raspberries and their juice through a nylon sieve into a bowl; discard the pips in the sieve. Stir in the rosewater and the crème de cassis, if using. Whisk in the yogurt until smoothly blended. Taste the mixture and sweeten with the icing sugar.

3 Pour into an ice-cream machine and freeze according to the manufacturer's instructions. When you have a smooth and creamy frozen mixture, spoon it into a rigid freezerproof container. Freeze for at least 1 hour. If you do not have an ice-cream machine, pour the mixture straight into a large freezerproof container and freeze for 1 hour or until set round the edges. Beat until the mixture is smooth, then return to the freezer. Freeze for 30 minutes, then beat again. Repeat the freezing and beating several times more until the frozen yogurt has a smooth consistency, then leave it to freeze for at least 1 hour.

4 If storing in the freezer for longer than 1 hour, transfer the frozen yogurt to the fridge 20 minutes before serving, to soften slightly. Decorate with raspberries and mint, if liked.

Some more ideas

• Use frozen raspberries instead of fresh.

• For a frozen yogurt flavoured with mango and orange-flower water, replace the raspberries and jam with 2 cans mangoes, 425 g each, drained and puréed, and use orange-flower water and Cointreau instead of the rosewater and cassis. There should be no need to sweeten the mixture. Mangoes are an excellent source of beta-carotene, which the body can convert into vitamin A.

Plus points

• Although Greek-style yogurt is regarded as extremely rich and creamy-tasting, it is surprising to find that it has just 17 kcal per level tbsp, while double cream has an amazing 67 kcal for the same amount.

• Raspberries are an excellent source of vitamin C, whether fresh or frozen. If freshly picked there may be more C, but it is not always easy to tell how long fruit has been sitting on the shelf, and vitamin C content will be going down steadily following picking. Frozen fruits are usually processed immediately after picking and may therefore be a richer source of this vital vitamin.

Fragrant mango cream in brandy-snap baskets

What could be quicker than luscious fresh fruit blended with Greek-style yogurt and lemon curd, spooned into ready-made brandy-snap baskets? This is a really special, creamy treat.

Serves 6

1 large ripe mango
2 passion fruit
2 tbsp good-quality lemon curd
300 g (10½ oz) Greek-style yogurt
6 brandy-snap baskets
1 tbsp chopped pistachio nuts
fresh mint leaves to decorate

Preparation time: 15 minutes

Each serving provides Ⓥ

kcal 220, protein 5 g, fat 11 g (of which saturated fat 3 g), carbohydrate 26 g (of which sugars 22 g), fibre 2 g

✓✓✓	C
✓✓	A
✓	B₂, B₁₂, calcium

1 Cut the peel from the mango and slice the flesh from the flat stone. Place half the mango flesh in a food processor or blender and process briefly until smooth. Spoon into a bowl. Chop the remaining mango flesh into pieces and set aside.

2 Cut the passion fruit in half and scoop out the seeds and pulp into the mango purée. Stir in the lemon curd. Add the yogurt and fold everything together until well combined.

3 Spoon the fruit and yogurt cream into the brandy-snap baskets and top with the chopped mango. Scatter a few chopped pistachio nuts over the top of each serving and decorate with fresh mint leaves. Serve immediately.

Some more ideas

● Orange curd, which is becoming more widely available, makes a delicious alternative to lemon curd.

● Substitute a papaya for the mango.

● For a raspberry and chocolate cream on panettone, add 2 tbsp chopped toasted hazelnuts and 4 tbsp chocolate ice cream sauce to 300 g (10½ oz) Greek-style yogurt, and swirl together until the chocolate sauce has marbled the yogurt. Cut 3 long slices of dried fruit panettone in half and toast under the grill until golden. Spoon the chocolate cream over the panettone and scatter on 125 g (4½ oz) fresh raspberries. Dust lightly with icing sugar and serve decorated with fresh mint leaves.

● Slice 2 bananas and divide them among the brandy-snap baskets. Top with the chocolate and hazelnut cream above and finish with a fine drizzle of warm chocolate sauce.

Plus points

● Greek-style yogurt tastes luxurious, but has a fraction of the fat and calories of double cream: double cream contains 449 kcal and 48 g fat per 100 g (3½ oz), while the same weight of Greek-style yogurt has just 115 kcal and 9 g fat.

● The ancient Indians believed that mangoes helped to increase sexual desire and prolong love-making. Whether or not this is true, mangoes are rich in carotenoid compounds and vitamin C, both antioxidants that can help to protect against damage by free radicals. Mangoes also provide useful amounts of fibre and copper.

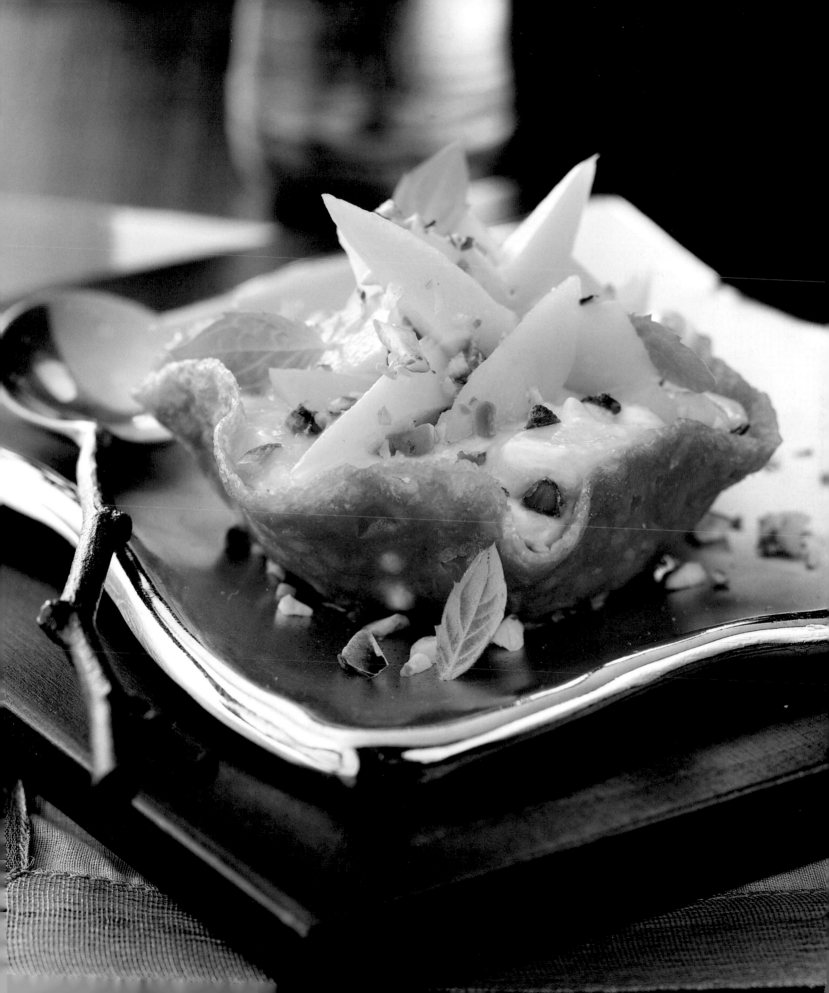

Summer pudding

What an amazing dish the British summer pudding is – simplicity itself, and as perfect as a midsummer's day. The peaches or nectarines add a slightly different dimension to this version, a marvellous way of eating a nice large portion of ripe fresh fruit, not cooked at all so as to retain all its nutrients.

Serves 6

600 g (1 lb 5 oz) mixed summer fruit
   (raspberries, blueberries, redcurrants,
   sliced strawberries)
2 ripe peaches or nectarines, stoned
   and diced
3 tbsp sugar, or to taste
150 ml (5 fl oz) cranberry juice
8 thin slices white bread, about 200 g (7 oz)
   in total, preferably 1–2 days old

To serve (optional)
reduced-fat crème fraîche

Preparation time: 20 minutes, plus 2 hours
   macerating and 8 hours chilling

Each serving (fruit alone) provides Ⓥ
kcal 130, protein 2 g, fat 0.5 g,
carbohydrate 30 g (of which sugars 26 g),
fibre 2 g

✓✓✓	C
✓	folate, potassium

1 Crush the different types of fruit individually, to be sure all the skins are broken and the fruit is pulpy. Put all the fruit in a large bowl with the sugar and cranberry juice and stir to mix. Leave to macerate for 2 hours.

2 Cut the crusts from the bread and cut the slices into strips or triangles. Fit the bread into a 1 litre (2 pint) pudding basin to line the bottom and sides, reserving enough bread to cover the top. Fill in any gaps with small bits of bread.

3 Reserve 3–4 tbsp of juice from the mixed fruit, then gently pour the fruit mixture into the bread-lined pudding basin. Top with the remaining bread. Cover with a plate that just fits inside the rim of the basin, setting it directly on top of the bread, and then place a heavy weight such as a can of food on top. Place the basin in the fridge to chill for 8 hours or overnight.

4 To serve, turn the pudding out onto a serving dish. Use the reserved fruit juice to brush or pour over any parts of the bread that have not been coloured. Serve with crème fraîche, if liked.

Some more ideas

• Use an enriched bread such as Jewish challah or brioche instead of white bread.
• For an autumn pudding, substitute raisin bread for white bread, and instead of the summer fruits and peaches, use 2 large dessert apples, diced, 2 pears, diced, 30 g (1 oz) sultanas, 30 g (1 oz) dried cranberries and 50 g (1¾ oz) dried apricots, chopped. Put the fruit in a saucepan with 300 ml (10 fl oz) apple juice and ½ tsp ground cinnamon. Bring to the boil, then poach gently for 5–7 minutes or until the apples are tender. Pour into the bread-lined mould and weight as in step 3. Serve decorated with diced sharon fruit and/or a scattering of pomegranate seeds, if you like.

Plus points

• Raspberries, redcurrants and strawberries are an excellent source of vitamin C (blueberries are a good source). This vitamin is not only an antioxidant with an important role in preventing heart disease, but is also essential for good wound-healing and resistance to infections.
• Low in fat and high in carbohydrate and fibre, this is a delicious dessert in a diet for a healthy heart.

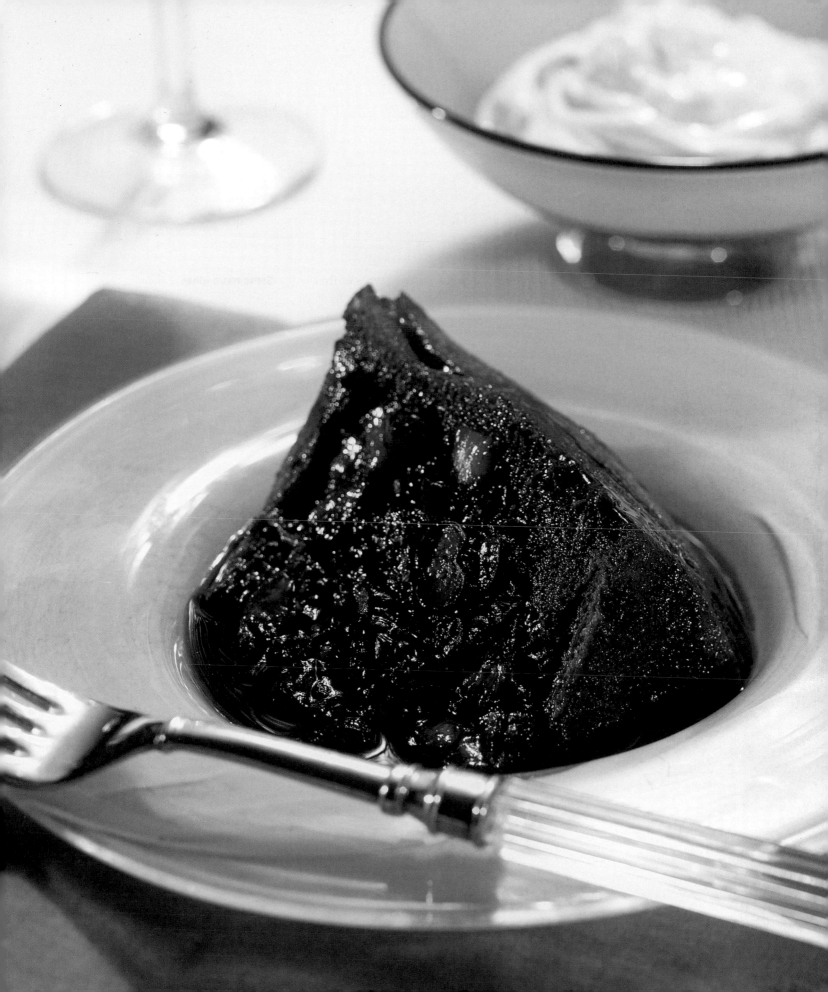

Raspberry and vanilla risotto

This sweet and creamy fruit risotto is a delicious way of introducing more grain into your diet, and can balance a meal when it follows a main course that does not contain much starchy carbohydrate. The fresh raspberries colour the pudding a lovely pale pink, as well as adding sweetness.

Serves 6

1 litre (1¾ pints) semi-skimmed milk

1 vanilla pod, split open in half

140 g (5 oz) risotto rice

1 strip lemon zest

3 tbsp golden caster sugar or light soft brown sugar

6 tbsp flaked almonds

200 g (7 oz) fresh raspberries

6 tbsp single cream

vanilla pods to decorate (optional)

Preparation and cooking time: 30 minutes

Each serving provides

kcal 320, protein 11 g, fat 14 g (of which saturated fat 4 g), carbohydrate 38 g (of which sugars 19 g), fibre 2 g

✓✓	C, E, calcium
✓	B₂, B₁₂, copper, iron, zinc

1 Pour the milk into a heavy-based saucepan and add the vanilla pod. Sprinkle in the rice, stirring constantly. Bring to the boil over a moderate heat, stirring, then reduce the heat so the mixture is gently simmering.

2 Add the lemon zest and sugar. Cook, stirring frequently, for 15–18 minutes or until the rice is suspended in the sauce and is tender, and the liquid is thick and creamy.

3 Meanwhile, put the almonds in a small non-stick frying pan and toast over a low heat for 4–5 minutes or until they are lightly browned.

4 When the risotto has finished cooking, remove the vanilla pod and lemon zest. Stir in half of the raspberries. Remove from the heat and continue stirring for 1–2 minutes or until the fruit softens and begins to turn the risotto pink.

5 Spoon the raspberry risotto into 6 warmed bowls and drizzle 1 tbsp cream over each serving. Sprinkle the almonds over the top and add the remaining berries. Decorate with vanilla pods, if wished, and serve at once – the risotto thickens as it cools.

Another idea

• Make a sweet pudding with quinoa, an ancient grain used by the Incas. Available from healthfood shops, quinoa is rich in nutrients and has a high amino acid content. Rinse 125 g (4½ oz) quinoa and drain well, then toast in a frying pan, without any fat, for about 4 minutes, stirring frequently. It will become a deeper golden colour and pop regularly. Sprinkle the quinoa into the hot milk (heated without the vanilla pod), stirring. When the milk boils, reduce the heat so the mixture is bubbling very gently. Cover and cook for 10 minutes. Instead of flaked almonds, use 45 g (1½ oz) ground almonds and stir them into the quinoa. Continue cooking for about 20 minutes or until most of the milk has been absorbed, stirring occasionally. (The quinoa will retain a slight crunchy texture and have a lovely toasted flavour.) Stir in 1 tbsp clear honey with half of the raspberries, or serve them all on top of the pudding.

Plus point

• Almonds are a good source of vitamin E, which helps to protect against heart disease. They also contribute useful amounts of phosphorus, copper and magnesium.

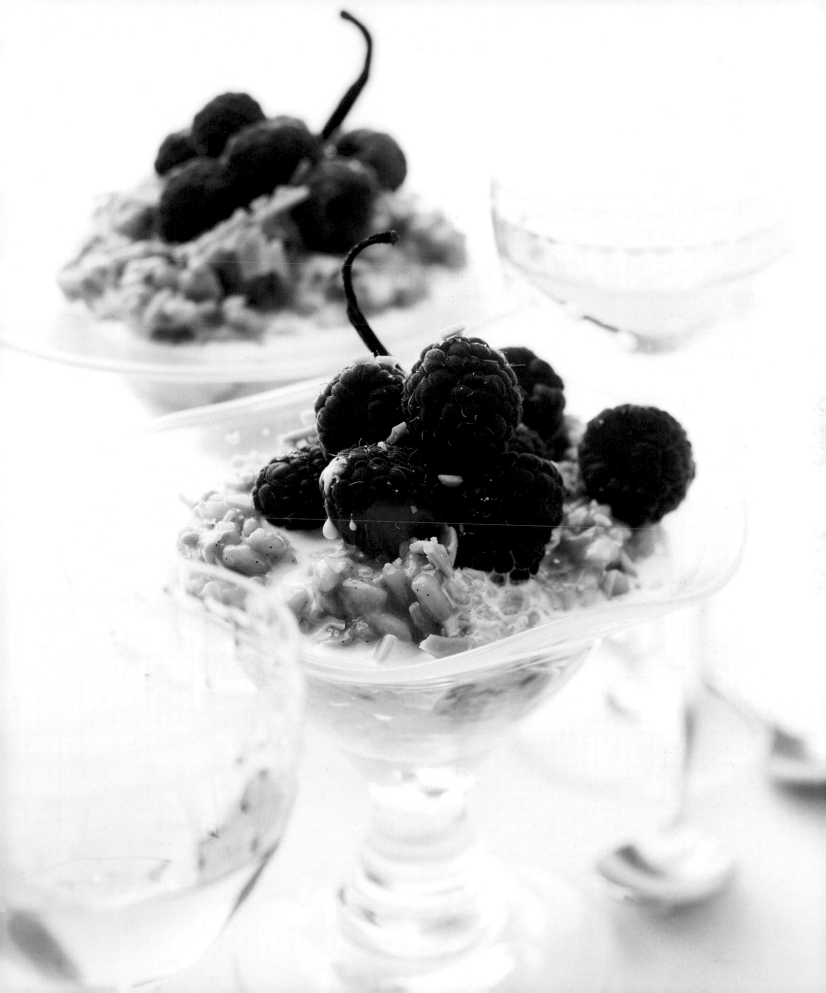

Cherry and almond strudel

Austria's famous melt-in-the-mouth pastry, here packed with juicy fresh cherries, looks very impressive, but is surprisingly easy to make. Ground almonds and breadcrumbs are added to the filling to absorb the fruit juices, so the layers of filo pastry bake wonderfully light and crisp.

Serves 6

3 sheets filo pastry, 30 x 50 cm (12 x 20 in) each, about 90 g (3¼ oz) in total

30 g (1 oz) butter, melted

15 g (½ oz) flaked almonds

1 tbsp icing sugar, sifted

Greek-style yogurt to serve (optional)

Cherry filling

30 g (1 oz) fresh white breadcrumbs

55 g (2 oz) ground almonds

45 g (1½ oz) soft light brown sugar

finely grated zest of 1 orange

675 g (1½ lb) fresh cherries, stoned and halved if large

Preparation time: 30–40 minutes

Cooking time: 20 minutes

Each serving provides Ⓥ

kcal 254, protein 5.5 g, fat 11 g (of which saturated fat 3 g), carbohydrate 36 g (of which sugars 24 g), fibre 2 g

✓✓	E
✓	C, copper

1 Preheat the oven to 200°C (400°F, gas mark 6). To make the filling, stir the breadcrumbs, almonds, brown sugar and orange zest together in a large bowl. Add the cherries and mix well.

2 Lay a sheet of filo pastry out on a clean tea-towel and brush very lightly with melted butter. Place a second sheet of filo on top and brush very lightly with butter. Place the third sheet of filo on top and brush again with butter.

3 Spoon the filling evenly over the stacked pastry, leaving a 2.5 cm (1 in) margin clear around the edges. Turn in the edges of the short sides.

4 With the help of the tea-towel, roll up from a long side to make a thick sausage shape. Transfer to a lightly greased, non-stick baking tray, curving the strudel slightly to fit, if necessary. The seam should be underneath. Brush with the remaining butter, then scatter over the flaked almonds.

5 Bake for 20 minutes or until the pastry and almonds are golden brown. Dust with the icing sugar and serve hot or warm, with a little Greek-style yogurt, if liked.

Another idea

• For a plum, rum and raisin strudel, soak 50 g (1¾ oz) raisins in 2 tbsp dark rum for 1 hour. Mix with 675 g (1½ lb) sliced ripe plums, 75 g (2½ oz) fresh white breadcrumbs, 30 g (1 oz) chopped walnuts, 45 g (1½ oz) soft light brown sugar and the finely grated zest of 1 small lemon. Spread this filling over the filo pastry, roll up and bake as in the main recipe. Dust the hot strudel with 2 tsp icing sugar sifted with ½ tsp ground cinnamon.

Plus points

• Cherries are used all over the world in many famous dishes as well as being a key ingredient in liqueurs such as Kirsch and Maraschino. Like other fruits they are rich in potassium and they also contain a small amount of iron.

• Almonds are a good source of vitamin E, a powerful antioxidant that helps to protect against heart disease.

• Butter contains useful amounts of the fat-soluble vitamins A and D. Vitamin A is needed for healthy skin and vision. Vitamin D is required for the absorption of calcium and therefore has a vital role in maintaining strong teeth and bones.

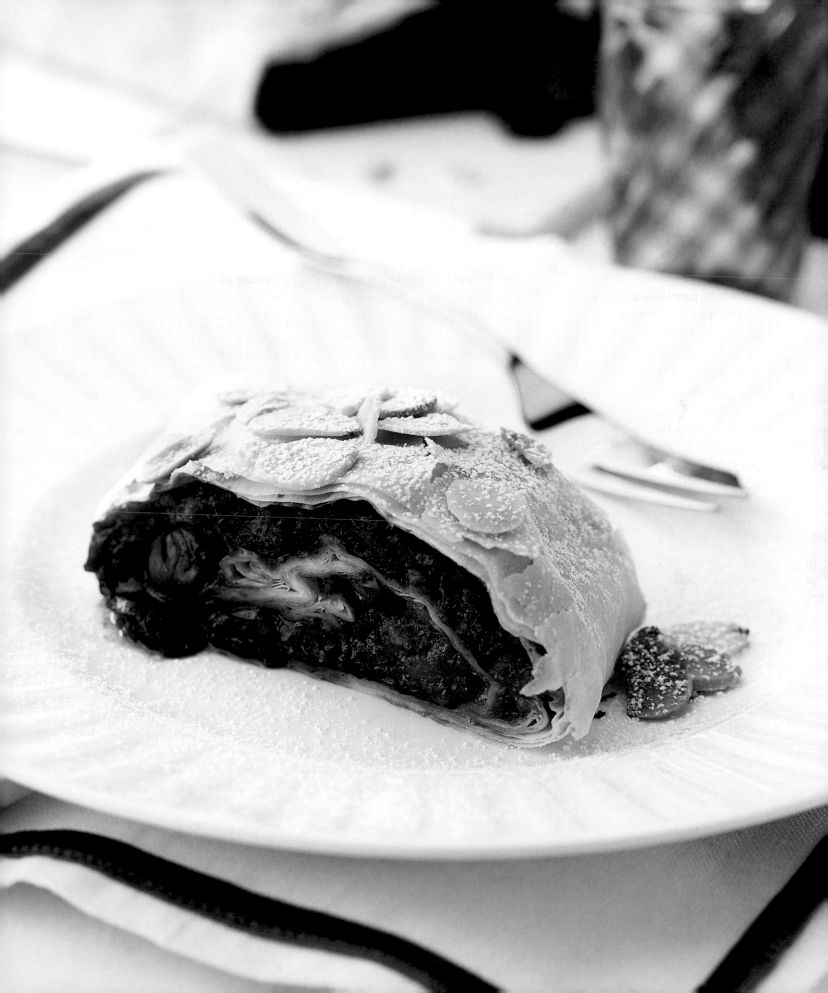

Spiced apple and blueberry pie

Here's the easiest fruit pie you could wish for – a crumbly, half wholemeal shortcrust pastry
simply wrapped around a spiced mixture of tangy apples and juicy blueberries,
to make a rough parcel with an open top. There's no flan tin to line or pie dish to cover,
so it's quick to make and looks sensational too.

Serves 6

Wholemeal shortcrust pastry
75 g (2½ oz) plain white flour
75 g (2½ oz) plain wholemeal flour
1b tsp ground mixed spice
75 g (2½ oz) cool unsalted butter, diced
30 g (1 oz) icing sugar, sifted
1 egg yolk

Apple and blueberry filling
550 g (1¼ lb) cooking apples
100 g (3½ oz) blueberries
45 g (1½ oz) light muscovado sugar
1 tsp ground cinnamon
½ tsp freshly grated nutmeg
1 egg white, whisked lightly to loosen

To serve (optional)
vanilla frozen yogurt or Greek-style yogurt

Preparation time: 20 minutes,
   plus at least 30 minutes chilling
Cooking time: 30–35 minutes

Each serving provides Ⓥ
kcal 261, protein 4 g, fat 12 g (of which
saturated fat 7 g), carbohydrate 38 g (of
which sugars 20 g), fibre 3 g

✓　A, C, copper, selenium

1 First make the pastry. Sift the white
and wholemeal flours and the spice
into a bowl, tipping in the bran left in
the sieve. Rub in the butter until the
mixture resembles fine breadcrumbs.
Stir in the sugar.

2 Mix the egg yolk with 1 tbsp cold
water, add to the flour mixture and
mix to form a soft dough, adding a few
drops more water if needed. Wrap the
dough in cling film and chill for at least
30 minutes.

3 Preheat the oven to 190°C (375°F,
gas mark 5). Peel and slice the
apples, and mix with the blueberries.
Stir together the sugar, cinnamon and
nutmeg. Reserve 1 tbsp of the mixture,
and stir the rest into the fruit.

4 Roll out the pastry dough thinly on
a non-stick baking sheet to make a
30 cm (12 in) round. Brush the dough
all over with egg white.

5 Pile the fruit mixture in the middle
of the pastry round, then draw up
the sides over the fruit, but leaving the
centre open. Brush the outside of the
case with the remaining egg white and
sprinkle with the reserved spiced sugar.

6 Bake for 30–35 minutes or until the
pastry is golden brown and the
apples are tender. Serve warm, with
vanilla frozen yogurt or Greek-style
yogurt, if liked.

Some more ideas
• For a pastry with more texture, roll out the
dough on a surface lightly sprinkled with fine
oatmeal.
• Make a deep dish apple and blackberry pie.
Replace the blueberries with blackberries, and
sprinkle the fruit with the sugar and 1 tsp
ground allspice. Place the fruit in a deep 23 cm
(9 in) pie dish. Brush the rim with water. Roll out
the pastry dough to a round or oval to cover the
dish. Lay the dough over the filling and press
the edges to the rim to seal. Crimp the edges.
Brush the pastry lid with egg white, and sprinkle
with ½ tsp caster sugar and a pinch of allspice.
Bake in a preheated 190°C (375°F, gas mark 5)
oven for 30–35 minutes or until golden brown.

Plus points
• Blueberries are rich in vitamin C and
beta-carotene, both powerful antioxidants
that help to mop up free radicals before
they can do harm to cells in the body.
• Apples provide good amounts of
potassium and of soluble fibre in the form
of pectin.
• Combining wholemeal flour with white
flour increases the fibre content without
making the pie crust too heavy.

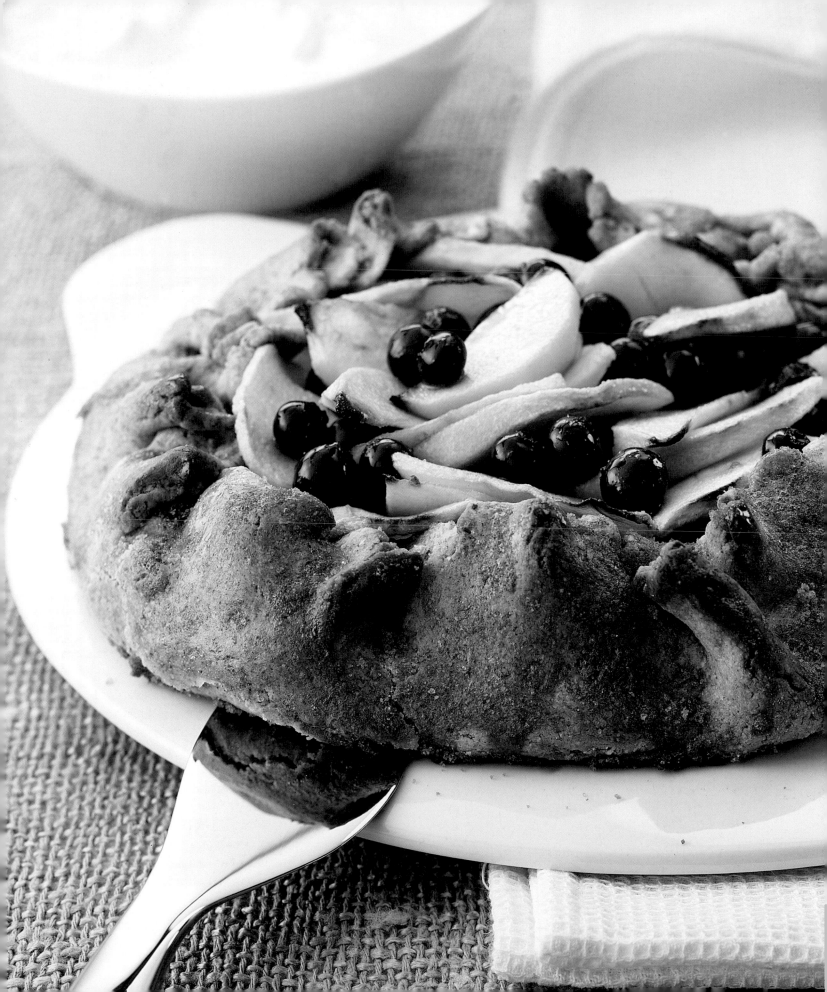

Fragrant gooseberry crumble

Crumbles are always a family favourite and gooseberries are one of the best fruit choices, as their slight tartness partners particularly well with a sweet crumble topping. Here, the flavour of the gooseberries is enhanced with fragrant elderflower cordial and fresh mint, and the crumble topping has oats, hazelnuts and wheatgerm added.

Serves 6

1 kg (2¼ lb) gooseberries, topped
 and tailed

2 sprigs of fresh mint

2 tbsp elderflower cordial

50 g (1¾ oz) caster sugar, or to taste

Crumble topping

55 g (2 oz) plain white flour

30 g (1 oz) plain wholemeal flour

55 g (2 oz) cool unsalted butter, diced

55 g (2 oz) light soft brown sugar

30 g (1 oz) jumbo oats

30 g (1 oz) hazelnuts, chopped

2 tbsp wheatgerm

Preparation time: 25 minutes
Cooking time: 20–25 minutes

1 Preheat the oven to 200°C (400°F, gas mark 6). Put the gooseberries in a saucepan with the mint sprigs and elderflower cordial. Cover and cook over a very low heat for 8–10 minutes or until the gooseberries start to soften and release their juices.

2 Stir in the caster sugar until it has dissolved, then transfer to a deep 1.7 litre (3 pint) baking dish, discarding the mint sprigs.

3 Sift the white and wholemeal flours into a mixing bowl, tipping in the bran left in the sieve. Rub the butter into the flour until the mixture resembles breadcrumbs. Stir in the sugar, oats, hazelnuts and wheatgerm. Sprinkle over 1 tbsp cold water and mix in to make a rough crumbly mixture. Spoon the topping evenly over the fruit.

4 Bake for 20–25 minutes or until the topping is golden brown and the fruit filling bubbling. Serve hot or warm, with custard, if liked.

Plus points

• This crumble has a lower proportion of fat than the traditional recipe; the crumbly texture is achieved by stirring in a little water. The water evaporates during cooking to give a deliciously crunchy texture.

• Gooseberries are an excellent source of vitamin C. Their high acid content protects the vitamin C, so little is lost during cooking.

• Mint has been used since Biblical times to relieve indigestion. Peppermint tea is still a favourite for relieving hiccups and nausea.

Each serving provides

kcal 278, protein 5 g, fat 13 g (of which saturated fat 6 g), carbohydrate 38 g (of which sugars 18 g), fibre 3 g

✓✓	A
✓	B₁, C, E, copper, iron, potassium

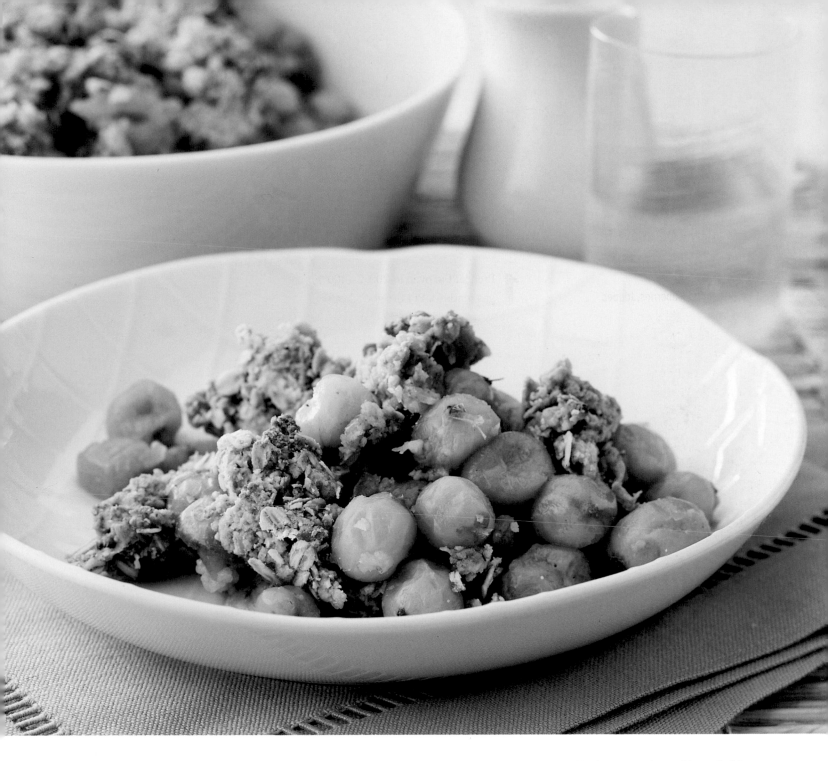

Some more ideas

• For a rhubarb and ginger crumble, cut 1 kg (2¼ lb) rhubarb into 2.5 cm (1 in) lengths and place in a wide, shallow saucepan with 4 tbsp ginger syrup from a jar of stem ginger. Cover and cook gently for 5–6 minutes or until the juices run and the rhubarb is just beginning to soften. Lift out the rhubarb with a draining spoon into the baking dish, leaving the juice in the pan. Sprinkle 45 g (1½ oz) light soft brown sugar over the rhubarb. Simmer the juices for 3–4 minutes or until reduced to about 4 tbsp. Drizzle over the rhubarb. Make the crumble topping with the flours and butter, but add 115 g (4 oz) sweetened muesli instead of the sugar, oats, hazelnuts and wheatgerm. Sprinkle over the fruit and bake as in the main recipe.

• To make a cinnamon plum crumble, quarter and stone 1 kg (2¼ lb) ripe plums and toss with 75 g (2½ oz) demerara sugar and 1 tsp ground cinnamon, then add the crumble topping.

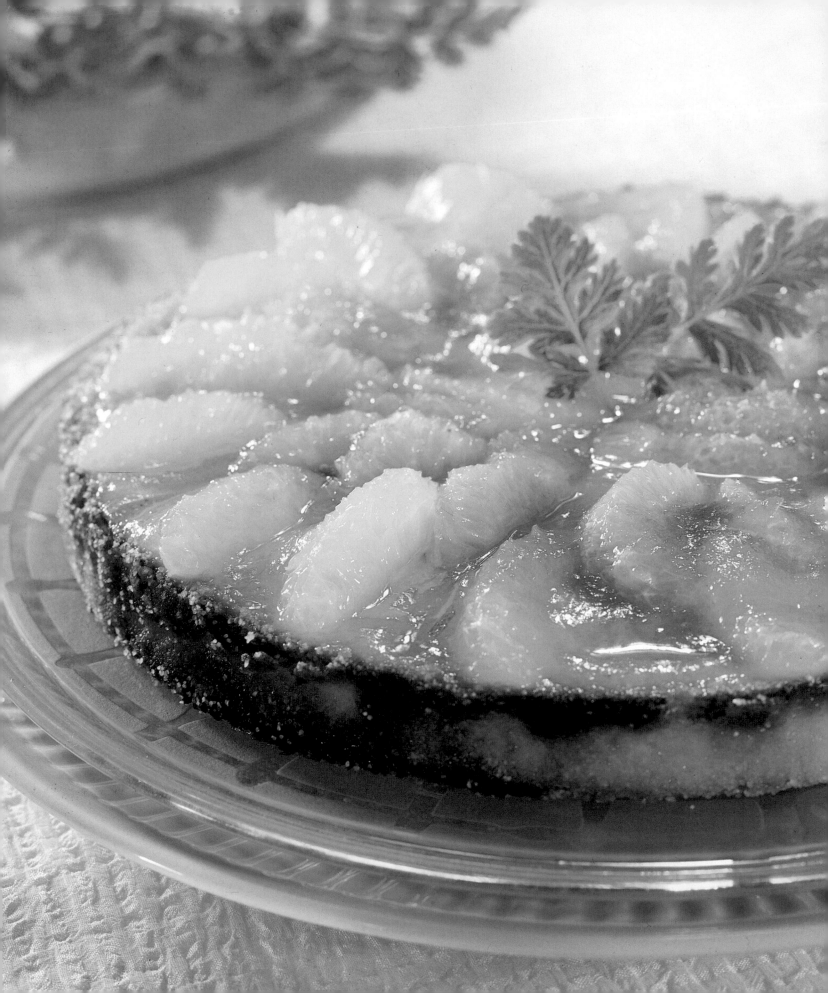

Sultana lemon cheesecake

Enjoy this thin but dense Italian-style cheesecake with its fresh lemon flavour with a cup of tea or as a dessert. Cheesecakes usually contain high levels of fat, but this recipe isn't baked with a butter-rich crust, and it uses lower-fat ricotta cheese rather than rich cream cheese, so the overall fat content is much reduced.

Serves 8

45 g (1½ oz) sultanas
3 tbsp brandy
3 tbsp semolina
340 g (12 oz) ricotta cheese
3 large egg yolks
85 g (3 oz) caster sugar
3 tbsp lemon juice
1½ tsp pure vanilla extract
finely grated zest of 2 large lemons

Topping

2 oranges
2 satsumas
1 lemon
4 tbsp lemon jelly marmalade

Preparation time: 20 minutes, plus 30 minutes soaking and 2–3 hours cooling
Cooking time: 35–40 minutes

Each scone provides

kcal 220, protein 7 g, fat 7 g (of which saturated fat 4 g), carbohydrate 32 g (of which sugars 26 g), fibre 1 g

✓✓	C
✓	A, B$_{12}$, calcium

1 Place the sultanas in a small bowl, add the brandy and leave to soak for at least 30 minutes or until most of the brandy has been absorbed.

2 Preheat the oven to 180°C (350°F, gas mark 4). Line the bottom of a non-stick, 20 cm (8 in) loose-bottomed sandwich tin with buttered baking parchment. Lightly butter the side of the tin. Sprinkle 1 tbsp of the semolina into the tin, turn and tilt the tin to coat the bottom and sides, then tap out any excess semolina. Set the tin aside.

3 Put the ricotta cheese into a fine sieve and press it through into a mixing bowl. Beat in the egg yolks, sugar, lemon juice, vanilla extract and remaining semolina. Stir in the lemon zest and the sultanas with any remaining brandy.

4 Spoon the mixture into the prepared tin and smooth the surface. Bake for 35–40 minutes or until the top is browned and the sides are shrinking from the tin. Leave to cool in the switched-off oven for 2–3 hours with the door ajar.

5 For the topping, peel the oranges, satsumas and lemon, removing all the white pith, then cut out the segments from between the membranes. Warm the marmalade very gently in a small saucepan until it has melted.

6 Carefully remove the cooled cheesecake from the tin and set on a serving platter. Brush with a layer of the melted marmalade. Arrange the citrus segments on top and glaze with the rest of the marmalade. Leave to set before serving.

Some more ideas

• Replace the sultanas with finely chopped dried apricots or sour cherries.

• For a mixed citrus flavour, add grated lime and orange zests, and soak the sultanas in orange juice. Replace the lemon juice with orange juice.

• Alternative fruit toppings include halved strawberries, blueberries and raspberries.

Plus points

• Many cheesecake recipes include finely ground nuts to help to bind the ingredients together. In this recipe the nuts have been replaced by semolina, which is finely ground durum wheat, thus omitting the fat that nuts would have supplied.

• The fresh citrus fruit topping provides lots of vitamin C.

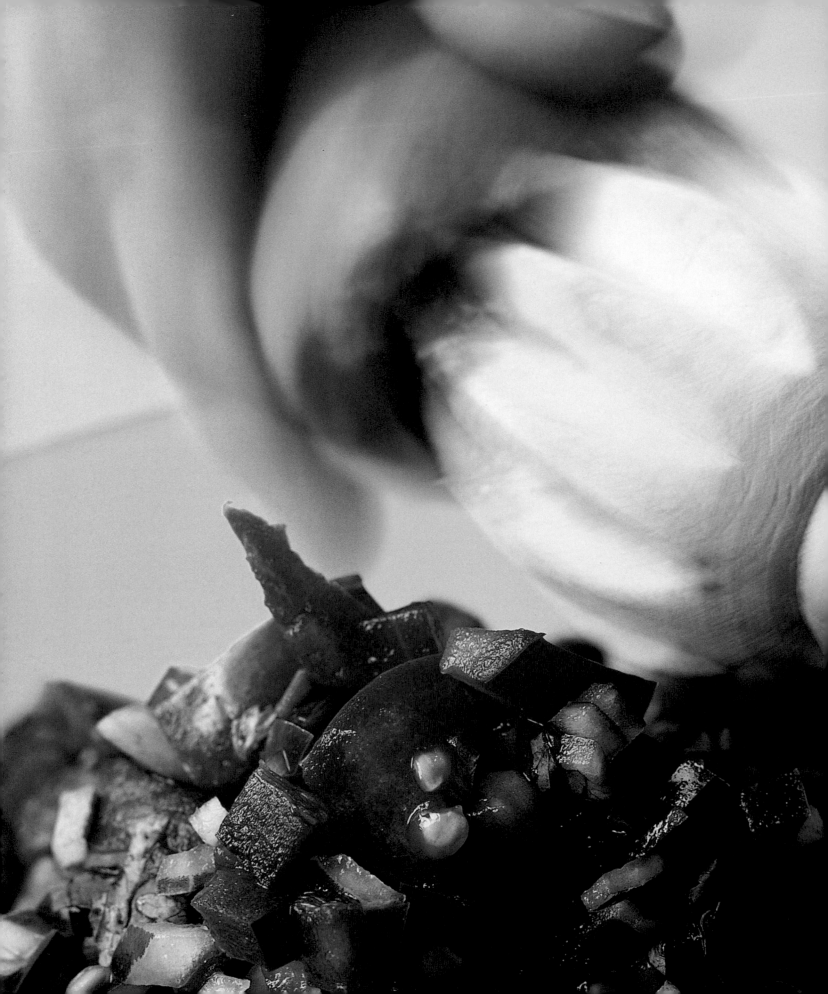

Food Facts

These charts allow you to compare what different food groups provide in the way of energy, protein, fat, carbohydrate and fibre (all figures are for raw weight unless otherwise specified). The list of foods is extensive but, of course, not every food could be included here. We have concentrated on including foods that seldom have their nutritional composition displayed on a label, such as fresh meat, fruit and vegetables. As well as comparing foods from different groups, it can be interesting to see how similar foods within a group can be – such as 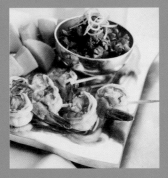 different types of pasta – so that you can make choices when shopping or preparing meals.

Vegetables and salads per 100g

Food	Energy kcals	Protein grams	Fat grams	Saturated fat grams	Carbohydrate grams	Sugars grams	Fibre grams
Alfalfa sprouts	30	3	0	0	3	0	3
Asparagus	25	2.9	0.6	0.1	2.0	1.9	1.7
Aubergine	15	0.9	0.4	0.1	2.2	2.0	2.0
Avocado	190	1.9	19.5	4.1	1.9	0.5	3.4
Beansprouts, mung	31	2.9	0.5	0.1	4.0	2.2	1.5
Beetroot	36	1.7	0.1	trace	7.6	7.0	1.9
Broad beans	81	7.9	0.6	0.1	11.7	1.3	6.5
Broccoli	33	4.4	0.9	0.2	1.8	1.5	2.6
Brussels sprouts	42	3.5	1.4	0.3	4.1	3.1	4.1
Cabbage	25	1.7	0.4	0.1	4.1	4.0	2.4
Carrots	35	0.6	0.3	0.1	7.9	7.4	2.4
Cauliflower	34	3.6	0.9	0.2	3.0	2.5	1.8
Celery	7	0.5	0.2	trace	0.9	0.9	1.1
Celeriac	42	1.3	0	0	9	1.3	1.9
Chicory	11	0.5	0.6	0.2	2.8	0.7	0.9
Courgettes	18	1.8	0.4	0.1	1.8	1.7	0.9
Cucumber	10	0.7	0.1	trace	1.5	1.4	0.6
Curly kale	33	3.4	1.6	0.2	1.4	1.3	3.1
Fennel	12	0.9	0.2	trace	1.8	1.7	2.4
Garlic	98	7.9	0.6	0.1	16.3	1.6	4.1
Green/French beans	24	1.9	0.5	0.1	3.2	2.3	2.2
Leeks	22	1.6	0.5	0.1	2.9	2.2	2.2
Lettuce, average	14	0.8	0.5	0.1	1.7	1.7	0.9
Mange-tout peas	32	3.6	0.2	trace	4.2	3.4	2.3
Marrow	12	0.5	0.2	trace	2.2	2.1	0.5
Mushrooms	13	1.8	0.5	0.1	0.4	0.2	1.1
Mustard and cress	13	1.6	0.6	trace	0.4	0.4	1.1
Okra	31	2.8	1.0	0.3	3.0	2.5	4.0
Onions	36	1.2	0.2	trace	7.9	5.6	1.4
Parsnips	64	1.8	1.1	0.2	12.5	5.7	4.6
Peas	83	6.9	1.5	0.3	11.3	2.3	4.7
Peppers, green	15	0.8	0.3	0.1	2.6	2.4	1.6
Peppers, red	32	1.0	0.4	0.1	6.4	6.1	1.6
Potatoes, new	70	1.7	0.3	0.1	16.1	1.3	1.0
Potatoes, maincrop	75	2.1	0.2	trace	17.2	0.6	1.3
Pumpkin	13	0.7	0.2	0.1	2.2	1.7	1.0
Radish	12	0.7	0.2	0.1	1.9	1.9	0.9
Runner beans	22	1.6	0.5	0.1	3.2	2.8	2.0
Spinach	25	2.8	0.8	0.1	1.6	1.5	2.1
Spring greens	33	3.0	1.0	0.1	3.1	2.7	3.4
Spring onions	23	2.0	0.5	0.1	3.0	2.8	1.5
Squash, butternut	45	0.7	0	0	11.4	2.1	2.1
Swede	24	0.7	0.3	trace	5.0	4.9	1.9
Sweet potato	87	1.2	0.3	0.1	21.3	5.7	2.4
Sweetcorn, on the cob	111	4.2	2.3	0.2	19.6	2.3	2.2
Tomatoes	17	0.7	0.3	trace	3.1	3.1	1.0
Turnips	23	0.9	0.3	trace	4.7	4.5	2.4
Watercress	22	3.0	1.0	0.3	0.4	0.4	1.5

Fish per 100g

Food	Energy kcals	Protein grams	Fat grams	Saturated fat grams	Carbohydrate grams	Sugars grams	Fibre grams
Anchovy	130	20.0	4.7	1.2	0	0	0
Bream, sea	96	17.5	2.9	0.3	0	0	0
Clam, cooked	148	25.9	2.4	0	4.7	0	0
Cod	80	18.3	0.7	0.1	0	0	0
Crab, boiled	128	19.5	5.5	0.7	trace	trace	0
Haddock	81	19.0	0.6	0.1	0	0	0
Hake	92	18.0	2.2	0.3	0	0	0
Halibut	110	20.6	2.5	0.3	0	0	0
Herring	190	17.8	13.2	3.3	0	0	0
Hoki	85	16.9	1.9	0.3	0	0	0
John Dory	89	19	1.4	0.4	0	0	0
Lobster, boiled	103	22.1	1.6	0.2	trace	0	0
Mackerel	220	18.7	16.1	3.3	0	0	0
Monkfish	66	15.7	0.4	0.1	0	0	0
Mullet red	109	18.7	3.8	0.1	0	0	0
Mussel, boiled	104	16.7	2.7	0.5	3.5	trace	0
Oyster	65	10.8	1.3	0.2	2.7	trace	0
Plaice	79	16.7	1.4	0.2	0	0	0
Prawn, shrimp boiled	99	22.6	0.9	0.2	0	0	0
Salmon	180	20.2	11.0	1.9	0	0	0
Sardine	165	20.6	9.2	2.7	0	0	0
Scallop, steamed	118	23.2	1.4	0.4	3.4	trace	0
Sea bass	100	19.3	2.5	0.4	0	0	0
Shark	130	21	5	1	0	0	0
Skate	64	15.1	0.4	trace	0	0	0
Sole, lemon	83	17.4	1.5	0.2	0	0	0
Squid	70	13.1	1.5	0.3	1.0	trace	0
Swordfish	109	18.0	4.1	0.9	0	0	0
Tilapia	85	17.8	1.5	0.3	0	0	0
Trout, rainbow, farmed	138	20.3	5.1	1.3	0	0	0
Trout, rainbow, wild	119	20.8	3.8	0.6	0	0	0
Tuna	136	23.7	4.6	1.2	0	0	0
Turbot	95	17.7	2.7	0.7	0	0	0
Whiting	81	18.7	0.7	0.1	0	0	0

Poultry and game per 100g

Food	Energy kcals	Protein grams	Fat grams	Saturated fat grams	Carbohydrate grams	Sugars grams	Fibre grams
Chicken	106	24.0	1.1	0.3	0	0	0
Turkey	105	24.4	0.8	0.3	0	0	0
Duck	137	19.7	6.5	2.0	0	0	0
Goose	161	22.7	7.0	2.7	0	0	0
Pheasant	133	23.6	3.7	1.2	0	0	0
Rabbit	137	21.9	5.5	2.1	0	0	0
Venison	157	22.0	7.0	3.0	0	0	0

Meat per 100g

Food	Energy kcals	Protein grams	Fat grams	Saturated fat grams	Carbohydrate grams	Sugars grams	Fibre grams
Bacon rashers, back	215	16.5	16.5	6.2	0	0	0
Bacon rashers, streaky	276	15.8	23.6	8.2	0	0	0
Ham, boiled	204	23.3	12.3	4.1	0	0	0
Beef, trimmed, lean	129	22.5	4.3	1.7	0	0	0
Lamb, trimmed, lean	153	20.2	8.0	3.5	0	0	0
Liver, calf	104	18.3	3.4	1.0	trace	0	0
Kidney, lamb's	91	17	2.6	0.9	0	0	0
Pork, trimmed, lean	123	21.8	4.0	1.4	0	0	0
Veal	106	22.7	1.7	0.6	0	0	0

Eggs, milk and cheese per 100g

Eggs	Energy kcals	Protein grams	Fat grams	Saturated fat grams	Carbohydrate grams	Sugars grams	Fibre grams
Chicken's	151	12.5	11.2	3.2	trace	trace	0
Duck's	163	14.3	11.8	2.9	trace	trace	0
Quail's	151	12.9	11.1	3.1	trace	trace	0
Milks							
Breakfast (Channel Island)	72	3.5	4.7	3.0	4.3	4.3	0
Buttermilk	37	3.4	0.5	0.3	5.0	5.0	0
Goats milk	62	3.1	3.7	2.4	4.4	4.4	0
Semi-skimmed	46	3.5	1.7	1.1	4.7	4.7	0
Sheep's milk	93	5.4	5.8	3.6	5.1	5.1	0
Skimmed	34	3.5	0.3	0.1	4.8	4.8	0
Soya, unsweetened	26	2.4	1.6	0.2	0.5	0.2	0.2
Whole milk	66	3.3	3.9	2.5	4.6	4.6	0
Cream							
Clotted	586	1.6	63.5	39.7	2.3	2.3	0
Crème fraîche, full fat	378	2.2	40.0	27.1	2.4	2.1	0
Crème fraîche, half fat	162	2.7	15.0	10.2	4.4	3.0	0
Double	496	1.6	53.7	33.4	1.7	1.7	0
Single	193	3.3	19.1	12.2	2.2	2.2	0
Soured	205	2.9	19.9	12.5	3.8	3.8	0
Whipping	381	2.0	40.3	25.2	2.7	2.7	0
Yogurt							
Greek, sheep's, plain	92	4.8	6.0	4.2	5.0	5.0	0
Low fat, plain	56	4.8	1.0	0.7	7.4	7.1	0
Whole milk, plain	79	5.7	3.0	1.7	7.8	7.8	0

Cheese	Energy kcals	Protein grams	Fat grams	Saturated fat grams	Carbohydrate grams	Sugars grams	Fibre grams
Brie	343	20.3	29.1	18.1	trace	trace	0
Camembert	290	21.5	22.7	14.2	trace	trace	0
Cheddar	416	25.4	34.9	21.7	0.1	0.1	0
Cheddar, half fat	175	15.0	9.5	9.9	7.9	trace	0
Cottage cheese, plain	101	12.6	4.3	2.3	3.1	3.1	0
Cottage cheese, reduced fat, plain	79	13.3	1.5	1.0	3.3	3.3	0
Danish Blue	342	20.5	28.9	19.1	trace	trace	0
Edam	341	26.7	26.0	15.8	trace	trace	0
Feta	250	15.6	20.2	13.7	1.5	1.5	0
Fromage frais, plain	113	6.1	8.0	5.5	4.4	4.1	0
Fromage frais, virtually fat free, plain	49	7.7	0.1	0.1	4.6	4.4	0
Gruyère	409	27.2	33.3	20.8	trace	trace	0
Goat's cheese	320	21.1	25.8	17.9	1.0	1.0	0
Mozzarella	257	18.6	20.3	13.8	trace	trace	0
Parmesan, fresh	415	36.2	29.7	19.3	0.9	0.9	0
Soft cheese	312	7.5	31.3	20.5	trace	trace	0
Soft cheese, reduced fat (light)	199	9.8	16.3	10.7	3.5	3.5	0
Stilton, blue	410	23.7	35.0	23.0	0.1	0.1	0

Uncooked rice, beans and grains per 100g

Rice	Energy kcals	Protein grams	Fat grams	Saturated fat grams	Carbohydrate grams	Sugars grams	Fibre grams
Basmati	359	7.4	0.5	0.2	79.8	trace	0.1
Brown	357	6.7	2.8	0.7	81.3	1.3	1.9
Red	354	7.4	1.6	0.7	76.0	trace	2.5
Risotto	349	7.0	1.0	0.2	78	0.2	0.1
White, easy cook	383	7.3	3.6	0.9	85.8	trace	0.4
White, polished	361	6.5	1.0	0.4	86.8	trace	0.5
Wild	357	15.0	1.2	0	75.0	2.5	6.3
Beans							
Aduki, dried	272	19.9	0.5	0.5	50.1	1.0	11.1
Black eyed, dried	311	23.5	1.6	0.5	54.1	2.9	8.2
Butter, dried	290	19.1	1.7	0.4	52.9	3.6	16.0
Haricot, dried	286	21.4	1.6	0.3	49.7	2.8	17.0
Pigeon, dried	317	20.0	1.9	0.4	58.6	1.7	15.1
Pinto, dried	327	21.1	1.6	0.2	57.1	2.1	15.5

Beans (continued)	Energy kcals	Protein grams	Fat grams	Saturated fat grams	Carbohydrate grams	Sugars grams	Fibre grams
Red kidney, dried	266	22.1	1.4	0.2	44.1	2.5	15.7
Soya, dried	370	35.9	18.6	2.3	15.8	5.5	15.7
Lentils and peas							
Chickpeas, whole, dried	320	21.3	5.4	0.5	49.6	2.6	10.7
Green lentils, whole, dried	297	24.3	1.9	0.2	48.8	1.2	8.9
Red lentils, whole, dried	318	23.8	1.3	0.2	56.3	2.4	4.9
Split peas, dried	328	22.1	2.4	0.4	58.2	1.9	6.3
Grains							
Bran	206	14.1	5.5	0.9	26.8	3.8	36.4
Buckwheat	364	8.1	1.5	0	84.9	0.4	2.1
Bulghur wheat	353	9.7	1.7	0	76.3	1.4	3.1
Hominy	362	8.7	0.8	0	77.7	1	5
Oatmeal	401	12.4	8.7	0	72.8	trace	6.8
Quinoa	309	13.8	5.0	0.5	55.7	6.1	5.9
Pearl barley	360	7.9	1.7	0	83.6	trace	less than 1
Wheatgerm	357	26.7	9.2	1.3	44.7	16.0	15.6

Pastas per 100g

Food	Energy kcals	Protein grams	Fat grams	Saturated fat grams	Carbohydrate grams	Sugars grams	Fibre grams
Macaroni	348	12.0	1.8	0.3	75.8	2.2	3.1
Noodles, egg	391	12.1	8.2	2.3	71.7	1.9	2.9
Pasta, plain, fresh	289	11.4	3.4	1.0	53.1	2.7	2.1
Spaghetti, white	342	12.0	1.8	0.2	74.1	3.3	2.9
Spaghetti, wholemeal	324	13.4	2.5	0.4	66.2	3.7	8.4

Fruit per 100g

Food	Energy kcals	Protein grams	Fat grams	Saturated fat grams	Carbohydrate grams	Sugars grams	Fibre grams
Apples, eating	47	0.4	0.1	Trace	11.8	11.8	1.8
Apricots	31	0.9	0.1	Trace	7.2	7.2	1.7
Bananas, flesh only	95	1.2	0.3	0.1	23.2	20.9	1.1
Blackberries	25	0.9	0.2	trace	5.1	5.1	3.1
Blackcurrants	28	0.9	trace	trace	6.6	6.6	3.6
Blueberries	30	0.6	0.2	trace	6.9	6.9	1.8
Cherries	48	0.9	0.1	trace	11.5	11.5	0.9

Food	Energy kcals	Protein grams	Fat grams	Saturated fat grams	Carbohydrate grams	Sugars grams	Fibre grams
Cranberries	15	0.4	0.1	0	3.4	3.4	3.0
Clementines, flesh only	37	0.9	0.1	trace	8.7	8.7	1.2
Currants	267	2.3	0.4	trace	67.8	67.8	1.9
Damsons	38	0.5	trace	trace	9.6	9.6	1.8
Dates, raw	124	1.5	0.1	trace	31.3	31.3	1.8
Dates, dried	270	3.3	0.2	0.1	68.0	68.0	4.0
Figs, semi-dried	209	3.3	1.5	trace	48.6	48.6	6.9
Gooseberries	19	1.1	0.4	trace	3.0	3.0	2.4
Grapefruit, flesh only	30	0.8	0.1	trace	6.8	6.8	1.3
Grapes	60	0.4	0.1	trace	15.4	15.4	0.7
Guava	26	0.8	0.5	trace	5.0	4.9	3.7
Kiwi, flesh and seeds	49	1.1	0.5	trace	10.6	10.3	1.9
Kumquats	43	0.9	0.5	trace	9.3	9.3	3.8
Lemons	19	1.0	0.3	0.1	3.3	3.2	4
Lychees, flesh only	58	0.9	0.1	trace	14.3	14.3	0.7
Mangoes, ripe, flesh	57	0.7	0.2	0.1	14.1	13.8	2.6
Melon, cantaloupe, flesh only	19	0.6	0.1	trace	4.2	4.2	1.0
Melon, Galia, flesh only	24	0.5	0.1	trace	5.6	5.6	0.4
Melon, honeydew, flesh only	28	0.6	0.1	trace	6.6	6.6	0.6
Nectarines	40	1.4	0.1	trace	9.0	0.0	1.2
Olives, green	103	0.9	11.0	1.7	trace	trace	2.9
Oranges, flesh only	37	1.1	0.1	trace	8.5	8.5	1.7
Passion fruit, flesh and pips	36	2.6	0.4	0.1	5.8	5.8	3.3
Papaya (paw paw) flesh only	36	0.5	0.1	trace	8.8	8.8	2.2
Peaches	33	1.0	0.1	trace	7.6	7.6	1.5
Pears	40	0.3	0.1	trace	10.0	10.0	2.2
Pineapple, flesh only	41	0.4	0.2	trace	10.1	10.1	1.2
Plums	36	0.6	0.1	trace	8.8	8.8	1.6
Pomegranate, whole	33	0.9	0.1	trace	7.7	7.7	2.2
Prunes, semi-dried, ready to eat	141	2.5	0.4	trace	34.0	34.0	5.7
Redcurrants	21	1.1	trace	trace	4.4	4.4	3.4
Raisins	272	2.1	0.4	trace	69.3	69.3	2.0
Raspberries	25	1.4	0.3	0.1	4.6	4.6	2.5
Rhubarb, stem only	7	0.9	0.1	trace	0.8	0.8	1.4
Satsumas, flesh only	36	0.9	0.1	trace	8.5	8.5	1.3
Strawberries	27	0.8	0.1	trace	6.0	6.0	1.1
Sultanas	275	2.7	0.4	trace	69.4	69.4	2.0
Tangerines, flesh only	35	0.9	0.1	trace	8.0	8.0	1.3
Watermelon, flesh only	31	0.5	0.3	0.1	7.1	7.1	0.1

Glossary

Antioxidants These are compounds that help to protect the body's cells against the damaging effects of free radicals. Vitamins C and E, beta-carotene (the plant form of vitamin A) and the mineral selenium, together with many of the phytochemicals found in fruit and vegetables, all act as antioxidants.

Calorie A unit used to measure the energy value of food and the intake and use of energy by the body. The scientific definition of 1 calorie is the amount of heat required to raise the temperature of 1 gram of water by 1 degree Centigrade. This is such a small amount that in this country we tend to use the term kilocalories (abbreviated to *kcal*), which is equivalent to 1000 calories. Energy values can also be measured in kilojoules (kJ): 1 kcal = 4.2 kJ.

A person's energy (calorie) requirement varies depending on his or her age, sex and level of activity. The estimated average daily energy requirements are:

Age (years)	Female (kcal)	Male (kcal)
1–3	1165	1230
4–6	1545	1715
7–10	1740	1970
11–14	1845	2220
15–18	2110	2755
19–49	1940	2550
50–59	1900	2550
60–64	1900	2380
65–74	1900	2330

Carbohydrates These energy-providing substances are present in varying amounts in different foods and are found in three main forms: sugars, starches and non-starch polysaccharides (NSP), usually called fibre.

There are two types of sugars: *intrinsic sugars*, which occur naturally in fruit (fructose) and sweet-tasting vegetables, and *extrinsic sugars*, which include lactose (from milk) and all the non-milk extrinsic sugars (NMEs) – sucrose (table sugar), honey, treacle, molasses and so on. The NMEs, or 'added' sugars, provide only calories, whereas foods containing intrinsic sugars also offer vitamins, minerals and fibre. Added sugars (*simple carbohydrates*) are digested and absorbed rapidly to provide energy very quickly. Starches and fibre (*complex carbohydrates*), on the other hand, break down more slowly to offer a longer-term energy source (see also Glycaemic Index). Starchy carbohydrates are found in bread, pasta, rice, wholegrain and breakfast cereals, and potatoes and other starchy vegetables such as parsnips, sweet potatoes and yams.

Healthy eating guidelines recommend that at least half of our daily energy (calories) should come from carbohydrates, and that most of this should be from complex carbohydrates. No more than 11% of our total calorie intake should come from 'added' sugars. For an average woman aged 19–49 years, this would mean a total carbohydrate intake of 259 g per day, of which 202 g should be from starch and intrinsic sugars and no more than 57 g from added sugars. For a man of the same age, total carbohydrates each day should be about 340 g (265 g from starch and intrinsic sugars and 75 g from added sugars).

See also Fibre and Glycogen.

Cholesterol There are two types of cholesterol – the soft waxy substance called blood cholesterol, which is an integral part of human cell membranes, and dietary cholesterol, which is contained in food. *Blood cholesterol* is important in the formation of some hormones and it aids digestion. High blood cholesterol levels are known to be an important risk factor for coronary heart disease, but most of the cholesterol in our blood is made by the liver – only about 25% comes from cholesterol in food. So while it would seem that the amount of cholesterol-rich foods in the diet would have a direct effect on blood cholesterol levels, in fact the best way to reduce blood cholesterol is to eat less saturated fat and to increase intake of foods containing soluble fibre.

Fat Although a small amount of fat is essential for good health, most people consume far too much. Healthy eating guidelines recommend that no more than 33% of our daily energy intake (calories) should come from fat. Each gram of fat contains 9 kcal, more than twice as many calories as carbohydrate or protein, so for a woman aged 19–49 years this means a daily maximum of 71 g fat, and for a man in the same age range 93.5 g fat.

Fats can be divided into 3 main groups: saturated, monounsaturated and polyunsaturated, depending on the chemical structure of the fatty acids they contain. *Saturated fatty acids* are found mainly in animal fats such as butter and other dairy products and in fatty meat. A high intake of saturated fat is known to be a risk factor for coronary heart disease and certain types of cancer. Current guidelines are that no more than 10% of our daily calories should come from saturated fats, which is about 21.5 g for an adult woman and 28.5 g for a man.

Where saturated fats tend to be solid at room temperature, the *unsaturated fatty acids* – monounsaturated and polyunsaturated – tend to be liquid. *Monounsaturated fats* are found predominantly in olive oil, groundnut (peanut) oil, rapeseed oil and avocados. Foods high in *polyunsaturates* include most vegetable oils – the exceptions are palm oil and coconut oil, both of which are saturated.

Both saturated and monounsaturated fatty acids can be made by the body, but certain polyunsaturated fatty acids – known as *essential fatty acids* – must be supplied by food. There are 2 'families' of these essential fatty acids: *omega-6*, derived from linoleic acid, and *omega-3*, from linolenic acid. The main food sources of the omega-6 family are vegetable oils such as olive and sunflower; omega-3 fatty acids are provided by oily fish, nuts, and vegetable oils such as soya and rapeseed.

When vegetable oils are hydrogenated (hardened) to make margarine and reduced-fat spreads, their unsaturated fatty acids can be changed into trans fatty acids, or '*trans fats*'. These artificially produced trans fats are believed to act in the same way as saturated fats within the body – with the same risks to health. Current healthy eating guidelines suggest that no more than 2% of our daily calories should come from trans fats, which is about 4.3 g for an adult woman and 5.6 g for a man. In thinking about the amount of trans fats you consume, remember that major sources are processed foods such as biscuits, pies, cakes and crisps.

Fibre Technically non-starch polysaccharides (NSP), fibre is the term commonly used to describe several different compounds, such as pectin, hemicellulose, lignin and gums, which are found in the cell walls of all plants. The body cannot digest fibre, nor does it have much nutritional value, but it plays an important role in helping us to stay healthy.

Fibre can be divided into 2 groups – soluble and insoluble. Both types are provided by most plant foods, but some foods are particularly good sources of one type or the other. *Soluble fibre* (in oats, pulses, fruit and vegetables) can help to reduce high blood cholesterol levels and to control blood sugar levels by slowing down the absorption of sugar. *Insoluble fibre* (in wholegrain cereals, pulses, fruit and vegetables) increases stool bulk and speeds the passage of waste material through the body. In this way it helps to prevent constipation, haemorrhoids and diverticular disease, and may protect against bowel cancer.

Our current intake of fibre is around 12 g a day. Healthy eating guidelines suggest that we need to increase this amount to 18 g a day.

Free radicals These highly reactive molecules can cause damage to cell walls and DNA (the genetic material found within cells). They are believed to be involved in the development of heart disease, some cancers and premature ageing. Free radicals are produced naturally by the body in the course of everyday life, but certain factors, such as cigarette smoke, pollution and over-exposure to sunlight, can accelerate their production.

Gluten A protein found in wheat and, to a lesser degree, in rye, barley and oats, but not in corn (maize) or rice. People with *coeliac disease* have a sensitivity to gluten and need to eliminate all gluten-containing foods, such as bread, pasta, cakes and biscuits, from their diet.

Glycaemic Index (GI) This is used to measure the rate at which carbohydrate foods are digested and converted into sugar (glucose) to raise blood sugar levels and provide energy. Foods with a high GI are quickly broken down and offer an immediate energy fix, while those with a lower GI are absorbed more slowly, making you feel full for longer and helping to keep blood sugar levels constant. High-GI foods include table sugar, honey, mashed potatoes and watermelon. Low-GI foods include pulses, wholewheat cereals, apples, cherries, dried apricots, pasta and oats.

Glycogen This is one of the 2 forms in which energy from carbohydrates is made available for use by the body (the other is *glucose*). Whereas glucose is converted quickly from carbohydrates and made available in the blood for a fast energy fix, glycogen is stored in the liver and muscles to fuel longer-term energy needs. When the body has used up its immediate supply of glucose, the stored glycogen is broken down into glucose to continue supplying energy.

Minerals These inorganic substances perform a wide range of vital functions in the body. The *macrominerals* – calcium, chloride, magnesium, potassium, phosphorus and sodium – are needed in relatively large quantities, whereas much smaller amounts are required of the remainder, called *microminerals*. Some microminerals (selenium, magnesium and iodine, for example) are needed in such tiny amounts that they are known as *'trace elements'*.

There are important differences in the body's ability to absorb minerals from different foods, and this can be affected by the presence of other substances. For example, oxalic acid, present in spinach, interferes with the absorption of much of the iron and calcium spinach contains.

• *Calcium* is essential for the development of strong bones and teeth. It also plays an important role in blood clotting. Good sources include dairy products, canned fish (eaten with their bones) and dark green, leafy vegetables.

• *Chloride* helps to maintain the body's fluid balance. The main source in the diet is table salt.

• *Chromium* is important in the regulation of blood sugar levels, as well as levels of fat and cholesterol in the blood. Good dietary sources include red meat, liver, eggs, seafood, cheese and wholegrain cereals.

• *Copper*, component of many enzymes, is needed for bone growth and the formation of connective tissue. It helps the body to absorb iron from food. Good sources include offal, shellfish, mushrooms, cocoa, nuts and seeds.

• *Iodine* is an important component of the thyroid hormones, which govern the rate and efficiency at which food is converted into energy. Good sources include seafood, seaweed and vegetables (depending on the iodine content of the soil in which they are grown).

• *Iron* is an essential component of haemoglobin, the pigment in red blood cells that carries oxygen around the body. Good sources are offal, red meat, dried apricots and prunes, and iron-fortified breakfast cereals.

• *Magnesium* is important for healthy bones, the release of energy from food, and nerve and muscle function. Good sources include wholegrain cereals, peas and other green vegetables, pulses, dried fruit and nuts.

• *Manganese* is a vital component of several enzymes that are involved in energy production and many other functions. Good dietary sources include nuts, cereals, brown rice, pulses and wholemeal bread.

• *Molybdenum* is an essential component of several enzymes, including those involved in the production of DNA. Good sources are offal, yeast, pulses, wholegrain cereals and green leafy vegetables.

• *Phosphorus* is important for healthy bones and teeth and for the release of energy from foods. It is found in most foods. Particularly good sources include dairy products, red meat, poultry, fish and eggs.

• *Potassium*, along with sodium, is important in maintaining fluid balance and regulating blood pressure, and is essential for the transmission of nerve impulses. Good sources include fruit, especially bananas and citrus fruits, nuts, seeds, potatoes and pulses.

• *Selenium* is a powerful antioxidant that protects cells against damage by free radicals. Good dietary sources are meat, fish, dairy foods, brazil nuts, avocados and lentils.

• *Sodium* works with potassium to regulate fluid balance, and is essential for nerve and muscle function. Only a little sodium is needed – we tend to get too much in our diet. The main source in the diet is table salt, as well as salty processed foods and ready-prepared foods.

• *Sulphur* is a component of 2 essential amino acids. Protein foods are the main source.

• *Zinc* is vital for normal growth, as well as reproduction and immunity. Good dietary sources include oysters, red meat, peanuts and sunflower seeds.

Phytochemicals These biologically active compounds, found in most plant foods, are believed to be beneficial in disease prevention. There are literally thousands of different phytochemicals, amongst which are the following:

• *Allicin*, a phytochemical found in garlic, onions, leeks, chives and shallots, is believed to help lower high blood cholesterol levels and stimulate the immune system.

• *Bioflavonoids*, of which there are at least 6000, are found mainly in fruit and sweet-tasting vegetables. Different bioflavonoids have different roles – some are antioxidants, while others act as anti-disease agents. A sub-group of these phytochemicals, called *flavonols*, includes the antioxidant *quercetin*, which is believed to reduce the risk of heart disease and help to protect against cataracts. Quercetin is found in tea, red wine, grapes and broad beans.

• *Carotenoids*, the best known of which are *beta-carotene* and *lycopene*, are powerful antioxidants thought to help protect us against certain types of cancer. Highly coloured fruits and vegetables, such as blackcurrants, mangoes, tomatoes, carrots, sweet potatoes, pumpkin and dark green, leafy vegetables, are excellent sources of carotenoids.

• *Coumarins* are believed to help protect against cancer by inhibiting the formation of tumours. Oranges are a rich source.

• *Glucosinolates*, found mainly in cruciferous vegetables, particularly broccoli, Brussels sprouts, cabbage, kale and cauliflower, are believed to have strong anti-cancer effects. *Sulphoraphane* is one of the powerful cancer-fighting substances produced by glucosinolates.

• *Phytoestrogens* have a chemical structure similar to the female hormone oestrogen, and they are believed to help protect against hormone-related cancers such as breast and prostate cancer. One of the types of these phytochemicals, called *isoflavones*, may also help to relieve symptoms associated with the menopause. Soya beans and chickpeas are a particularly rich source of isoflavones.

Protein This nutrient, necessary for growth and development, for maintenance and repair of cells, and for the production of enzymes, antibodies and hormones, is essential to keep the body working efficiently. Protein is made up of *amino acids*, which are compounds containing the 4 elements that are necessary for life: carbon, hydrogen, oxygen and nitrogen. We need all of the 20 amino acids commonly found in plant and animal proteins. The human body can make 12 of these, but the remaining 8 – called *essential amino acids* – must be obtained from the food we eat.

Protein comes in a wide variety of foods. Meat, fish, dairy products, eggs and soya beans contain all of the essential amino acids, and are therefore called first-class protein foods. Pulses, nuts, seeds and cereals are also good sources of protein, but do not contain the full range of essential amino acids. In practical terms, this really doesn't matter – as long as you include a variety of different protein foods in your diet, your body will get all the amino acids it needs. It is important, though, to eat protein foods every day because the essential amino acids cannot be stored in the body for later use.

The RNI of protein for women aged 19–49 years is 45 g per day and for men of the same age 55 g. In the UK most people eat more protein than they need, although this isn't normally a problem.

Reference Nutrient Intake (RNI) This denotes the average daily amount of vitamins and minerals thought to be sufficient to meet the nutritional needs of almost all individuals within the population. The figures, published by the Department of Health, vary depending on age, sex and specific nutritional needs such as pregnancy. RNIs are equivalent to what used to be called Recommended Daily Amounts or Allowances (RDA).

Vitamins These are organic compounds that are essential for good health. Although they are required in only small amounts, each one has specific vital functions to perform. Most vitamins cannot be made by the human body, and therefore must be obtained from the diet. The body is capable of storing some vitamins (A, D, E, K and B_{12}), but the rest need to be provided by the diet on a regular basis. A well-balanced diet, containing a wide variety of different foods, is the best way to ensure that you get all the vitamins you need.

Vitamins can be divided into 2 groups: *water-*

soluble (B complex and C) and *fat-soluble* (A, D, E and K). Water-soluble vitamins are easily destroyed during processing, storage, and the preparation and cooking of food. The fat-soluble vitamins are less vulnerable to losses during cooking and processing.

• *Vitamin A* (retinol) is essential for healthy vision, eyes, skin and growth. Good sources include dairy products, offal (especially liver), eggs and oily fish. Vitamin A can also be obtained from *beta-carotene*, the pigment found in highly coloured fruit and vegetables. In addition to acting as a source of vitamin A, beta-carotene has an important role to play as an antioxidant in its own right.

• *The B Complex vitamins* have very similar roles

to play in nutrition, and many of them occur together in the same foods.

Vitamin B_1 (thiamin) is essential in the release of energy from carbohydrates. Good sources include milk, offal, meat (especially pork), wholegrain and fortified breakfast cereals, nuts and pulses, yeast extract and wheat germ. White flour and bread are fortified with B_1 in the UK.

Vitamin B_2 (riboflavin) is vital for growth, healthy skin and eyes, and the release of energy from food. Good sources include milk, meat, offal, eggs, cheese, fortified breakfast cereals, yeast extract and green leafy vegetables.

Niacin (nicotinic acid), sometimes called vitamin B_3, plays an important role in the release of energy within the cells. Unlike the other B vitamins it can be made by the body from the essential amino acid tryptophan. Good sources include meat, offal, fish, fortified breakfast cereals and pulses. White flour and bread are fortified with niacin in the UK.

Pantothenic acid, sometimes called vitamin B_5, is involved in a number of metabolic reactions, including energy production. This vitamin is present in most foods; notable exceptions are fat, oil and sugar. Good sources include liver, kidneys, yeast, egg yolks, fish roe, wheat germ, nuts, pulses and fresh vegetables.

Vitamin B_6 (pyridoxine) helps the body to utilise protein and contributes to the formation of haemoglobin for red blood cells. B_6 is found in a wide range of foods including meat, liver, fish, eggs, wholegrain cereals, some vegetables, pulses, brown rice, nuts and yeast extract.

Vitamin B_{12} (cyanocobalamin) is vital for growth, the formation of red blood cells and maintenance of a healthy nervous system. B_{12} is unique in that it is only found in foods of animal origin. Vegetarians who eat dairy products will get enough, but vegans need to ensure they include food fortified with B_{12} in their diet. Good sources of B_{12} include liver, kidneys, oily fish, meat, cheese, eggs and milk.

Folate (folic acid) is involved in the manufacture of amino acids and in the production of red blood cells. Recent research suggests that folate may also help to protect against heart disease. Good sources of folate are green leafy vegetables, liver, pulses, eggs, wholegrain cereal products and fortified breakfast cereals, brewers' yeast, wheatgerm, nuts and fruit, especially grapefruit and oranges.

Biotin is needed for various metabolic reactions and the release of energy from foods. Good sources include liver, oily fish, brewers' yeast, kidneys, egg yolks and brown rice.

• *Vitamin C* (ascorbic acid) is essential for growth and vital for the formation of collagen (a protein needed for healthy bones, teeth, gums, blood capillaries and all connective tissue). It plays an important role in the healing of wounds and fractures, and acts as a powerful antioxidant. Vitamin C is found mainly in fruit and vegetables.

• *Vitamin D* (cholecalciferol) is essential for growth and the absorption of calcium, and thus for the formation of healthy bones. It is also

Nutritional analyses

The nutritional analysis of each recipe has been carried out using data from *The Composition of Foods* with additional data from food manufacturers where appropriate. Because the level and availability of different nutrients can vary, depending on factors like growing conditions and breed of animal, the figures are intended as an approximate guide only.

The analyses include vitamins A, B_1, B_2, B_6, B_{12}, niacin, folate, C, D and E, and the minerals calcium, copper, iron, potassium, selenium and zinc. Other vitamins and minerals are not included, as deficiencies are rare. Optional ingredients and optional serving suggestions have not been included in the calculations.

involved in maintaining a healthy nervous system. The amount of vitamin D occurring naturally in foods is small, and it is found in very few foods – good sources are oily fish (and fish liver oil supplements), eggs and liver, as well as breakfast cereals, margarine and full-fat milk that are fortified with vitamin D. Most vitamin D, however, does not come from the diet but is made by the body when the skin is exposed to sunlight.

• *Vitamin E* is not one vitamin, but a number of related compounds called tocopherols that function as antioxidants. Good sources of vitamin E are vegetable oils, polyunsaturated margarines, wheatgerm, sunflower seeds, nuts, oily fish, eggs, wholegrain cereals, avocados and spinach.

• *Vitamin K* is essential for the production of several proteins, including prothombin which is involved in the clotting of blood. It has been found to exist in 3 forms, one of which is obtained from food while the other 2 are made by the bacteria in the intestine. Vitamin K_1, which is the form found in food, is present in broccoli, cabbage, spinach, milk, margarine, vegetable oils, particularly soya oil, cereals, liver, alfalfa and kelp.

Index

EAT YOURSELF HEALTHY

was published by The Reader's Digest Association Limited, London from material first published in the Reader's Digest, *Eat Well, Live Well* series.

First edition Copyright © 2005
The Reader's Digest Association Limited
11 Westferry Circus, Canary Wharf,
London E14 4HE
www.readersdigest.co.uk

We are committed both to the quality of our products and the service we provide to our customers. We value your comments so please feel free to contact us on 08705 113366 or via our web site at **www.readersdigest.co.uk**.

If you have any comments or suggestions about the content of our books you can contact us at **gbeditorial@readersdigest.co.uk**

Originated by **Amazon Publishing Limited**, 7, Old Lodge Place, Twickenham, TW1 1RQ

Editors Susannah Blake, Bridget Jones, Jill Steed
Editorial Assistant Ella Fern
Designers Colin Goody, Vivienne Brar
Nutritionist Jane Griffin

FOR READER'S DIGEST, LONDON
Editor Lisa Thomas

FOR READER'S DIGEST GENERAL BOOKS
Editorial Director Cortina Butler
Art Director Nick Clark
Executive Editor Julian Browne
Managing Editor Alastair Holmes
Picture Resource Manager Martin Smith
Pre-press Account Manager Penny Grose

Origination Colour Systems Ltd
Printing and binding Tien Wah Press Ltd., Singapore

Book code 400-249-01
ISBN 0 276 44048 X
Oracle code 250009712S.00.24